# Adolescent Health Screening: An Update in the Age of Big Data

# Adolescent Health Screening: An Update in the Age of Big Data

*Edited by*

VINCENT MORELLI, MD
Professor Meharry Medical College
Professor Adjunct Vanderbilt University
Department of Family and Community Medicine
Meharry Medical College
Nashville, TN, United States

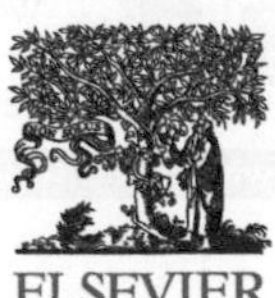

ELSEVIER

ADOLESCENT HEALTH SCREENING: AN UPDATE IN THE AGE OF BIG DATA
ISBN: 978-0-323-66130-0


*Publisher:* Taylor Ball
*Acquisition Editor:* Jessica L. McCool
*Editorial Project Manager:* Pat Gonzalez
*Production Project Manager:* Kiruthika Govindaraju
*Cover Designer:* Alan Studholme

3251 Riverport Lane
St. Louis, Missouri 63043

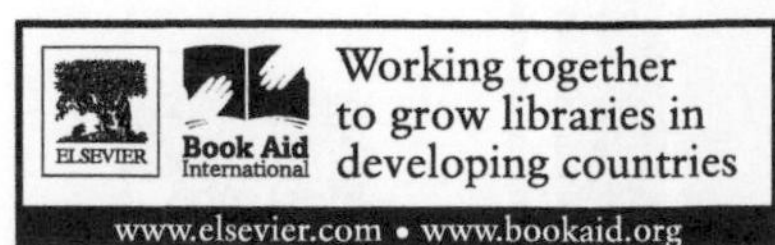

# List of Contributors

**Roger Apple, PhD**
Psychologist
Department of Pediatric and Adolescent Medicine
Western Michigan University, Homer Stryker School of Medicine
Kalamazoo, MI, United States

**Debra Kristen Braun-Courville, MD**
Assistant Professor
Pediatrics, Adolescent Medicine
Vanderbilt University Medical Center
Nashville, TN, United States

**Nicholas Conley, MD**
Resident Physician
Family and Community Medicine Resident
Meharry Medical College
Nashville, TN, United States

**Neerav Desai, MD**
Assistant Professor
Pediatrics
Vanderbilt University Medical Center
Nashville, TN, United States

**Gina Frieden, PhD**
Assistant Professor of the Practice
Department of Human and Organizational Development
Vanderbilt University
Nashville, TN, United States

**Sandra J. Gonzalez, MSSW, PhD**
Assistant Professor
Family and Community Medicine
Baylor College of Medicine
Houston, TX, United States

**Leslie Greenberg, MD, FAAFP**
Family Physician
Family and Community Medicine
University of Nevada School of Medicine
Reno, NV, United States

Associate Professor
Family and Community Medicine
University of Nevada Reno School of Medicine
Reno, NV, United States

**Zachary M. Hood, MD**
Department of Sports and Family Medicine
Meharry Medical College
Nashville, TN, United States

**Heidi Joshi, PsyD, MS, BMUS**
Assistant Professor, Behavioral Medicine Clinician/Educator
Medical Education
Western Michigan University Homer Stryker, M.D. School of Medicine
Kalamazoo, MI, United States

**Paul D. Juarez, PhD**
Professor, Department of Family & Community Medicine
Meharry Medical College
Nashville, TN, United States

**Medhat Kalliny, MD, PhD, FAAFP**
Vice-Chair for Clinical Affairs & Family Medicine Residency Program Director
Family & Community Medicine
Meharry Medical College
Nashville, TN, United States

**Alicia Kowalchuk, DO**
Assistant Professor
Department of Family and Community Medicine
Baylor College of Medicine
Houston, TX, United States

Medical Director
InSight Program
Harris Health System
Houston, TX, United States

Medical Director
CARE Clinic
Santa Maria Hostel
Houston, TX, United States

Medical Director
Sobering Center
Houston Recovery Center
Houston, TX, United States

**David Kurtmen, MD**
Resident Physician
Family and Community Medicine
University of Nevada Reno School of Medicine
Reno, Nevada, United States

**Maria C. Mejia de Grubb, MD, MPH**
Assistant Professor
Family and Community Medicine
Baylor College of Medicine
Houston, TX, United States

**Richard Milner, MD, PhD**
Associate Professor
Molecular and Experimental Medicine
Scripts Research Institute
CA, United States

**Vincent Morelli, MD**
Family & Community Medicine/Sports Medicine
Meharry Medical College/Adjunct Vanderbilt
Nashville, TN, United States

**Tamasyn Nelson, DO**
Assistant Professor of Pediatrics
Medical Director of Pediatric Obesity Services
Division of General Pediatrics
Monroe Carell Jr. Children's Hospital at Vanderbilt
Nashville, TN, United States

**Chenai Nettey, MD**
Family Medicine
Meharry Medical College
Nashville, TN, United States

**Heather O'Hara, MD, MSPH**
Associate Professor
Family and Community Medicine
Meharry Medical College
Nashville, TN, United States

**Gregory Plemmons, MD, MFA**
Associate Professor
Pediatric Hospital Medicine
Vanderbilt University Medical Center
Nashville, TN, United States

**Daljeet Rai, MD**
Adjunct Associate Clinical Professor
Division of Family and Community Medicine
Stanford University School of Medicine
San Jose, CA, United States

**Navdeep Rai, MD**
Resident in Family and Community Medicine
Stanford University School of Medicine
Palo Alto, CA, United States

**Mary E. Romono, MD, MPH**
Associate Professor
Department of Pediatrics – Division of Adolescent Medicine/Young Adult Health
Children's Hospital at Vanderbilt
Nashville, TN, United States

**Brittany D. Rudolph, MS**
PhD Candidate
Clinical Psychology
Palo Alto University
Palo Alto, CA, United States

**Emmy Sobieski, BA, MBA, CFA, CNC, DVA**
Senior Analyst
Nicholas Investment Partners
Rancho Santa Fe, CA, United States

Certified Nutritional Consultant
EMJS LLC
Carlsbad, CA, United States

Domestic Violence Victims Advocate
Women's Shelter
Community Resource Center
Encinitas, CA, United States

**James Sobieski, NREMT, NAEMT-I (Nutrition, Mathematics, Biology Chemistry)**
Director of Training and Emergency
Transport- Physicians Ambulance.
Emergency Medical Services
Case Western Reserve University
Cleveland, OH, United States

**Sarah Spinner, PsyD**
Clinical Psychologist
Private Practice
Sarah Spinner, Psy.D.
Mill Valley, CA, United States

Documentation Manager
Quality Improvement
Seneca Family of Agencies
San Leandro, CA, United States

**Ali Stuhl, MTS, BA**
Master of Theological Studies
Divinity School
Vanderbilt University
Nashville, TN, United States

**Brenda G. Vaccaro, PsyD**
Founder & Executive Director
Child, Adolescent, & Family Services
Spark Center for Self Development
Sacramento, CA, United States

**Roger Zoorob, MD, MPH**
Professor and Chair
Department of Family Medicine
Baylor School of Medicine
Houston, Texas, United States

# Contents


1 **Adolescent Health Screening: Toward A More Holistic Approach,** *1*
*Vincent Morelli, MD and Chenai Nettey, MD*

2 **Holistic Health Screening,** *7*
*Mary Romono, MD, MPH*
*Debra Kristen Braun-Courville, MD and Neerav Desai, MD*

3 **Dietary Screening—Questioning Adolescent Dietary Trends and Providing Evidence-Based Dietary Recommendations,** *21*
*Emmy Sobieski, CNC, CFA, MBA, DVA, James Sobieski, NREMT, NAEMT-I and Richard Milner, MD, PhD*

4 **Obesity Screening in Adolescents,** *33*
*Tamasyn Nelson, DO*

5 **Sleep Disorders,** *43*
*Medhat Kalliny, MD, PhD, FAAFP*

6 **Adolescent Exercise Screening,** *57*
*Zachary M. Hood, MD and Vincent Morelli, MD*

7 **ACES: Screening for Adverse Childhood Experiences,** *75*
*Heather O'Hara, MD, MSPH and Vincent Morelli, MD*

8 **Adolescent Educational Assessment: Risk Factors Associated With Academic Achievement and Indicators of Learning Challenges,** *83*
*Sarah Spinner, PsyD, Brenda G. Vaccaro, PsyD and Brittany D. Rudolph, MS*

9 **Screening Adolescents for ADHD, Oppositional Defiant Disorder, and Conduct Disorder in Primary Care,** *107*
*Heidi Joshi, PsyD, MS, BMUS and Roger Apple, PhD*

10 **Screening for Violent Tendencies in Adolescents,** *115*
*Paul D. Juarez, PhD*

11 **Depression and Suicide Screening,** *135*
*Gregory Plemmons, MD, MFA*

12 **Screening for Body Image Concerns, Eating Disorders, and Sexual Abuse in Adolescents: Concurrent Assessment to Support Early Intervention and Preventative Treatment,** *151*
*Sarah Spinner, PsyD and Brittany D. Rudolph, MS*

13 **Addressing Substance Use with the Adolescent in Primary Care: the SBIRT Model,** *165*
*Alicia Kowalchuk, DO, Maria Mejia de Grubb, MD, MPH, Sandra Gonzalez, MSSW, PhD and Roger Zoorob, MD, MPH*

14 **Screening for Leading Indicators of Juvenile Delinquency,** *179*
*Vincent Morelli, MD*

15 **Screening for Resilience in Adolescents,** *191*
*Vincent Morelli, MD*

16 **Spiritual Screening in Adolescents,** *207*
*Daljeet Rai, MD, Ali Stuhl, MTS, BA, Vincent Morelli, MD and Navdeep Rai, MD*

17 **Screening for Strengths and Assets in Adolescents,** *227*
*Gina Frieden, PhD*

18 **Screening for Screen Time,** *245*
*Leslie Greenberg, MD, FAAFP and David Kurtmen, MD*

19 **Putting It All Together: A Role for Big Data in Health and Adolescent Health Screening,** *251*
*Vincent Morelli, MD and Nicholas Conley, MD*

**INDEX,** *257*

CHAPTER 1

# Adolescent Health Screening: Toward A More Holistic Approach

VINCENT MORELLI, MD • CHENAI NETTEY, MD

## INTRODUCTION

Adolescence is a critical time of transition and identity formation[1] that lays the foundation for healthy adulthood. This period of physical, cognitive, social, and emotional change can be stressful for both adolescents and those around them. It can be a trying time of learning to navigate new emotions, changes in school or home life, increased responsibility, and a new sense of autonomy. It can also mark the beginning of a youth's search for meaning and spiritual evolution (see the chapter on spirituality). Importantly, the values, behaviors, and habits developed in adolescence can significantly impact adult health, life satisfaction, and overall long-term quality of life.[2]

Also important, when discussing adolescence, is that adolescence can generally be divided into three development phases: early adolescence (ages 10–13 years old), middle adolescence (ages 14–17), and late adolescence (ages 17–21).[3] As we will see later, any biopsychosocial assessment of the adolescent should consider these developmental stages, probing appropriate areas of health and development and eliciting age-relevant health information.

This book's focus is on adolescent health screening, our intent being to identify adolescent health risks early and, if possible, to address them before the untoward effects are manifest.

In the remainder of this chapter, we will first review the general principles of screening, then look at our current method of health screening in adolescents (the biopsychosocial model), and finally draw some conclusions and steer the reader into the chapters that follow.

## PRINCIPLES OF SCREENING

There are two main reasons for screening: early detection and prevention.[4] "Detection screening" should have acceptable sensitivity, specificity, and predictive value and should be judged in terms of measurable outcome (i.e., does screening for cancer accurately detect cancer and will this detection actually improve survival rates). "Prevention screening" is held to similar standards, with the intent to intervene to prevent some future harmful health outcome (i.e., screening for alcohol use to prevent liver disease).

As set out by the World Health Organization (WHO)[5] screening is optimal when

- patients are given clear information regarding the risks and benefits of screening;
- the health issues screened for are significant—meaning issues with high incidence or high morbidity;
- the tools themselves are well validated; and
- the illuminated health issues benefit more from early intervention than delayed treatment.

Naturally, the benefits of screening should outweigh any potential for harm brought on by screening, and the costs should be considered acceptable. Finally, screening is only useful when it can be disseminated outside of the academic setting and takes hold in the larger population.

In the chapters that follow we will sometimes talk of screening for detection and sometimes of screening for prevention. Our emphasis, however, will be on prevention, hoping to highlight leading indicators of affliction so that the primary care provider may intervene, educate, and prevent.

It is important to note that the gold standard for verifying and validating screening—the prospective randomized trial—is often lacking in the adolescent literature. The current state of adolescent screening often relies instead on observational or epidemiologic studies or on small studies with methodological shortcomings—flaws that can lead to potential biases such as selection bias, statistical lead-time bias, and over diagnosis bias. Although all of this can become

Adolescent Health Screening: An Update in the Age of Big Data. https://doi.org/10.1016/B978-0-323-66130-0.00001-6

statistically complicated, the authors of this issue have attempted to simplify the data and make the information accessible to primary care providers.

## SCREENING VIA THE BIOMEDICAL MODEL

In 1977, internist and psychoanalysis George Engel wrote an impassioned article on what he called the "crisis of medicine".[6] He wrote that the current medicine management model of that time (the biomedical model) was "no longer adequate for the scientific tasks and social responsibilities of medicine or psychiatry." He believed that the biomedical model, which focused solely on the "somatic parameters" of disease, was inadequate. Instead, he held that psychosocial issues were also significant contributors that should be considered in approaching illness.[6] According to his writing, the biomedical model "interferes with patient care" by ignoring other factors that could also be contributing to a person's disease or response to medical management.[6]

During that period, psychiatry as a profession was battling to win acceptance, fighting to be included as part of conventional somatic medicine. Engel's stance was that by taking into account a patient's social and psychological factors, medical diagnosis and management would be more encompassing, resulting in legitimizing the field of psychiatry in modern medicine and leading to improved diagnosis and treatment of medical ailments. Thus, Engel proposed the biopsychosocial model (BPS model)—a model would look at disease from multiple angles: genetic, biochemical, psychological (e.g., mood, personality, and behavior), and social (e.g., cultural, familial, socioeconomic, and medical), acknowledging that there are other elements besides the "science of the body" affecting patient disease states.

## CRITICISM OF THE BPS MODEL

Several psychiatrists have since responded to Engel's BPS model to either criticize or praise it. Nassir Ghaemi's "The rise and fall of the biopsychosocial model" stated that the "evidence-based practices," used by pharmaceutical, insurance, and national health industries favored the biomedical model, and that opponents only embraced the BPS model as a way to combat the oppression of industry.[7] He believed that the BPS model was only designed as a way to legitimize the failing field of psychoanalysis (Engel's specialty) not, as Engel had stated, to incorporate biology and sociology into a more holistic approach. He supported this view by pointing out that even Engel's later research was devoid of mentioning biological or social issues in the face of psychological diagnoses. He also mentioned that for many, the BPS model was a means to justify one's "unscientific" management of a patient. In essence, he felt that the BPS model was being used to allow practitioners to manage their patients however they wanted to manage them. Instead of Engel's comprehensive, holistic approach, Ghaemi believed in allowing the practitioner to choose which aspect of the three (biological, psychological, or social) to focus on when treating the patient.[7]

Benning furthered Ghaemi's criticism by writing that for many, the BPS model was an idea and not a method to be followed. He did not believe that the BPS model's theories gave a list of organized steps for practitioners to follow to give proper weight to biological, psychological, or social factors in a patient's disease process. He too felt that not all diseases were grounded in all three BPS categories It seemed to him that a sore throat would not require a full psychosocial evaluation.

In more of an academic argument, Benning pointed out that the BPS model received its roots in the general systems theory (GST), which broadly applied concepts and principles to more than one domain of knowledge. However, he states, "Engel himself fails to live up to some of the central tenets of GST" by neglecting the psychopathology of large social units (e.g., community, culture, subculture, and society-nation).[8]

Despite such critics, proponents of the BPS model have praised and embraced the idea—especially in adolescent healthcare where changing factors—growth, and development, family environment, school environment, etc., can be more fully assessed and factored into a more holistic approach to treatment.

## APPLICATION OF THE BPS MODEL IN ADOLESCENT MEDICINE

The BPS model should address the many health risks encountered in adolescence. For example, according to the World Health Organization, "more than 3000 adolescents die every day, totaling 1.2 million deaths a year from largely preventable causes".[9] The BPS model should help to screen for and address such preventable causes of adolescent death.

It should help identification of comorbid conditions (e.g., mental health disorders, sexual health, and substance use disorders) as well as help to provide focused patient education and appropriate referral for mental health services, social support, and other needed interventions. It should also help to address barriers to adolescent healthcare.[9,10]

## EXAMPLES OF THE BPS MODEL IN ACTION

In the field of adolescent medicine, the BPS model has been studied in areas such as pain management, and preventive medicine.

In pain management, biopsychosocial acceptance has been shown to be crucial in helping to improve the management of pediatric and adolescent pain. Factors such as the influence of their guardian(s), social beliefs, coping in school, and the ability to manage stress have been studied in relation to chronic pain in adolescents. The general consensus has been that adolescents who are unable to manage stress are more likely to have higher rates of complications and worsened outcomes with pain, thus leading to distrust of pain management techniques. Often, this leads to noncompliance with prescribed medicine regimens.[11–13] In one study, Guite et al. found that parents and adolescents who were less willing to accept the biopsychosocial perspective were less likely to be ready for change and less willing to self-manage their pain.[14] Conversely, those who were *more* willing to look at and address biopsychosocial factors were more likely to be satisfied with pain management and were more compliant. Interestingly, the study also showed that parents were also better at accepting a self-management approach and in recognizing the need to establish care with a multidisciplinary pain management group.[14]

In adolescent preventive medicine, there are many different interview techniques that have been devised to identify areas of biopsychosocial need in the patient's life. These interview techniques are aimed at helping to draw out psychosocial health information from adolescents who are famous for clamming up when approached by an adult. Some of these are as follows: the HEEADSSS (Home, Education/Employment, Eating, Activities, Drugs and Alcohol, Sexuality, Suicide and Depression, Safety) assessment and questions to identify adverse childhood experiences (ACEs). The HEEADSSS assessment is a guideline of topics to address during the adolescent visit that examines the following:

1. Home (environment, sleep)
2. Education/Employment
3. Eating (food groups, barriers to obtaining food)
4. Activities (screen time, outdoor playtime)
5. Drugs (exposure, experimentation)
6. Sexuality (sexual identification, experimentation, exposure)
7. Suicidal/Homicidal thoughts and actions (low mood)
8. Safety (home, school, work)

Using the HEEADSSS assessment has been proposed as a "gold standard" for getting a psychosocial history from adolescents and identifying deficient and potentially problematic areas.[15] The HEEADSSS assessment is designed to be used in any medical environment that requires interviewing adolescents (e.g., in preventive and chronic illness clinics, the emergency room, and mental health visits). It is supposed to help the adolescent understand that the practitioner asking the questions truly cares about the answers. It is performed with the assumption that the adolescent understands that the practitioner is not judgmental and can offer meaningful discussion on any problems that arise in a safe and confidential environment.[15]

Identification of childhood stress(es) can also be performed by inquiring about ACEs. (See chapter on ACEs in this publication.) As will be discussed in several chapters (see those on ACEs, Resilience), many children are able to adapt to stress, cope well, and self-manage. However, many others are less able to cope and may have stress that affects all aspects of their lives (e.g., mental, biological, social, creativity, and the ability to work). The importance of screening for ACEs as part of the biopsychosocial history is evidenced by the fact that more than three ACEs have been linked to suicide attempts,[16] poor academic outcomes, future health issues, high health care utilization (in adolescence and adulthood), substance abuse, sexual deviances, adult aggression[17–19] and, in later life, premature morbidity and mortality.[20] All of this to say that ACEs are a critical part of a biopsychosocial intake history.

Besides using the HEEADSSS examination to expose the ACEs, it has been proposed that guardian(s) and adolescents fill out questionnaires designed specifically for directly identifying ACEs. Studies have shown that most adults are not aware of the effects that ACEs can have in their child's life, as well as a future generation's lives[16] and such involvement allows for an educational opportunity. As clinicians, we are sorely lacking in addressing these adverse events. Kerker et al.'s study of 302 pediatricians on their use of ACEs screening demonstrated that only "4% of pediatricians usually asked about all 10 ACEs and 32% did not usually ask about any. Less than 11% of pediatricians reported being very or somewhat familiar with the ACE study".[17]

We mention the earlier shortcomings of pediatricians in screening for ACEs only to highlight the ever-expanding data pool that is relevant in screening for, preventing, and treating disease. As we continue in this publication, we will highlight several other areas that might be examined in a more comprehensive health assessment of the adolescent.

## LIMITATIONS TO IMPLEMENTING THE BPS MODEL IN ADOLESCENTS HEALTHCARE

Unfortunately, although there are methods in place to help implement the BPS model in adolescent healthcare, many feel that the BPS model is not achievable. Why? According to some, time, lack of facilities, availability of resources, discomfort with addressing sensitive topics with teens, lack of parental education, and unfamiliarity on what to do after problems are identified are just some of the reasons that have been listed.[9,18] Lawrence et al. point out in *"Adolescent Health Services—Missing Opportunities"* that even though primary care may be available to most adolescents, the services can be highly dependent on "fee-based reimbursement" making it difficult for those teens who are "uninsured or underinsured" to get access to all services. Some facilities may also be unskilled at fostering relationships or "addressing risky behaviors" in adolescents. Others simply lack the resources to offer specialty services even after identifying that there is a problem.[10]

Lack of time is a common constraint. Typically, healthy adolescents are seen in the clinic once or twice a year. The first visit being the school physical, and the next a sick visit. Because of these spare, sporadic and time constrained visits, many practitioners, even if they use the HEEADSSS exam or ask questions to determine ACEs, have difficulty establishing trust, assessing and addressing many issues. This "lack of relationship" will often lead to discomfort when sensitive topics are eventually broached. (One retrospective study of 11−18-year-olds found that 40% had only a single preventive visit and 33% had NO preventive visits).[21]

Thus, many factors contribute to the failure of the healthcare system to adequately address adolescent health issues. This is a critical shortcoming because so many adult health habits are established during adolescence and because failure to address these issues will eventually lead to health problems later in their adult lives.

## CONCLUSIONS

Critiques, such as Ghaemi and Benning, felt that implementation of the BPS model was not possible in practical terms. The information PCPs needed to extract was too expensive and difficult to extract during short, infrequent PCP adolescent visits. They were also put off by the model's failure to provide a specific set of steps a PCP could easily follow in the clinical setting. The critics were correct. Time restraints and infrequent visits are real barriers to its usefulness. However, we do think that incorporating Engel's biological, psychological, and social parameters can help practitioners reach a fuller understanding of both the patient and their health risks. Thus, while we embrace the BPS model in adolescent care, we realize in practice it is difficult to implement.

With this in mind, in the chapters that follow, we will do two things. First, we will review the screening methods used to assess health risks in many underappreciated areas of adolescent health. Following this, we will present a concluding chapter where we will offer insights gleaned from our review. In this concluding chapter, we will consider ways to surmount the barriers to implementation of the BPS model—hopefully contributing to risk reduction, adolescent disease prevention, and health promotion. In doing so, we will propose a "new and improved" expansion of the BPS model—a model appropriate for practitioners caring for adolescents in the age of big data.

## REFERENCES


1. Erikson EH. *Identity: Youth and Crisis.* New York: Norton; 1968.
2. Arnett JJ. Emerging adulthood. a theory of development from the late teens through the twenties. *Am Psychol.* 2000;55(5):469−480.
3. Neinstein L. *Adolescent Health Care.* 2008.
4. Bretthauer M, Kalager M. Principles, effectiveness and caveats in screening for cancer. *Br J Surg.* 2013;100(1): 55−65. https://doi.org/10.1002/bjs.8995. Review. PMID: 23212620.
5. Wilson JMG, Junger G. *Principles and Practice of Screening for Disease.* Geneva: World Health Organization; 1968.
6. Engel G. The need for a new medical model: a challenge for biomedicine. *Science.* 1977;196:129−135.
7. Ghaemi SN. The rise and fall of the biopsychosocial model. *British J Psychiatry.* 2009;195:3−4.
8. Benning T. Limitation of the biopsychosocial model in psychiatry. *Adv Med Educ Pract.* 2015;6:347−352.
9. World Health Organization. *More Than 1.2 Million Adolescents Die Every Year, Nearly all Preventable.* News Release; May 16, 2017. Retrieved from: http://www.who.int/en/news-room/detail/16-05-2017-more-than-1-2-million-adolescents-die-every-year-nearly-all-preventable; Accessed October 28.10.2018.
10. National Research Council and Institute of Medicine. *Adolescent Health Services: Missing Opportunities.* Washington, DC: The National Academies Press; 2009. https://doi.org/10.17226/12063.
11. Crushell E, Rowland M, Doherty M, et al. Importance of parental conceptual model of illness in severe recurrent abdominal pain. *Pediatrics.* 2003;112:1368−1372.
12. Jensen MP, Nielson WR, Kerns RD. Toward the development of a motivational model of pain self-management. *J Pain.* 2003;4:477−492.

13. Palermo TM, Chambers CT. Topical review: parent and family factors in pediatric chronic pain and disability: an integrative approach. *Pain*. 2005;119:1–4.
14. Guite JW. Pain beliefs and readiness to change among adolescents with chronic musculoskeletal pain and their parents before an initial pain clinic evaluation. *Clin J Pain*. 2014;30:1–18.
15. Doukrou M, Segal TY. Fifteen-minute consultation: communicating with young people-how to use HEEADSSS, a psychosocial interview for adolescents. *Arch Dis Child Educ Pract Ed*. 2018;103(1):15–19.
16. Hughes K, Bellis MA, Hardcastle KA, et al. The effect of multiple adverse childhood experiences on health: a systematic review and meta-analysis. *Lancet Public Health*. 2017;2:356–366.
17. Kerker B, Storfer-Isser A, Szilagyi M, et al. Do pediatricians ask about adverse childhood experiences in pediatric primary care? *Acad Pediatr*. 2016;16(2):154–160.
18. American Academy of Pediatrics. *Addressing Adverse Childhood Experiences and Other Types of Trauma in the Primary Care Setting*; 2014. Available at: https://www.aap.org/en-us/Documents/ttb_addressing_aces.pdf.
19. Chartier MJ, Walker JR, Naimark B. Separate and cumulative effects of adverse childhood experiences in predicting adult health and health care utilization. *Child Abuse Negl*. 2010;34:454–464.
20. Shalev I, Moffitt TE, Sugden K, et al. Exposure to violence during childhood is associated with telomere erosion from 5 to 10 years of age: a longitudinal study. *Mol Psychiatry*. 2013;18(5):576–581.
21. Nordin J, Solberg L, Parker E. Adolescent primary care visit patters. *Ann Fam Med*. Nov/Dec 2010;8(6):511–516.


## FURTHER READING


1. Katzenellenbogen R. HEADSS: the "review of systems" for adolescents. *AMA J Ethics*; March 2005. https://journalofethics.ama-assn.org/article/headss-review-systems-adolescents/2005-03; Accessed October 28.10.2018.

CHAPTER 2

# Holistic Health Screening

MARY ROMANO, MD, MPH • DEBRA KRISTEN BRAUN-COURVILLE, MD • NEERAV DESAI, MD

## INTRODUCTION

This chapter will focus on complementary and alternative medicine (CAM) therapy, as it relates to adolescents. We will first review the epidemiology of CAM in this age group, then focus on provider opportunities to screen for CAM, followed by a section on specific medical conditions that are commonly associated with CAM use in adolescents. For these medical conditions, we will emphasize the literature on the most common practices and those that have evidence for use in adolescents. Finally, we will discuss regulation of CAM and the potential risks of CAM in adolescents.

More than 1 out of every 10 children utilize complementary medicine as part of their healthcare plan.[1] Complementary medicine may include mind–body medicine practices, dietary and herbal supplements, dietary eliminations, homeopathy, acupuncture, chiropractic care, massage, or holistic functional medicine approaches. The 2012 Centers for Disease Control and Prevention National Health Interview Survey (NHIS) included a section on Child Complementary and Alternative Medicine. Overall, 44.2% of children aged 4–17 years report using some complementary health approach.[2] Adolescents (ages 12–17 years) are more likely to utilize complementary medicine than children (ages 4–11 years). A 2006 study looking exclusively at adolescent use of complementary medicine found that 79% of adolescents (>12 years) had used at least one form of complementary medicine in their lifetime and almost one-third had used it in the past 30 days.[3] The most commonly used modalities include homeopathy, hypnosis, chiropractic or osteopathic manipulation, energy healing, and acupuncture. Although the NHIS data have shown that the numbers of those using complementary medicine are unchanged between 2007 and 2012, there have been shifts in what modalities and supplements are being used most often.[2] In the 2012 survey, among all pediatric users aged 4–17 years, the most commonly used supplements were (1) fish oil, (2) melatonin, (3) pro-/prebiotics, and (4) echinacea.[2] In the 2007 survey, echinacea had been the most frequently used dietary supplement.[2] Of note, most individuals who reported dietary supplement use are obtaining it on their own rather at the discretion of a medical provider.

When queried about reasons for complementary medicine use, most children report using it for a specific problem, rather than for general health and well-being.[1] The most common conditions for which complementary medicine is used include back/neck/musculoskeletal pain, URI symptoms (common cold), anxiety/stress, attention-deficit/hyperactivity disorder/attention deficit disorder (ADHD/ADD), and difficulty with sleep. Use of complementary medicine increases significantly in children/adolescents living with a chronic illness. Rates of use in this population are reported at greater than 50%.[2] This also includes those with a psychiatric diagnosis. The most commonly used modalities in patients with chronic illness included dietary supplements, massage, and homeopathy.[2] Adolescent use of complementary medicine is slightly different in terms of reasons for use and the most common supplements used. When asked about reasons for use, adolescents have typically reported using supplements to lose weight, increase energy, or improve their athletic performance/stamina.[2] Girls report weight loss as the most common reason for use, whereas boys most commonly cite desire for increased muscle mass as their reason for use.[3] The most commonly used supplements in adolescents differ from those used in adults and young children. Commonly used supplements in adolescents include ginseng, echinacea, ginkgo, weight loss supplements, and creatine.[3]

Parental use of complementary medicine has been shown to be the most consistent factor associated with its use in children.[1] Other consistently associated factors include a higher level of education and income. A study showed that children whose parents were

Adolescent Health Screening: An Update in the Age of Big Data. https://doi.org/10.1016/B978-0-323-66130-0.00002-8

educated with "more than an HS diploma" were seven times more likely to report the use of complementary medicine when compared with those who had "less than an HS diploma" as their education level.

Adolescent-specific studies have demonstrated that overall use of complementary medicine is higher in girls, and those who were 16–17 years of age reported the highest use.[3] Among adolescents, ethnic variations are also reported—Caucasian adolescents were more likely to have used herbal remedies, African Americans were more likely to have used faith healing or prayer and Hispanics were more likely to have used chiropractic manipulation.[3] Complementary medicine may be used on its own, but it is often used in combination with usual allopathic medical practices. Among adolescents, 10% reported the concurrent use of prescription medications AND dietary supplements.[3]

Given the fact that many adolescents and their families utilize complementary medicine, it is important that providers regularly ask about use. The National Center for Complementary and Integrative Health (NCCIH), a part of the National Institutes of Health, has resources for patients, families, and providers.[4] Included in these resources are "tips" on how to approach this topic with patients. The mnemonic the NCCIH uses is "ARMED."[1]

A-ASK which complementary medicine modalities patients and families are using. Patients may be reluctant to disclose use, as they may be unsure of a provider's attitude and/or knowledge about this topic. Providers might obtain more information if they ask WHAT (not IF) patients and families are utilizing in terms of complementary medicine.

R-RESPECT the patient's and family beliefs regarding this topic. As with all areas of medicine where families and providers disagree, keeping an open dialogue will make sure that the provider is able to provide the family with evidence-based information and gather the appropriate information from patients and families about use.

M-MONITOR the patient's response to therapy. Documenting improvement as well as any negative side effects is an important part of the dialogue with families about the ongoing use.

E-EDUCATE yourself and D-DISTRIBUTE evidence-based information. Providers should be open to critical evaluation of the literature on the efficacy of complementary medicine use and to discuss this literature with families. Knowing that patients and families will often seek out complementary medicine options, it is helpful for providers to discuss and review this as part of their anticipatory guidance when appropriate.

Providers should consider asking about complementary health practices at routine medical visits as well as during acute care or sick visits. Another time healthcare practitioners can screen for CAM use is at the sports physical examination. The primary purpose of the sports physical examination is to identify and screen for possible illness, injury, or conditions that may adversely affect the student athlete's health. Therefore the preparticipation sports physical examination is an ideal time to address nutritional the intake of supplements and performance-enhancing substances in athletes.[5] This may be the practitioner's only chance for provision of anticipatory guidance and assessment of health risk behaviors. The American Academy of Pediatrics preparticipation physical evaluation form (www.aafp.org/dam/AAFP/documents/patient_care/fitness/ppephysicalexamform2010.pdf) contains at least two questions targeted on supplement use and abuse by adolescents: (1) Have you ever taken anabolic androgenic steroids or used any other performance supplements? and (2) Have you ever taken any supplements to help you gain or lose weight or improve your performance? If patients report supplement use, further questioning should assess the specific supplements used and providers should be sure to discuss the risks and benefits of dietary supplements, including a review of the evidence-based medicine. As will be discussed later in this chapter, many of these products are deemed safe by the consumer, but the healthcare provider should address the limited data and often unknown short- and long-term consequences.

Thus far we have outlined the epidemiology of and the reasons for the use of complementary health practices in adolescents. We will now turn our attention to prevalent adolescent medical conditions that are commonly associated with complementary and alternative medical treatment modalities.

## MEDICAL CONDITIONS FOR WHICH ADOLESCENTS COMMONLY USE COMPLEMENTARY AND ALTERNATIVE MEDICINE

### Dysmenorrhea

Dysmenorrhea is the most common gynecologic complaint and its prevalence rates range from 67% to 90% in adolescent girls and young adult women.[4] Dysmenorrhea is one of the main causes of school absence among adolescent girls.[6] Despite its common occurrence, less than 20% of adolescents report having asked their provider about treatment options.[4] This means that many adolescents are self-medicating and potentially utilizing complementary medicine. The reasons for which a patient may utilize complementary medicine are many—they might be opposed to conventional medical treatments or might prefer complementary medicine options, traditional medical options may be contraindicated in certain patients, or they might not realize that the issue at hand can be treated by a medical provider. It is incumbent on the provider to ask about menstrual symptoms and about ALL treatment modalities that may already be in use by patients and families.

The two complementary medicine modalities most commonly used to treat dysmenorrhea are acupuncture and dietary and/or herbal supplements.[6] A 2016 Cochrane database review found that there was no evidence to demonstrate consistent efficacy of acupuncture or acupressure in the treatment of primary dysmenorrhea. In this review, acupuncture/pressure was compared with nonsteroidal anti-inflammatory drugs (NSAIDs), placebo, and no treatment.[7]

There have been several small studies looking at numerous vitamins and their effects on dysmenorrhea. The following supplements have been shown to have some effect on reducing dysmenorrhea symptoms: magnesium, vitamin E, vitamin D, vitamin $B_1$, fish oil supplements, and ginger; however, none of those studies measured the efficacy of these supplements against that of NSAIDs or hormonal therapy. Furthermore, no studies have shown a difference of effect between supplements. Whatever effect was noted was shown when supplements were compared with placebo and/or no treatment.[8] Although all studies show a measurable effect on symptoms, these studies are all limited by their small sample size and inconsistent methods.[6,7] In addition, there are no studies looking at the safety and/or adverse effects of supplement use in larger doses.[8]

Another supplement commonly used to treat dysmenorrhea is Chinese herbal medicine (CHM). A review of the literature showed that CHM showed an effect on pain symptoms that was superior to no treatment, placebo, NSAIDs, oral contraceptive pills (OCPs), and acupuncture.[9] The most commonly found herbs in menstrual formulations of CHM include angelica root, fennel fruit, licorice root, cinnamon bark, and red peony root. These herbs are thought to have anti-inflammatory and sedating properties.[10] However, these studies were poorly designed and were of a small sample size, which was not large enough to detect any clinically significant adverse effects.[9]

In sum, dysmenorrhea is a common ailment in adolescent girls and young adult women. There is no evidence to support acupuncture for the treatment of primary dysmenorrhea. Dietary and vitamin supplements may be helpful in reducing pain symptoms, but they are not superior to conventional treatment modalities such as NSAIDs and hormonal contraception. Studies are small and not well-designed to evaluate for adverse effects, but CHM, with its anti-inflammatory and sedation qualities, may have a role in the treatment of dysmenorrhea.

## Psychiatric Disorders

A large-scale survey in 2012 found that among youth with a psychiatric diagnosis, 5% had received mental health services in a complementary medicine setting.[11] Among patients and parents, there are often concerns about the safety of psychotropic medications, and for this reason, complementary medicine, particularly dietary and herbal supplements, is considered a "safer" option by patients and families.[11] Some therapeutic interventions, considered "alternatives" to traditional medicine, are often with little risk and should be discussed with patients and families: exercise, light therapy, and music therapy. However, some CAM treatments are not without risk. Given the potential for interactions with other medications, it is important that clinicians who are treating adolescents with a mental health diagnosis query specifically about the use of complementary medicine. Table 2.1 lists the complementary medicine supplements most commonly used in the treatment of depression, anxiety, and ADHD.[12] There is little to no data on the effects of CAM on psychiatric disorders in adolescent patients. Therefore most recommendations are extrapolated from the limited data available in the adult population.

**TABLE 2.1**

| Supplement | Psychiatric Diagnosis |
|---|---|
| Omega 3 Fatty Acids | Depression, ADHD |
| St John's wort (*Hypericum*) | Depression |
| S-Adenosyl-L-Methonine (SAMe) | Depression |
| Kava root (*Piper methysticum*) | Generalized Anxiety Disorder |
| Valerian root (*Valeriana officinalis*) | Generalized Anxiety Disorder |
| Passionflower root (*Passiflora incarnata*) | Generalized Anxiety Disorder |

## Depression

St. John's wort (*Hypericum perforatum*) is one of the more commonly used supplements to treat depression. In Europe, St. John's wort is regularly prescribed to patients with a diagnosis of depression.[13] The active ingredients are thought to be hypericin and hyperforin. Both seem to decrease serotonin uptake therefore increasing serotonin levels, and hypericin has been shown to decrease cortisol production.[13] Studies on the efficacy of St. John's wort have been inconsistent. A 2005 Cochrane review looked at double-blind, randomized controlled trials (RCTs) that utilized a standardized scale to study outcomes.[14] In this review, St. John's wort had no effect when compared with placebo in adult patients with a diagnosis of major depression. In patients with a diagnosis of mild to moderate depression, St. John's wort seemed to have a slightly greater effect than placebo, but this did not have a statistically significant or clinically relevant effect. When compared with specific pharmacologic antidepressant therapy (tricyclic antidepressants [TCAs] and selective serotonin reuptake inhibitor [SSRI] medications), St. John's wort improved symptoms at a similar rate in adult patients with mild to moderate depression. However, a 2017 meta-analysis showed that SSRIs and serotonin-norepinephrine reuptake inhibitors only had a small benefit over placebo and their effect was significantly greater in patients with anxiety disorder than in those with depressive disorder, thus demonstrating that the placebo effect does play a role in the treatment of depression.[15] Patients taking St. John's wort stopped therapy less often than patients on TCAs. Dropout rates were similar in patients taking SSRI medication. In general, most studies seem to show a greater benefit in patients with mild to moderate depression than in those with major depression or a chronic course of illness. One of the biggest confounding factors in these studies is that there is no standardized preparation of St. John's wort, which means there is no way of knowing how much of the "active" component patients are receiving. This may contribute to the heterogeneity of results.

Another issue with St. John's wort is its potential for adverse drug interactions. A few side effects have been reported in patients taking St. John's wort as monotherapy. However, because of metabolism by the liver enzyme cytochrome P450 3A4, St. John's wort can decrease levels of warfarin, cyclosporine, OCPs (Oral contraceptive pills), digoxin, and several antiretroviral medications. This should be discussed with patients who may be taking or considering initiation of St. John's wort therapy. There have also been reports of serotonin syndrome in patients who have combined St. John's wort with SSRI medication.[14]

S-adenosyl-L-methionine (SAMe) is thought to play a role in the treatment of depression by affecting the synthesis of serotonin and the metabolic pathways of folate and vitamin $B_{12}$. Patients with depression are routinely screened for folate and $B_{12}$, as there has been some evidence that patients who are deficient in these have a poor response to antidepressants.[13] A 2016 Cochrane review looked at RCTs that compared SAMe with placebo and antidepressant therapy in patients with a diagnosis of major depression. The only antidepressants studied were escitalopram, imipramine, and desipramine. The quality of evidence was rated low or very low in all included studies. The efficacy of SAMe as monotherapy did not show any difference in treatment effect from that of TCAs or escitalopram.[16] There was also no evidence of a difference between SAMe and placebo in improving depressive symptoms. SAMe showed a small benefit versus placebo when taken in combination with an SSRI. In most studies, SAMe has demonstrated few side effects and drug interactions. There have been isolated reports of mania in patients with bipolar disorder who have taken SAMe and these patients should be appropriately cautioned about its use.[13] As with St. John's wort, variations in SAMe preparations as well as variations in the severity of depressive symptoms may play a role in the varying results reported in most studies. As is the case with most data available, the abovementioned studies were on adult patients, and the effects and risks specific to adolescent patients are as of yet unstudied.

ω-3 Fatty acids, typically found in seafood and fatty fish, are found at low levels in a typical Western diet. This "deficiency" has been blamed for a variety of conditions that seem to occur at higher rates in the Western world, including cardiovascular disease and major depression. The mechanism of action is thought to be the role that ω-3 fatty acids play in regulating neurotransmitter signaling through membrane-bound receptors. They are also thought to decrease levels of cortisol and inflammatory cytokines.[13] A 2015 Cochrane review was on RCTs comparing ω-3 fatty acids to placebo and antidepressants and their effects on depressive symptoms. All the studies included were deemed as "low-quality" evidence and only one small study compared antidepressants with ω-3 fatty acids. This review found that ω-3 fatty acids seem to have a small benefit over placebo and no difference in effect when compared with antidepressant therapy. A few side effects or drug interactions are reported, with the most common side effect being gastrointestinal distress or upset.[17]

## Generalized Anxiety Disorder

Anxiety disorders are one of the most common mental health diagnoses, although less than half of those affected report receiving treatment. Anxiety is the most common mental health diagnosis for which patients report using complementary medicine. At least one-third of patients receiving treatment for anxiety report using complementary medicine as part of their treatment regimen.[2] The most commonly employed treatments use include yoga and meditation. There is no evidence to support consistent benefits in patients with anxiety and no data specific to its use in the adolescent population. However, given the minimal risk associated with these interventions, it is appropriate for providers to discuss these options and encourage their use in patients, particularly for patients and families seeking treatment options in the realm of complementary medicine.

The most commonly used complementary medicine supplements to target anxiety symptoms are kava, valerian, and passion fruit root. As with many other supplements, high-quality evidence is limited and inconclusive. These dietary supplements are thought to affect γ-aminobutyric acid activity in the brain. A 2003 Cochrane review compared kava root with placebo and found that kava root did reduce anxiety symptoms. However, both the measured effect and sample size were small and safety data was lacking.[18] There have been several case reports of hepatotoxicity and liver failure in patients using kava root. The Food and Drug Administration (FDA) has subsequently issued a warning for patients in whom liver disease is already a concern.[19] Only one small study compared valerian root and its effects on anxiety symptoms with placebo and the benzodiazepine, diazepam. Given the small size of the study, no conclusions could be made on the effect of valerian root.[20] Passion fruit root is not available as monotherapy and is typically included in a supplement marketed as an "anxiety preparation." To date, there are no studies with adequate data to support its use in reducing anxiety symptoms. Also, given its combination preparation, little is known about the role that passion fruit root alone plays in mitigating anxiety symptoms.[21]

## Attention-Deficit/Hyperactivity Disorder

ADD and/or ADHD are common diagnoses in children and adolescents. Often the side effects and/or efficacy of stimulant medications can cause patients and parents to seek out complementary medicine options as either adjuvants or monotherapy. ADHD is also the only diagnosis for which there is significant data on the use of complementary medicine in children and adolescents, as this is the age range in which diagnosis and treatment commonly occur. One dietary supplement of interest is polyunsaturated fatty acids (PUFAs). These include ω-3 and ω-6 fatty acids. Both are thought to play a role in brain development and function, given their abundance in brain tissue. A 2014 meta-analysis studied the blood levels of ω-3 fatty acids in children with ADHD and found that the fatty acid levels were reduced in these patients when compared with controls.[22] A 2018 review studied the nonpharmacologic treatments for ADHD, specifically PUFAs and dietary or herbal approaches that have been advertised to reduce ADHD symptoms. This review found that PUFAs have little to no effect on ADHD symptoms when compared with placebo or pharmacologic therapy with nonstimulants.[23] A 2012 Cochrane review evaluated ADHD symptoms in patients treated with PUFAs as compared with placebo, medication, behavior therapy, and psychotherapy.[24] It also evaluated the activity of PUFA alone or in combination with medication, behavior therapy, or psychotherapy. Overall, there was no significant evidence that fatty acid supplementation had any significant effect on ADHD symptoms. Although isolated studies showed some effect when ω-3 and ω-6 fatty acids were used in combination, data quality was low and sample size was too small to be of statistical significance. No significant side effects were reported. Additional reviews have studied acupuncture and meditation as potential complementary treatment modalities for ADHD. There is insufficient data and there are no well-designed studies that support these options. However, given their minimal risk, use of fatty acid supplementation should certainly be encouraged in patients who perceive symptom benefits.

## Sleep Disorders

Insomnia is a common problem of adolescence and approximately 1.8% of youth use CAM for trouble sleeping.[25] There are limited data on the comparison of CAM to behavioral sleep modifications in adolescents. Melatonin has moved from the arena of CAM to conventional therapy because of the large amount of evidence claiming that it improves sleep latency and is safe in low doses.[25] Valerian root appears to be safe and improves sleep latency and sleep length in some limited pediatric studies.[26] Chamomile tea and acupuncture have not been studied in pediatric populations for sleep. Hypnosis and music therapy have been shown to be beneficial for insomnia in children.[25]

## Headaches

Patients have used CAM for the treatment and prevention of headaches for a variety of reasons including because "their provider recommended it, conventional treatment was ineffective, and conventional treatment was too expensive."[27] Literature comparing benefits is divided into two categories: one for migraines and the other for tension-type headaches.[28] In general, however, patients utilizing CAM for headaches do not differentiate between the two, so we will review the major categories of treatment together.

A few small studies in adults and children have demonstrated the benefits of butterbur (*Petasites hybridus*) oral supplementation in the prevention of migraines; however, there has been a historical risk of liver injury associated with certain formulations of this compound.[29] Magnesium supplementation for headache prophylaxis in adolescents has a weak recommendation owing to its very minimal benefit and well-delineated side effect of diarrhea.[29] Based on the evidence in the adult and pediatric literature, ginkgolide B, PUFAs, and riboflavin are not recommended for pediatric migraine prophylaxis.[29] The evidence for using coenzyme $Q_{10}$ for headache prevention in children and adolescents has not been well established.[29]

Other methods for management of pediatric headache include acupuncture, transcutaneous electric nerve stimulation, transcranial magnetic stimulation, massage, and a host of biofeedback and neurofeedback techniques.[30] The effectiveness of these modalities in adolescents has not been studied.

## Acne

Acne vulgaris is one of the most common conditions of adolescence and many patients use complementary and alternative methods to improve skin lesion outcome, minimize scarring, and prevent new lesions. Adolescents cite turning to CAM due to both lack of improvement in, or adverse reactions associated with, conventional acne treatment.[31] A Cochrane review summarized and reviewed clinical trials that used a variety of complementary and alternative methods for treatment and prevention of acne. They focused on objective measurements of change in skin lesion numbers and change in acne severity over time.[32]

A low-glycemic-load diet has been proposed and studied as a treatment for prevention of acne lesions because of the reduction in circulating androgen levels. Although one study showed a decrease in skin lesion numbers over 12 weeks, no other studies have effectively been able to reproduce this end outcome.[32] The evidence trends toward benefit but further data is needed.

Others have turned to complementary dietary supplements for benefit. Bovine lactoferrin (a multifunctional protein present in milk and other secretions that can be purified from human or cow's milk or produced recombinantly) may have some benefit as a dietary supplement by acting as an effective anti-inflammatory agent, without reported side effects.[33] ω-3 Fatty acid supplementation has not been fully evaluated for acne management and no data is available.[31]

Patients have also used unconventional topical therapies for acne management and prevention. Tea tree oil, which has some antibacterial and antifungal properties, has shown significant improvement in acne treatment when compared with placebo, with the minimal side effects of pruritus and burning sensation. Cosmetics containing purified bee venom also showed benefit when compared with placebo in reducing the number of skin lesions. Resveratrol gel has shown some benefit as compared with controls in acne count reduction. Importantly, tea tree oil, purified bee venom, or resveratrol was not compared with conventional therapy.[31] Other cosmeceutical topical agents containing either retinoic acid derivatives, niacinamide, or glycolic acid have shown no benefit when compared with conventional treatment controls.[34]

The Cochrane review from 2016 also demonstrated no benefit from acupuncture, moxibustion, or wet-cupping for reducing the number of acne lesions when compared with controls who were untreated or given conventional therapy. Other herbal remedies for acne, either Ayurvedic or Chinese in origin, have not been supported by this systematic review of evidence and may have worse side effect profiles.[32]

## Atopic Dermatitis

A variety of complementary methods have emerged over the years to improve atopic dermatitis (AD) or to alleviate its symptoms. Patients have cited steroid phobia as a major reason for turning to CAM in AD therapy.[35] Here we will review CAM therapies that are utilized for AD while focusing on objective outcome improvements, such as improvement in the Scoring Atopic Dermatitis (SCORAD) scale.

Some therapies for AD involve ingesting or supplementing dietary additives, whereas others focus on removal of certain substances from the diet. The potential benefit of prebiotics and probiotics has been demonstrated in AD; however, the exact organisms and their dosages have not been clearly determined.[36] A few studies have shown objective improvement with vitamin D supplementation.[37] Evening primrose oil, black currant seed oil, and borage oil supplementation all failed to show objective improvement when compared with placebo.[38] The removal of foods or substances, such as gluten, from the diet has not shown to be beneficial in AD to this point.[37]

For many years, topical oils and emollients have been used in one form or another as moisturizing or antiseptic agents for AD. Coconut oil has been studied in patients with AD and shown to be beneficial in improving SCORAD indexes and in lowering bacterial colonization, with minimal reported side effects.[35] Sunflower seed oil also significantly reduced the SCORAD index and allowed steroid-sparing regimens in several studies, with no reported adverse effects.[35] Olive oil, on the other hand, showed detriment to the skin barrier and resulted in much more contact dermatitis, so it is not recommended.[37] Both colloidal oatmeal and glycerin-based emollients have also shown benefit in a few clinical trials as adjunct therapies to conventional treatment.[39]

Other modalities such as dilute bleach baths have shown improvement in treating AD, and they are an example of alternative therapy that has moved into conventional recommended use.[37] Balneotherapy (bathing in 10% mineral bath followed by ultraviolet light exposure) has been shown to be beneficial in treating AD. Acupuncture has been used successfully to reduce pruritus in patients with AD.[40] Other therapies such as CHM and homeopathy have not shown any demonstrable improvement in patients with AD.[37]

## NUTRITION, PHYSICAL HEALTH, AND COMPLEMENTARY AND ALTERNATIVE MEDICINE

Puberty is marked by a rapid growth in height and weight. As a result, one of the tasks of adolescence is adapting to a new sense of physical and emotional health. Early and mid-adolescents (those aged 12–17 years) are particularly prone to peer pressure and often start to critically look at themselves and their self-image during puberty. This may be even more likely for adolescents who are overweight or obese. Conventional and traditional medical treatment plans for weight loss include increasing physical activity, reducing caloric intake, and adopting healthy dietary habits. However, the need for immediate and more proximal results may lead adolescents and young adults to consider complementary healthcare approaches to lose weight and/or improve sports performance.

### Obesity and Eating Disorders (see also chapter 3 on nutrition and chapter 12 on screening for body image and sexual abuse).

The role of mindfulness (which includes yoga, meditation, and present-moment self-awareness) has been studied for a variety of health-related topics, including obesity and eating disorders. Yoga has been shown to have several positive health effects: weight reduction, decreased body mass index, healthier food choices, and slower eating.[41] However, there has been insufficient evidence for yoga in the treatment of eating disorders. Although yoga may not be specifically helpful in eating disorder behaviors per se, it may help with the anxiety, obsessive-compulsive traits, or attitudes that are often associated with eating disorders. One particular study found that fifth-grade girls who were introduced to yoga as a stress reduction strategy, had improved self-body satisfaction and fewer eating disorder attitudes when compared with controls.[42] In general, overall studies suggest that yoga is a low-risk, possibly beneficial mind–body practice for stress reduction and anxiety, which can improve psychologic functioning.[43]

### Weight Loss and Diet Pills

Nutritional supplements may be marketed to improve physical and mental performance, but they can have a broader appeal as well to improve overall nutrition and fitness. As such, dietary supplements may be marketed for weight loss or appetite suppression. Weight loss product sales are big business, and the 2014 worldwide estimates are close to $600 billion spent.[44] Data from Monitoring the Future 2014 has shown that more than 10% of high-school girls report any lifetime use of nonprescription diet pills and approximately 4% of boys report a similar lifetime prevalence.[45] Over-the-counter diet pills often contain stimulants such as caffeine in addition to laxatives. Guarana is a plant extract that contains variable levels of caffeine and is often marketed for weight loss.[46] Taurine is an amino acid commonly found in energy drinks and weight loss products that can potentiate the effects of caffeine.[46] Kola nut and green tea are naturally derived caffeine products that may also be found in dietary weight loss supplements.[46] Several herbal products with mild diuretic properties (such as uva ursi or buchu leaf) may also be found in diet pills.[46] Garcinia is a plant-derived product that contains hydroxycitric acid and is marketed for weight loss product.[46] The proposed mechanism of action involves increased fat oxidation; however, there have been no definitive studies to support its use in weight loss treatment.

*Hoodia gordonii* is another plant-derived product that has anorectic activity in animals and has been studied for appetite suppression. Some small studies have shown decreased calorie intake in adult men who consumed *Hoodia*, but there is a paucity of evidence for adolescents and young adults.[46] None of the aforementioned products have substantiated use or medical research to support use. Most studies have found a very small improvement in short-term weight loss, which is unable to be sustained. Bulk-forming or stimulant laxatives may also be found in diet pills. Studies have found that adolescents and young adults who display body image and weight dissatisfaction may be at risk for unhealthy weight loss practices, including use of diet pills.[47] Medical providers should screen for these behaviors and discourage the use of such products, as they may lead to other health problems such as eating disorders or substance use. There is insufficient evidence to suggest that they are helpful, not even in the short term. The risks of use and abuse generally outweigh the benefits, as will be discussed shortly.

## Performance-Enhancing Substances

More than 50% of middle-school and high-school students play organized sports. With growing sports participation comes competition and striving for the competitive advantage, which may come in the form of performance-enhancing substances. Performance-enhancing substances are commonly used by US adolescents: in 2012, more than 1 million teens admitted to have taken a sports-related performance-enhancing dietary supplement in the past month.[48] These substances are marketed as safe and natural products to alter body composition and improve speed, endurance, or strength. Vitamins and mineral supplements are most commonly reported, but protein powder and creatine use are also on the rise, particularly by young adults.[48,49] Adolescent male athletes are more likely to use performance-enhancing products than female athletes and nonathletes. In fact, previous studies have found that up to 50% of high-school male athletes have taken dietary supplements or made significant dietary changes to improve their sports performance.[48] The common reasons for use among adolescent boys include building muscle mass or increased energy, whereas adolescent girls frequently cite that they use dietary supplements to increase energy or avoid illness. Adolescents and young adults who are overweight or obese may be more likely to use dietary supplements in order to lose weight and improve sports performance. It is a slippery slope; adolescents who use dietary supplements for weight loss or to enhance sports performance may engage in other at-risk health behaviors such as illicit substance use or use of performance-enhancing drugs such as anabolic steroids, stimulants, and hormone manipulators. Practitioners who uncover dietary supplement use in their adolescent athletes should therefore screen for these additional at-risk behaviors.

### *Creatine*

Creatine is a naturally occurring compound derived from the amino acids glycine and arginine. About 95% of bodily stores of creatine are found in skeletal muscles. Creatine is essential for the biochemical metabolic process of phosphorylation of adenosine diphosphate to adenosine triphosphate (ATP), the basis of energy. The phosphorylation process is critical in conditions with high ATP demand (such as exercise), as it provides increased energy to fast-twitch muscle fibers and aids in metabolic recovery. The resting human body requires 1–2 g/day of creatine to maintain health, much of which is endogenously produced or acquired from dietary sources such as meat and other animal products. Athletes who engage in brief, high-intensity exercises (such as weight lifting or football) may benefit from more creatine and therefore ingest it as an ergogenic aid; this is the basis for creatine supplementation.[50] Supplementation has been found to improve anaerobic muscle performance in high-intensity exercisers, albeit this has only been studied in adults.[5,51] RCTs have found very small benefits, and creatine use is limited only to short-duration resistance training.[50] There is no evidence to support use in the athlete participating in endurance sports. Owing to the possible risks associated with creatine use, the American Academy of Pediatrics and American College of Sports Medicine discourage individuals less than 18 years of age from using it.[48] Previous studies have reported that overuse of creatine can result in gastrointestinal complaints, fluid retention, and weight gain, as well as muscle cramps. There are also case reports of kidney injury associated with creatine supplementation. As there is little regulatory oversight of these products, accepted doses are unknown.

### *Prohormones*

Although androgenic anabolic steroids are not available as dietary supplements, androgen precursors in the form of dehydroepiandrosterone (DHEA) are widely available over the counter. DHEA is a hormone produced by the adrenal cortex and then peripherally converted to other sex-hormone steroids such as testosterone. As an anabolic steroid, testosterone is important in muscle and bone metabolism. As a steroid precursor, physiologic findings would suggest that more DHEA could lead to increased testosterone levels, with its performance-enhancing metabolic effects. However, studies have not found this to be true.[48] There have been no evidence-based studies to date to show that DHEA increases serum testosterone levels, improves muscle mass, or enhances sports performance in athletes.[48,49] Female athletes who ingest testosterone precursors may experience adverse androgenizing side effects with increased facial hair, deepening of the voice, acne, and clitoromegaly. Endogenous testosterone production may be downregulated in men who ingest these products leading to impaired growth, gynecomastia, and testicular atrophy. The risks of oral ingestion of these steroid precursors therefore outweigh the unfounded benefits.

### Stimulants

Performance-enhancing substances may also fall into the category of stimulants, which are ergogenic products marketed to improve focus and energy. Stimulants are sympathomimetic drugs that can theoretically improve performance by stimulating the central nervous system, activating muscles, and reducing fatigue. Stimulants may include caffeine, ephedrine, or amphetamine derivatives. It is not just athletic aerobic performance that may be improved with stimulants, there are possible neurocognitive effects as well. Caffeine can be easily ingested by adolescents and young adults, as it is commonly found in beverages, energy drinks, and over-the-counter pills. More than 70% of adolescents and young adults ingest caffeine on a daily basis.[5] The caffeine content of soft drinks and coffee is routinely monitored; however, there is less regulation with regard to energy drinks and dietary supplements. There is some data to show improved performance in endurance activities and reduction in time to exhaustion with caffeine intake. A meta-analysis in 2010 found small but statistically significant improvements in maximal volitional muscle contraction strength and endurance, primarily in knee extensors for adults.[52] However, these results are variable and have not been replicated in other muscle groups, or in adolescents. Experts warn that caffeine overuse can have untoward side effects such as palpitations, increased blood pressure, headaches, irritability, and cardiac arrhythmia.[5] Ephedra is probably one of the more well-known stimulants, but it is no longer legally sold in the United States as a result of more than 800 reports of serious side effects, including death.[53]

### β-Hydroxy-β-Methylbutyrate

β-Hydroxy-β-methylbutyrate (HMB) is one of the newer performance-enhancing substances to reach the market.[5] It is a leucine metabolite, with reported anticatabolic effects that slow protein breakdown after exercise. Two small studies conducted with adolescents and young adults have found that HMB can improve muscular strength and power during resistance training and reduce muscle damage after exercise.[5] To date, no adverse effects of HMB have been identified. In fact, HMB may have cholesterol-lowering properties as well, which may be cardioprotective.

### Additional products

Other dietary performance products that should be screened for in the adolescent athlete include nitrates, protein powders, and growth hormone stimulators. Nitric oxide boosters (commonly found in arginine, beetroot juice, and citrulline) have been associated with cardiovascular health, particularly as vasodilators. Performance results with these products are mixed, and minimal at best in healthy young athletes.[5] Protein powders reportedly contain amino acids, which are essential for muscle and tissue growth. If ingested soon after exercise, protein can also help with muscle recovery. However, if the adolescent diet contains adequate and well-balanced nutrition, there is no added benefit from protein supplementation.[54] In fact, most US youth who consume an omnivorous diet have excessive dietary protein intake and eat more than the recommended 1.2–2.0 g/kg daily allowance.[48] Therefore protein powders and supplements are unnecessary. While human growth hormone is a highly regulated substance (except in cases of actual growth hormone deficiency), dietary supplements that are advertised as growth hormone stimulators may contain amino acids or other substances that are known to increase endogenous growth hormone production. While there is evidence for athletic performance enhancement with human growth hormone, the benefits of use do not outweigh the serious risks of carpal tunnel syndrome, fluid retention, and acromegaly.[5,48]

### Energy drinks

Up to 50% of youth have consumed energy drinks.[55] Energy drinks are flavored beverages that commonly contain caffeine, vitamins, sugar, taurine, ginseng, herbs, and other additives that are marketed to teens to build stamina, improve physical performance, and improve mental alertness. The American Academy of Pediatrics Committee on Nutrition and the Council on Sports

Medicine and Fitness have repeatedly stated that energy drinks have no role in the diet of children and adolescents.[54] As energy drinks more often contain stimulants, the purported effects are due to activation of the cardiovascular and central nervous system, as mentioned earlier. However, it is often difficult to determine the actual drink ingredients. The total caffeine content of energy drinks may not be easily identified, so overingestion may occur. Caffeine is an addictive substance, so there is a real risk of physical dependence. Energy drinks may be consumed solo, but they are often used in combination with alcohol or other prescription and nonprescription drugs. As a stimulant, the energy drink may mask the untoward and sedating effects of alcohol, such that the individual is unaware of his or her level of intoxication. In 2011, more than 20,000 emergency room visits were attributed to overconsumption in the form of energy drinks, often in combination with other drugs or alcohol. Almost 9000 of these visits were in adolescents and young adults aged less than 25 years.[55]

## ADDITIONAL COMPLEMENTARY AND ALTERNATIVE MEDICINE PRACTICES

Thus far, this chapter has addressed herbal supplements, dietary approaches, topical oils, and mindfulness practices. Two additional complementary health practices that may be used by adolescents include homeopathy and functional medicine.

### Homeopathy

Homeopathic products are often described as safe and natural, particularly because they are diluted substances and only contain minute traces of the initial substance. Previous surveys from the NHIS have found that individuals self-prescribe homeopathic remedies for cold and musculoskeletal pain.[2] However, homeopathy is often regarded as one of the more controversial complementary therapies. According to the National Center for Complementary and Alternative Medicine, homeopathic remedies are based on imprinting, that is, serial dilutions of substances that leave a "memory" in the water (https://nccih.nih.gov/health/homeopathy). Previous meta-analyses have found weak evidence to support homeopathy (as compared with conventional medicine practices), and most of the available positive results are likely due to placebo effect.[56]

### Functional Medicine

Functional medicine is an individualized, holistic approach to disease management, focusing on identifying and addressing the immediate causes, root causes, and mediators of illness.[57] Functional medicine proponents believe that it is the interaction between an individual's bodily systems and his or her environment that result in disease. Therefore identifying and treating triggers and mediators of illness instead of symptoms are the basis of functional medicine management. Opponents argue that this identification approach often results in an extensive and exhaustive battery of laboratory examinations to isolate the cause, at considerable expense. There is limited evidence-based literature to argue for or against functional medicine. In 2016, one of the advisory bodies of the American Academy of Family Physicians conducted a medical literature review of functional medicine and was unable to find sufficient evidence to support the use of functional medicine in family medicine practice.[57]

## SAFETY OF COMPLEMENTARY AND ALTERNATIVE MEDICINE IN ADOLESCENTS

Although there is a plethora of information about the use of complementary medicine, some of which is evidence based, there is little evidence regarding safety and medical side effects. Much of the available literature focuses on use and efficacy in adults. Overall safety and efficacy literature on CAM practices is limited, particularly for children and adolescents. In general, as has been described throughout this chapter, evidence-based medicine is lacking with regard to complementary health practices in adolescents and young adults; we have little to go on in terms of what does and does not work. As we know that the most common CAM modality used by adolescents are nonvitamin, nonmineral dietary supplements, practitioners should be aware of possible side effects from these products. Manufacturers of dietary supplements are required to report adverse events only if they are deemed serious (inpatient hospitalization, significant disability, or death). Voluntary postmarketing reporting of less severe events is likely grossly underestimated. In fact, an FDA report indicated that they are notified of less than 1% of all adverse events related to dietary supplements.[58]

## RISKS VERSUS BENEFITS

When evaluating complementary and integrative medicine practices, there are several factors that patients, providers, and families should consider before deciding whether they are beneficial or harmful: (1) How acute is the illness? (2) Is the condition treatable or curable with traditional medical practices? (3) How invasive is the product or treatment? (4) What does the safety evidence show? (5) Are the studies of high quality? (6) What does the family and patient understand as the

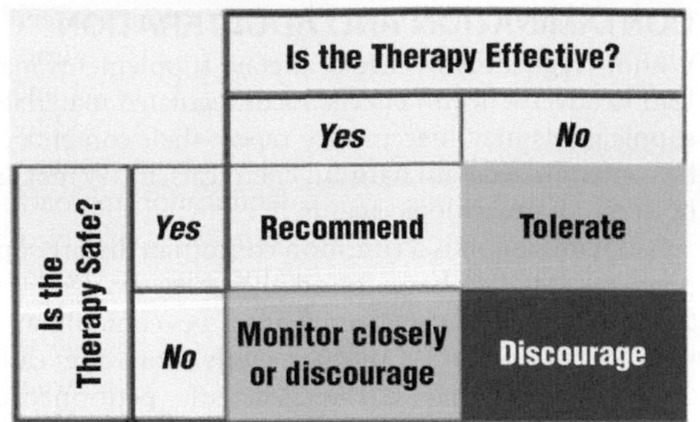

Is the Therapy Effective?
Yes
No
Is the Therapy Safe?
Yes
No
Recommend
Tolerate
Monitor closely or discourage
Discourage


FIG. 2.1 Guide to complementary and alternative medicine treatment recommendations.[59]

risks and benefits of using this modality as compared with traditional medicine?[1] Fig. 2.1 can help illustrate these principles and guide the practitioner.

Although dietary supplements are often marketed as safe and natural, they have been implicated in a variety of adverse health effects, particularly related to cardiovascular complications such as potentially fatal arrhythmias.[5] Other common cardiac complications of dietary and nutritional supplements (particularly those used for bodybuilding, weight loss, or energy) include palpitations, chest pain, or tachycardia.[48] Known dietary supplements with proarrhythmic potential include ephedra, caffeine, phenylpropanolamine, cesium, and others.

Just because products are dilute, herbal, natural, or marketed as safe, it does not mean that they are free of adverse effects. Zinc is a naturally occurring element. However, intranasal zinc products (brand name Zicam) were removed from the market 10 years ago because of consumer reports of anosmia.[60] Similarly, Hydroxycut dietary supplements (which previously contained ephedra, but now primarily contain a green coffee extract) were found to be associated with liver damage, seizures, rhabdomyolysis, and myocardial infarctions.[60]

## RISKS

It is not only the use of homeopathic and complementary practices but also the nonuse of conventional medical practices poses a risk. A study in Australia identified four deaths over a 3-year period that were attributed to failure to use conventional medical practices in favor of complementary medicine.[61] It is often the use of complementary practices at the expense of traditional allopathic medicine that may be problematic. This is particularly true when individuals choose complementary or integrative medical practices instead of traditional primary prevention such as vaccination. Individuals who consult naturopathic and/or chiropractic providers are less likely to adhere to vaccination guidelines and are therefore at risk for and can potentially acquire otherwise preventable diseases.[62]

Dietary and nutritional supplement use is underreported by patients and underidentified by healthcare providers. Important considerations for health providers include supplement–drug interactions, contamination, and direct toxicities from ingestion. There is a lengthy list of herbal supplements that have anticoagulant effects, most prominently when taken in combination with prescription warfarin.[14] A similar list of supplements can significantly interact with digoxin, which is often used in heart failure patients.[46]

There are a number of drug–drug interaction applications and web-based platforms to identify possible interactions with prescription medications. These same entities do not necessarily exist for dietary or nutritional supplements. However, there are several important herb–pharmaceutical interactions that healthcare providers should be aware of, and there are online accessible charts for reference (the NCCIH or www.standardprocess.com/MediHerb-Document-Library/Catalog-FIles/herb-drug-interaction-chart.pdf). Another aspect to consider is possible allergies. Echinacea has been touted as helpful for treatment or prevention of upper respiratory infections; however, it is a type of ragweed, so individuals with environmental and ragweed allergies may be sensitive to, and even allergic to, echinacea.

## ADVERSE EVENTS

Geller et al.[63] surveyed clinical data from 63 emergency departments within the United States and found that more than 23,000 adverse events annually are related to the use of dietary supplements (which were defined as oral or topically administered herbal products, complementary nutritionals such as amino acids, and micronutrients). Young adults (less than 34 years of age) and children comprised more than 40% of affected individuals. Slightly less than 10% of those annual events required inpatient hospitalization because of their severity. Among all age groups, the top three herbal or complementary nutritional products associated with emergency department visits for adverse events were those advertised for weight loss, energy, and sexual enhancement. Weight loss and energy products were accountable for more than one-third of adverse events among all age groups (excluding unintentional ingestion by children) and accounted for more than 50% of visits for those between the ages of 5 and 34 years. Performance-enhancing and bodybuilding products were the proximal cause of adverse events among male patients. The most commonly described adverse events related to micronutrients such as multivitamins, iron, calcium, and potassium are allergic reactions, abdominal pain, and swallowing problems.

## REGULATION

Unlike prescription or over-the-counter products, nutritional and dietary supplements have few safety regulations and package inserts do not need to provide information on possible adverse health effects. The Dietary Supplement Health and Education Act (DSHEA) was enacted in 1994 to regulate dietary and nutritional supplements. Regulation is a limited term; there is no premarketing oversight of these products, and there is no quality control or research into the instructions for use. These products are considered food substances and not drugs and are therefore not under the safety purview of the FDA. The DSHEA allows manufacturers to determine how the listed ingredients affect bodily function or support health but cannot explicitly state that the product can be used for prevention or treatment of a specific disease. The FDA similarly has no ability to regulate or authorize premarket approval for dietary and nutritional supplements. Most information regarding adverse effects comes from the aftermarket and only when serious side effects are reported by consumers or, rarely, manufacturers. Select products that are labeled United States Pharmacopeia have had some premarket validation, verifying product accuracy and potency. In general, postmarketing data submission is voluntary from both consumers and health professionals but is regarded as the primary source of safety information.[58] Less than 10% of adverse event reports come directly from manufacturers. One of the prototypical examples of postmarketing adverse effects comes from the historically used weight loss supplement ephedra. Ephedra is a naturally occurring plant substance that has been used in traditional Chinese medicine for more than 2000 years. Ephedra alkaloids were sold as performance-enhancing substances and weight loss products in the United States in the late 1980 and 1990s. The bestselling brand of ephedra in the 1990s was Metabolife. In 2002, it was revealed that more than 14,000 individual reports of adverse events associated with ephedra were reported to Metabolife manufacturers.[53] Based on postmarketing reports of adverse reactions (including seizures, sudden cardiac death, and stroke), it came to light as a harmful supplement. Ephedra and ephedrine substances were later banned by the FDA in 2004 because of the unreasonable risk of injury or illness, most prominently fatal side effects.

## CONTAMINATION AND ADULTERATION

Without regulatory oversight, dietary supplements may lead to adverse health effects. As unregulated materials, supplements may inaccurately report their contents or be contaminated with harmful chemicals, heavy metals, or other pharmacologic agents.

Contamination is a common concern in dietary supplements. Studies have found that between 8% and 20% of protein supplements may be contaminated with heavy metals.[64] Another study from the early 2000s found that 10%–25% of performance-enhancing dietary substances were tainted with stimulants and anabolic steroids, which were not listed as approved ingredients.[64] Herbal preparations may also be contaminated with microbial products (bacteria and/or fungi) in the manufacturing or storage processes. Ayurvedic medicine is a traditional Indian medical practice that uses herbal products often combined with metals such as zinc, lead, iron, and mercury. More than 80 cases of lead poisoning worldwide have been attributed to Ayurvedic medicine, and more than 20% of Ayurvedic products sold on the Internet (manufactured in both the United States or India) or available in US ethnic markets contain detectable levels of mercury, lead, or arsenic.[65] If taken as directed, these metal-containing Ayurvedic products would exceed published standards for an individual's acceptable daily intake, raising concerns for possible toxicity.

In the absence of premarket analysis, there may be lack of product verification and consistency. In 2015, the New York Times reported that 80% of herbal supplements tested at four different national retailers did not contain any of the herbs listed on the ingredient labels. Although the product labels listed gingko biloba, ginseng, and St. John's wort (in addition to others), independent analyses found that most of them did not contain any of those herbs but instead were composed of powdered rice, wheat, beans, and houseplants.[5]

## CONCLUSION

Given the overwhelming use of CAM therapies by adolescents and young adults, healthcare practitioners should familiarize themselves with available therapies, patient-perceived benefits, and risks of use. Most individuals use CAM in addition to traditional allopathic medical practices, but often without provider knowledge. Clinicians should take an open approach and ask patients in a nonjudgmental manner about their use of CAM in order to establish a therapeutic rapport. Primary care providers need to be sure they are screening for complementary medicine/supplement use by including it as part of routine history-taking procedure. It could be as simple as asking about general use or it could include questions about diagnoses known to be associated with CAM/supplement use. Asking about specific supplements or modalities known to be used to treat disorders such as anxiety or dysmenorrhea might be more likely to yield positive and accurate data. Asking specifically about weight or body image concerns might also trigger providers to question about supplements commonly used for weight loss and/or athletic performance enhancement. Healthcare professionals should be willing to provide evidence-based information in an effort to facilitate mutual decision-making. Unfortunately, the overall safety and efficacy literature with respect to complementary and integrative medicine is limited, particularly for children and adolescents. Most studies are small, and not well-designed to evaluate for adverse effects. However, there are some complementary health approaches that can be considered for the treatment of mental health disorders (particularly St. John's wort, ω-3 fatty acids, and mind–body practices such as yoga or meditation) as long as they are accompanied by a discussion of benefits and potential risks. Including CAM screening in our adolescent population would help us educate patients and families and separate fact from fiction.

## REFERENCES


1. McClafferty H, et al. Pediatric integrative medicine. *Pediatrics*. 2017;140(3).
2. Black LI, et al. Use of complementary health approaches among children aged 4–17 years in the United States: National Health Interview Survey, 2007–2012. *Natl Health Stat Report 78*. 2015:1–19.
3. Wilson KM, et al. Use of complementary medicine and dietary supplements among U.S. adolescents. *J Adolesc Health*. 2006;38(4):385–394.
4. Ryan SA. The treatment of dysmenorrhea. *Pediatr Clin North Am*. 2017;64(2):331–342.
5. LaBotz M, et al. Use of performance-enhancing substances. *Pediatrics*. 2016;138(1).
6. Doty E, Attaran M. Managing primary dysmenorrhea. *J Pediatr Adolesc Gynecol*. 2006;19(5):341–344.
7. Smith CA, Zhu X, et al. Acupuncture for dysmenorrhea. *Cochrane Database Syst Rev*. 2016.
8. Pattanittum P, Kunyanone N, Brown J, et al. Dietary supplements for dysmenorrhea. *Cochrane Database Syst Rev*. 2016;3.
9. Zhu X, Proctor M, Bensoussan A, et al. Chinese Herbal medicine for primary dysmenorrhea. *Cochrane Database Syst Rev*. 2007;(2):CD005288.
10. Pan JC, et al. The traditional Chinese medicine prescription pattern of patients with primary dysmenorrhea in Taiwan: a large-scale cross sectional survey. *J Ethnopharmacol*. 2014; 152(2):314–319.
11. Deborah S. Complementary and integrative medicine in Child and adolescent psychiatric disorders: fact, fiction, and challenges in clinical education and residency training. *J Am Acad Child Adolesc Psychiatry*. 2017;56(10):S116.
12. Rey JM, Walter G, Soh N. Complementary and alternative medicine (CAM) treatments and pediatric psychopharmacology. *J Am Acad Child Adolesc Psychiatry*. 2008;47(4):364–368.
13. Mischoulon D. Update and critique of natural remedies as antidepressant treatments. *Psychiatr Clin North Am*. 2007; 30(1):51–68.
14. Linde K, Berner MM, Kriston L. St John's wort for major depression. *Cochrane Database Syst Rev*. 2008;(4): CD000448. https://doi.org/10.1002/14651858.CD000448.pub3.
15. Locher C, et al. Efficacy and safety of selective serotonin reuptake inhibitors, serotonin-norepinephrine reuptake inhibitors, and placebo for common psychiatric disorders among children and adolescents: a systematic review and meta-analysis. *JAMA Psychiatry*. 2017;74(10):1011–1020.
16. Galizia I, Oldani L, Macritchie K, et al. S-adenosyl methionine (SAMe) for depression in adults. *Cochrane Database Syst Rev*. 2016;10:CD011286.
17. Appleton K, Sallis H, Perry R, et al. Omega-3 fatty acids for depression in adults. *Cochrane Database Syst Rev*. 2015; (11):CD004692.
18. Pittler MH, Ernst E. Kava extract versus placebo for treating anxiety. *Cochrane Database Syst Rev*. 2003;(2): CD003383.
19. Campo JV, et al. Kava-induced fulminant hepatic failure. *J Am Acad Child Adolesc Psychiatry*. 2002;41(6):631–632.
20. Miyasaka LS, Atallah ÁN, Soares B. Valerian for anxiety disorders. *Cochrane Database Syst Rev*. 2006;(4):CD004515. https://doi.org/10.1002/14651858.CD004515.pub2.
21. Miroddi M, et al. *Passiflora incarnata* L.: ethnopharmacology, clinical application, safety and evaluation of clinical trials. *J Ethnopharmacol*. 2013;150(3):791–804.
22. Hawkey E, Nigg JT. Omega-3 fatty acid and ADHD: blood level analysis and meta-analytic extension of supplementation trials. *Clin Psychol Rev*. 2014;34(6):496–505.
23. Goode AP, et al. Nonpharmacologic treatments for attention-deficit/hyperactivity disorder: a systematic review. *Pediatrics*. 2018;141(6).
24. Gillies D, Sinn J, Lad S, et al. Polyunsaturated fatty acids (PUFS) for attention deficit hyperactivity disorder (ADHD) in children and adolescents. *Cochrane Database Syst Rev*. 2012;(7):CD007986.
25. Sawni A, Breuner CC. Complementary, holistic, and integrative medicine: depression, sleep disorders, and substance abuse. *Pediatr Rev*. 2012;33(9):422–425.
26. Taibi DM, et al. A systematic review of valerian as a sleep aid: safe but not effective. *Sleep Med Rev*. 2007;11(3):209–230.
27. Wells RE, et al. Complementary and alternative medicine use among adults with migraines/severe headaches. *Headache*. 2011;51(7):1087–1097.

28. Schetzek S, et al. Headache in children: update on complementary treatments. *Neuropediatrics*. 2013;44(1): 25–33.
29. Orr SL, Venkateswaran S. Nutraceuticals in the prophylaxis of pediatric migraine: evidence-based review and recommendations. *Cephalalgia*. 2014;34(8):568–583.
30. Kedia S. Complementary and integrative approaches for pediatric headache. *Semin Pediatr Neurol*. 2016;23(1): 44–52.
31. Sawni A, Singh A. Complementary, holistic, and integrative medicine: acne. *Pediatr Rev*. 2013;34(2):91–93.
32. Cao H, Yang G, Wang Y, et al. Complementary therapies for acne vulgaris. *Cochrane Database Syst Rev*. 2016;1: CD009436.
33. Mueller EA, et al. Efficacy and tolerability of oral lactoferrin supplementation in mild to moderate acne vulgaris: an exploratory study. *Curr Med Res Opin*. 2011;27(4): 793–797.
34. Barros BS, Zaenglein AL. The use of cosmeceuticals in acne: help or hoax? *Am J Clin Dermatol*. 2017;18(2):159–163.
35. Karagounis TK, et al. Use of "natural" oils for moisturization: review of olive, coconut, and sunflower seed oil. *Pediatr Dermatol*. 2018.
36. Kim SO, et al. Effects of probiotics for the treatment of atopic dermatitis: a meta-analysis of randomized controlled trials. *Ann Allergy Asthma Immunol*. 2014; 113(2):217–226.
37. Goddard AL, Lio PA. Alternative, complementary, and forgotten remedies for atopic dermatitis. *Evid Based Complement Alternat Med*. 2015;2015:676897.
38. Bamford J, Ray S, Musekiwa A, et al. Oral evening primrose oil and borage oil for eczema. *Cochrane Database Syst Rev*. 2013;(4):CD004416.
39. Silverberg NB. Selected active naturals for atopic dermatitis: atopic dermatitis part 1. *Clin Dermatol*. 2017;35(4): 383–386.
40. Lee KC, et al. Effectiveness of acupressure on pruritus and lichenification associated with atopic dermatitis: a pilot trial. *Acupunct Med*. 2012;30(1):8–11.
41. Godsey J. The role of mindfulness based interventions in the treatment of obesity and eating disorders: an integrative review. *Complement Ther Med*. 2013;21(4): 430–439.
42. Scime M, Cook-Cottone C. Primary prevention of eating disorders: a constructivist integration of mind and body strategies. *Int J Eat Disord*. 2008;41(2):134–142.
43. Rosen L, et al. Complementary, holistic, and integrative medicine: yoga. *Pediatr Rev*. 2015;36(10):468–474.
44. *Global Market for Weight Loss Worth US$586.3 Billion by 2014*; 2014. Available from: https://www.marketsandmarkets.com/PressReleases/global-market-for-weight-loss-worth-$726-billion-by-2014.asp.
45. Miech RA, et al. *Monitoring the Future National Survey Results on Drug Use, 1975–2014*. Vol. 1. Secondary School Students; 2015:640.
46. Neinstein LS, Katzman D, Callahan T. *Neinstein's Adolescent and Young Adult Health Care: A Practical Guide*. 6th ed. Philadelphia, PA: Wolters Kluwer; 2016:690. xxviii.
47. Hazzard VM, Hahn SL, Sonneville KR. Weight misperception and disordered weight control behaviors among U.S. high school students with overweight and obesity: associations and trends, 1999–2013. *Eat Behav*. 2017;26: 189–195.
48. Chorley JN, Anding RH. Performance-enhancing substances. *Adolesc Med State Art Rev*. 2015;26(1):174–188.
49. Breuner CC. Performance-enhancing substances. *Adolesc Med State Art Rev*. 2014;25(1):113–125.
50. Metzl JD, et al. Creatine use among young athletes. *Pediatrics*. 2001;108(2):421–425.
51. Momaya A, Fawal M, Estes R. Performance-enhancing substances in sports: a review of the literature. *Sports Med*. 2015;45(4):517–531.
52. Warren GL, et al. Effect of caffeine ingestion on muscular strength and endurance: a meta-analysis. *Med Sci Sports Exerc*. 2010;42(7):1375–1387.
53. Fontanarosa PB, Rennie D, DeAngelis CD. The need for regulation of dietary supplements–lessons from ephedra. *JAMA*. 2003;289(12):1568–1570.
54. Committee on, N., M. the Council on Sports, and Fitness. Sports drinks and energy drinks for children and adolescents: are they appropriate? *Pediatrics*. 2011;127(6): 1182–1189.
55. Mattson ME. Update on emergency department visits involving energy drinks: a continuing public health concern. *CBHSQ Rep*. 2013:1–7. Rockville (MD).
56. Shang A, et al. Are the clinical effects of homoeopathy placebo effects? comparative study of placebo-controlled trials of homoeopathy and allopathy. *Lancet*. 2005; 366(9487):726–732.
57. Crawford C. AAFP credit system reconsiders functional medicine topics. *Ann Fam Med*. 2018;16(4):373–374.
58. *Adverse Event Reporting for Dietary Supplements: An Inadequate Safety Valve*; 2001. Available from: https://oig.hhs.gov/oei/reports/oei-01-00-00180.pdf.
59. Kemper K, Cohen M. Ethics meet complementary and alternative medicine: new light on old principles. *Contemporary Pediatrics*. 2004;21(3):61.
60. Kuehn BM. Despite health claims by manufacturers, little oversight for homeopathic products. *JAMA*. 2009; 302(15):1631–1632, 1634.
61. Lim A, Cranswick N, South M. Adverse events associated with the use of complementary and alternative medicine in children. *Arch Dis Child*. 2011;96(3):297–300.
62. Downey L, et al. Pediatric vaccination and vaccine-preventable disease acquisition: associations with care by complementary and alternative medicine providers. *Matern Child Health J*. 2010;14(6):922–930.
63. Geller AI, et al. Emergency department visits for adverse events related to dietary supplements. *N Engl J Med*. 2015;373(16):1531–1540.
64. Maughan RJ. Quality assurance issues in the use of dietary supplements, with special reference to protein supplements. *J Nutr*. 2013;143(11):1843S–1847S.
65. Saper RB, et al. Lead, mercury, and arsenic in US- and Indian-manufactured ayurvedic medicines sold via the internet. *JAMA*. 2008;300(8):915–923.

CHAPTER 3

# Dietary Screening—Questioning Adolescent Dietary Trends and Providing Evidence-Based Dietary Recommendations

EMMY SOBIESKI, CNC, CFA, MBA, DVA • JAMES SOBIESKI, NREMT, NAEMT-I • RICHARD MILNER, MD, PhD

Many nutritional studies are limited by their epidemiologic nature (self-reporting, compliance) and the expense of creating an environment of full compliance. Frequent advancements are being made in the field of nutritional research. Most nutritional studies are conducted on adults and do not take into account the impact of ongoing mental and physical development of adolescents. Where adult conditions are considered similar to those of adolescents, we refer to the adult studies.

Understanding the correlations between nutrition and health is critical to create an accurate and comprehensive public health perspective. The following sections discuss how nutrition plays into major community health concerns.

## NEUROCOGNITIVE EFFECTS OF NUTRITION

When looking at the nutritional status of the planet, it is particularly difficult to identify the accurate prevalence of adolescent undernutrition. However, a survey[1] of seven African countries shows malnutrition rates ranging from 12.6% (Egypt) to 31.9% (Djibouti). This prevalence of undernutrition directly relates to neurocognitive performance. Data from the National Longitudinal Study of Adolescent Health (a study using a sample of same-sex twin pairs) and others show that multiple nutritional and exercise factors during adolescence influence adult verbal intelligence and verbal, visuospatial, and memory tasks, as well as other neurocognitive performance metrics.[2,3] These findings suggest that inadequate nutrition, and the associated mental health and developmental consequences, will continue to challenge these countries until conditions can be ameliorated.

## DEPRESSION AND NUTRITION

Mental health impacts communities around the globe, with many of the impacts happening early in life. In 2016, 12.8% of the US population aged 12–17 years had at least one major depressive episode and clinical depression was the primary cause of disability in children aged 5 years and over.[4] Nutrition may have an important role to play in the prevalence of depression. A 2012 study found that consumption of fast foods and processed pastries was linked to depression in a dose-dependent manner.[5]

Diet has also been seen to play an important role in the production of serotonin. Serotonin not only plays its well-known role in depression but also plays significant roles in the regulation of executive functions, sensory gating, and behavior disorders such as attention-deficit/hyperactivity disorder (ADHD), bipolar disorder, schizophrenia, and impulsive behavior. Up to 90% of serotonin is synthesized in the digestive tract and both ω-3 fatty acids (especially the two marine ω-3 fatty acids, eicosapentaenoic acid [EPA] and docosahexaenoic acid [DHA]) and vitamin D have been shown to help control serotonin synthesis and action.[6] Foods containing ω-3 fatty acids can be "brain protective" by helping to maintain the blood–brain barrier. However, these protections are reversed when the

Adolescent Health Screening: An Update in the Age of Big Data. https://doi.org/10.1016/B978-0-323-66130-0.00003-X

misbehavior were drastically reduced when the ultra-processed foods were replaced with "nonprocessed" items.[52] Reducing adolescent intake of processed foods in favor of whole foods can decrease the levels of added sugars and trans fats, while raising the levels of protein, fiber, and many micronutrients in the diet.

### Fast Foods

Much like processed foods, fast foods are prepared to maximize profits for companies and fast food preparation and ingredients can be risky to adolescent nutrition and health. Thermally induced oxidation of polyunsaturated fatty acids (PUFAs) in foods and culinary oils during frying or cooking forms alkoxyl radicals that generate a wide range of toxic aldehydic products.[53] These hydrogenated oils have a wide range of untoward effects including gastropathic,[54] proinflammatory,[55] and genotoxicologic[56] properties. High-temperature wok cooking with unrefined Chinese rapeseed oil may increase lung cancer risk, the highest risk from unrefined Chinese rapeseed oil (canola oil).[57–59] The fatty acid composition of inflammatory and immune cells is sensitive to dietary composition, linking oxidized dietary PUFA intake with inflammation and immunity.[60] A study of 8544 fifth-grade children showed fast-food consumption as a dose-dependent inverse predictor of subsequent academic performance (reading, math, and science) in eighth grade.[61]

### *Implications of Excessive ω-6 Polyunsaturated Fatty Acids in Diets via Processed and Fast Foods*

The optimal dietary n-6 to n-3 PUFA ratio is 2:1 or lower, whereas in the current Western diet, with its aforementioned prevalence of fast foods and processed foods, the ratio is typically in the range of 10:1 to 25: 1.[62] The shift in modern diets toward reduced ω-3 (n-3) PUFA intake and increased n-6 PUFA consumption has had a detrimental impact on the development of cognitive function. DHA (an ω-3 PUFA) likely played an important role in the evolution of the human brain, as significant gains in cognitive abilities coincided with the incorporation of fish into the human diet.[63] Maintaining optimal lipid composition in the brain, specifically DHA levels, is important during the development and maturation of the brain from gestation through childhood and adolescence.[64,65]

DHA, the predominant ω-3 (n-3) PUFA found in the brain, comprises 8% of brain volume and can modulate signaling pathways and synapses, generation of new neurons, membrane integrity, membrane receptor function, neuroinflammation, and membrane organization.[66] DHA also alters gene expression in mammalian brain tissues that influences learning and memory.[64,67–69] DHA is deposited within the cerebral cortex at an accelerated rate during the last trimester of gestation and during the first 2 years after birth.[70] DHA is important for neurologic health; however, animal data shows that it is physiologically difficult to entirely reverse the effects of early brain DHA depletion.[71] Primate studies show that low DHA levels are associated with visual and motor deficits.[72] The reduction of dietary n-3 PUFAs levels negatively affects DHA concentrations within the brain.[73] Animal models provide solid evidence that the consequences of dietary DHA deficiency are a high n-6: n-3 PUFA ratio in brain fatty acid composition and deficiencies in learning and memory behaviors,[74,75] possibly due to negative impacts on neurite outgrowth and myelination.[76]

Although the above studies show the importance of DHA as well as the difficulty in reversing low DHA levels through supplementation, in the DHA Oxford Learning and Behavior (DOLAB) study, significant results were observed with the poorest reading subgroup (lowest quintile) experiencing an 8-month improvement in reading age after DHA supplementation. Moreover, parent-rated behavior problems (ADHD-type symptoms) were significantly reduced by DHA supplementation. The DOLAB study showed that DHA can affect brain function well beyond early development in healthy children.[77] Benefits from dietary supplementation with ω-3 PUFA found for ADHD, dyspraxia, dyslexia, and related conditions might extend to the general school population.[78] A medical review of 14 intervention studies showed some aggression-/hostility-controlling effects of fish oils in 11 of the studies via activation of the serotonergic neuron system.[79] Thus although most DHA deposition happens in the first 2 years of childhood, supplementation in adolescents may be beneficial.

## WHEAT, GLYPHOSATE (ROUNDUP), GLUTEN, AND CELIAC DISEASE

Although no genetically modified (GMO) wheat is being grown (as of 2015), glyphosate, a key ingredient in Monsanto's Roundup herbicide, is often sprayed on wheat crops just before harvest, killing the crop so that uniform drying and harvest can take place in a predictable fashion. Glyphosate has come under increased scrutiny with the World Health Organization's classifying it as a probable carcinogen. It has also been documented to kill beneficial gut bacteria and to damage the DNA in human embryonic cells and is linked to birth defects and reproductive problems in laboratory animals. For our purposes, here it has been implicated in increasing gluten sensitivity and permeability.

Gluten intolerance appears to be a growing epidemic in the United States. Celiac disease is a more specific disorder characterized by gluten intolerance along with production of autoantibodies to the protein transglutaminase.[80] A growing body of literature suggests that the spraying of crops with glyphosate (an active component of Roundup) correlates with an increased prevalence of gluten intolerance.[81] Both celiac disease and glyphosate exposure share these common symptoms: (1) disrupting the shikimate pathway; (2) altering the balance between pathogens and beneficial biota in the gut; (3) chelating transition metals, as well as sulfur and selenium; and (4) inhibiting cytochrome P450 enzymes. Glyphosate is a metal chelator that impairs sulfate supply to tissues and is correlated with proportional deficiencies in multiple trace metals and micronutrients, including iron, copper, cobalt, calcium, zinc, and sodium.[82,83]

Glyphosate may also be a contributor to the obesity and autism epidemics in the United States.[84] Glyphosate exposure in carnivorous fish revealed remarkable adverse effects throughout the digestive system,[85] including "disruption of mucosal folds and disarray of microvilli structure" in the intestinal wall and an exaggerated secretion of mucin throughout the alimentary tract. Evidence of disruption of gut bacteria by glyphosate is available in poultry,[86] cattle,[87] and swine.[88] Although such alterations have not been documented in the human digestive tract, such findings in animal studies merit mention and may fuel future human research.

Glyphosate can also be linked causally to depression and functional dyspepsia through its ability to severely impair methionine and tryptophan synthesis, via interference with the shikimate pathway in plants.[89] Reducing the bioavailability of these nutrients in derived foods could lead to decreased synthesis of serotonin in the brain, which is associated with behavior disorders in children, such as depression.[90]

## DAIRY

Data collected over 12 years in the Framingham Children's Study was used to evaluate usual dairy consumption and adolescent bone health. Subjects were aged from 3 to 5 years at the beginning of the 12-year study. The study found that consuming ≥2 servings/day of dairy (vs. less) was associated with significantly higher mean bone mineral content (BMC) and bone area (BA) at 15–17 years of age. Higher intakes of meats/other proteins (≥4 servings per/day) were also associated with higher mean BMC and BA values.[91]

Lactose intolerance can be dose-dependent and is a clinical syndrome of one or more of the following: abdominal pain, diarrhea, nausea, flatulence, and/or bloating after the ingestion of lactose-containing food substances. Primary lactase deficiency is attributable to relative or absolute absence of lactase and is the most common cause of lactose malabsorption and lactose intolerance. Approximately 70% of the world's population has primary lactase deficiency.[92] In populations with a predominance of dairy foods in the diet, particularly northern European people, as few as 2% of the population has primary lactase deficiency. In contrast, the prevalence of primary lactase deficiency is 50%–80% in Hispanic people and almost 100% in Asian and American Indian people.[93,94] Most lactase-deficient individuals experience onset of symptoms in late adolescence and adulthood,[95] although this varies. Evidence indicates that dietary lactose enhances calcium absorption and, conversely, that lactose-free diets result in lower calcium absorption.[96] Lactose intolerance may predispose patients to inadequate bone mineralization, especially in pediatric patients.[97] Calcium homeostasis is also affected by protein intake, vitamin D status, salt intake, and other factors and can be supplemented to maintain adequate calcium absorption.[98]

## FUTURE CONSIDERATIONS: CUTTING-EDGE DIETARY BREAKTHROUGHS

### Microbiome

A human fetus is thought to develop in a largely sterile uterus.[99] Colonization of the gut begins during or immediately after delivery, depending on the delivery method.[100–103] Babies born vaginally are colonized initially by vaginal bacteria, whereas those born by C-section are colonized by skin microbiota.[101] Microbiota diversity increases with time and exposure to microbes,[104] and this colonization is quite varied based on exposure to diet, illnesses, environment, and chemicals. Although gut microbiomes differ among human populations,[104] the intestinal microbiota of the young resembles that of the adult by approximately the age of 3 years,[104] thus many adult studies are relevant. Factors affecting the composition of the microbiome include malnutrition, stress, and exposure to antibiotic agents.[105]

About 70%–80% of the body's immune cells are contained within the gut-associated lymphoid tissue and they help maintain gut homeostasis.[106] The gut adjust to a more regular and balanced intake of nutrition. Eating a healthy whole-food diet can help equip teens to resist drug and alcohol cravings through feelings of self-care and well-being.

2. *Sugar*: Reduce as much as possible, watch out for hidden sources (soda, processed foods), screen for adverse effects of too much sugar (high blood glucose, fatty liver disease), and consider types and amounts of fruits (low glycemic vs. high glycemic index).
3. *Processed foods*: These drive up inflammatory ω-6 PUFA levels. Reduce their intake as much as possible and substitute with natural alternatives
4. *Fast foods*: Reduce overall; recommend healthier options such as salads at fast-food establishments. Reducing fast-food intake helps reduce ω-6 PUFA levels.
5. *Fats*: Reduce intake of ω-6 PUFAs. Encourage eating natural fats from healthy whole foods.
6. *Wheat*: Although specific recommendations on the amount of "glyphosate wheat products" that adolescents may consume are lacking, it may be worth limiting its intake, especially if an adolescent is experiencing symptoms associated with gluten intolerance
7. *Dairy*: Data on children (not adolescents) support a minimum of two servings per day of dairy. Screen for lactose intolerance so healthy alternatives can be suggested. Focus on the most natural, least processed sources of dairy.
8. *Microbiome/Epigenetics*: Nutritional history of an adolescent and his/her family, especially any nutritional deficiencies experienced during gestation or the first few years of life, is vital to understand the current nutritional status. Potential epigenetic interventions still require research to unravel the interrelations of genetic, environmental, nutritional, and epigenetic factors.
9. *Discourage* fad diets and weight-loss supplements, weight-loss pills, or meal replacement. Teenagers should be encouraged to accept a realistic, healthy weight for themselves. Where available, referral to a multidisciplinary pediatric obesity program may be beneficial.

## REFERENCES


1. Manyanga T, et al. The prevalence of underweight, overweight, obesity and associated risk factors among school-going adolescents in seven African countries. *BMC Public Health*. 2014;14:887.
2. Nyaradi A, et al. Diet in the early years of life influences cognitive outcomes at 10 years: a prospective cohort study. *Acta Paediatrica*. 2013;102:1165–1173.
3. Ruiz JR, et al. Physical activity, fitness, weight status, and cognitive performance in adolescents. *J Pediatr*. 2010; 157:917–922.
4. https://www.nimh.nih.gov/health/statistics/major-depression.shtml#part_155031.
5. Sánchez-Villegas A, et al. Fast-food and commercial baked goods consumption and the risk of depression. *Public Health Nutr*. 2012;15(3):424–432.
6. Patrick RP, Ames BN, et al. Vitamin D and the Omega-3 fatty acids control serotonin synthesis and action, part 2: relevance for ADHD, bipolar disorder, schizophrenia, and impulsive behavior. *FASEB J*. 2015;29(6): 2207–2222.
7. Rahal A, et al. Oxidative stress, prooxidants, and antioxidants: the interplay. (Review). *Bio Med Res Int*. 2014; 2014, 761264.
8. Gesch CB1, et al. Influence of supplementary vitamins, minerals and essential fatty acids on the antisocial behaviour of young adult prisoners. Randomised, placebo-controlled trial. *Br J Psychiatry*. 2002;181:22–28.
9. Zaalberg A1, et al. Effects of nutritional supplements on aggression, rule-breaking, and psychopathology among young adult prisoners. *Aggress Behav*. 2010;36(2):117–126.
10. Suglia SF, et al. Soft drinks consumption is associated with behavior problems in 5-year-olds. *J Pediatr*. 2013; 163(5):1323–1328.
11. Moore SC1, et al. Confectionery consumption in childhood and adult violence. *Br J Psychiatry*. 2009;195(4): 366–367.
12. Janesick A, Blumberg B. Endocrine disrupting chemicals and the developmental programming of adipogenesis and obesity. *Birth Defects Res C Embryo Today*. 2011; 93(1):34–50.
13. Heindel JJ, et al. Metabolism disrupting chemicals and metabolic disorders. *Reprod Toxicol*. 2017;68:3–33.
14. Das UN. Obesity: genes, brain, gut, and environment. *Nutrition*. 2010;26(5):459–473.
15. Exley MA, et al. Interplay between the immune system and adipose tissue in obesity. *J Endocrinol*. 2014;223(2): R41–R48.
16. Volkow ND, et al. Obesity and addiction: neurobiological overlaps. *Obes Rev*. 2013;14(1):2–18.
17. Jager G, Witkamp RF. The endocannabinoid system and appetite: relevance for food reward. *Nutr Res Rev*. 2014; 27(1):172–185.
18. Schellekens H, et al. Ghrelin signalling and obesity: at the interface of stress, mood and food reward. *Pharmacol Ther*. 2012;135(3):316–326.
19. Dieting. Information for teens. *Paediatr Child Health*. 2004;9(7):495–496.
20. Project EAT, University of Minnesota, http://www.sphresearch.umn.edu/epi/project-eat/.
21. Crow S, et al. Psychosocial and behavioral correlates of dieting among overweight and non-overweight adolescents. *J Adolesc Health*. 2006;38(5):569–574.
22. Grotzkyj-Giorgi M. Nutrition and addiction: can dietary changes assist with recovery? *Drugs Alcohol Today*. 2009; 9(2):24–28. (Review).

23. Ross LJ, et al. Prevalence of malnutrition and nutritional risk factors in patients undergoing alcohol and drug treatment. *Nutrition*. 2012;28(7–8):738–743.
24. Baer D, Nietert PJ. Patterns of fruit, vegetable, and milk consumption among smoking and nonsmoking female teens. *Am J Prev Med*. 2002;22(4):240–246.
25. Alberg A. The influence of cigarette smoking on circulating concentrations of antioxidant micronutrients. *Toxicology*. 2002;180(2):121–137.
26. Preson AM. Cigarette Smoking-Nutritional Implications Department of Biochemistry and Nutrition. San Juan: University of Puerto Rico, School of Medicine, 00936-5067.
27. Research Society on Alcoholism. *Drunkorexia 101: Increasing Alcohol's Effects Through Diet and Exercise Behaviors*. ScienceDaily; June 27, 2016. https://www.sciencedaily.com/releases/2016/06/160627100223.htm.
28. Putnam JJ, Allshouse JE. *Food Consumption, Prices, and Expenditures, 1970–1997*. Statistical Bulletin No. (SB-965). Food and Consumers Economics Division, Economics Research Service. Washington, D.C: US Department of Agriculture; 1999.
29. Bray G, et al. Consumption of high-fructose corn syrup in beverages may play a role in the epidemic of obesity. *Am J Clin Nutr*. 2004;79(4):537–543.
30. Sanger-Katz M. *The Decline of Big Soda*. New York Times; October 2, 2015.
31. DiNicolantonio J, Berger A. Added sugars drive nutrient and energy deficit in obesity: a new paradigm. *Open Heart*. 2016;3(2):e000469.
32. Bode JC, et al. Depletion of liver adenosine phosphates and metabolic effects of intravenous infusion of fructose or sorbitol in man and in the rat. *Eur J Clin Invest*. 1973;3: 436–441.
33. Vartanian LR, et al. Effects of soft drink consumption on nutrition and health: a systematic review and meta-analysis. *Am J Public Health*. 2007;97:667–675.
34. Beck-Nielsen H, et al. Impaired cellular insulin binding and insulin sensitivity induced by high-fructose feeding in normal subjects. *Am J Clin Nutr*. 1980;33: 273–278.
35. Taubes G. *Why We Get Fat and what to Do about it*. Anchor Books; 2011.
36. Taubes G. *Good Calories, Bad Calories*. New York City: Knopf; 2007.
37. Younossi Z, Anstee QM, Marietti M, et al. Global burden of NAFLD and NASH: trends, predictions, risk factors and prevention. *Nat Rev Gastroenterol Hepato*. 2017;15(1): 11–20.
38. Welsh JA, et al. Increasing prevalence of nonalcoholic fatty liver disease among United States adolescents, 1988–1994 to 2007–2010. *J Pediatr*. 2013;162(3), 496.e1– 500.e1.
39. van der Crabben SN, et al. Early endotoxemia increases peripheral and hepatic insulin sensitivity in healthy humans. *J Clin Endocrinol Metabl*. 2009;94(2):463–468.
40. Wagnerberger S, et al. Toll-like receptors 1–9 are elevated in livers with fructose-induced hepatic steatosis. *Br J Nutr*. 2012;107(12):1727–1738.
41. Jin R, Willment A, Patel SS, et al. Fructose induced endotoxemia in pediatric nonalcoholic fatty liver disease. *Int J Hepatol*. 2014;2014, 560620, 8 pages.
42. Avena NM, Hoebel BG. A diet promoting sugar dependency causes behavioral cross-sensitization to a low dose of amphetamine. *Neuroscience*. 2003;122:17–20.
43. Liester MB, Moore JD. Is sugar a gateway drug? *J Drug Abuse*. 2015;1:1.
44. Colantuoni C, et al. Evidence that intermittent, excessive sugar intake causes endogenous opioid dependence. *Obesity Res*. 2002;10:478–488.
45. O'Keefe Jr JH, Cordain L. Cardiovascular disease resulting from a diet and lifestyle at odds with our Paleolithic genome: how to become a 21st-century hunter-gatherer. *Mayo Clin Proc*. 2004;79:101–108.
46. Ludwig DS. The glycemic index: physiological mechanisms relating to obesity, diabetes, and cardiovascular disease. *JAMA*. 2002;287:2414–2423.
47. Westman EC. Is dietary carbohydrate essential for human nutrition? *Am J Clin Nutr*. 2002;75, 951–3; author reply 953–4.
48. Louzada ML, et al. Ultra-processed foods and the nutritional dietary profile in Brazil. *Rev Saude Publica*. 2015a; 49:38.
49. Monteiro CA. Nutrition and health. The issue is not food, nor nutrients, so much as processing. *Public Health Nutr*. 2009;12(5):729–731.
50. Vandevijvere S, et al. Monitoring and benchmarking population diet quality globally: a step-wise approach. *Obes Rev*. 2013;(suppl 1):135–149.
51. Steele EM, et al. The share of ultra-processed foods and the overall nutritional quality of diets in the US: evidence from a nationally representative cross-sectional study. *Popul Health Metr*. 2017;15:6.
52. Keeley J. *Case Study: Appleton Central Alternative Charter High School's Nutrition and Wellness Program*. Michael Fields Agricultural Institute; December 2004.
53. Esterbauer H, et al. Separation and characterization of the aldehydic products of lipid peroxidation stimulated by ADP-Fe2+ in rat liver microsomes. *Biochem J*. 1982; 208(1):129–140.
54. Jayaraj AP, Rees RK, Tovey F, White JS. A molecular basis of peptic ulceration due to diet. *Br J Exp Pathol*. 1986;67: 149–155.
55. Benedetti A, Mancini R, Marucci L, Paolucci F, Jezequel AM, Orlandi F. Quantitative study of apoptosis in normal rat gastroduodenal mucosa. *J Gastroenterol Hepatol*. 1990;5:369–374.
56. Esterbauer H, Cheeseman KH, Dianzani MU, Poli G, Slater TF. Separation and characterization of the aldehydic products of lipid peroxidation stimulated by ADP-Fe2+ in rat liver microsomes. *Biochem J*. 1982; 208(1):129–140.
57. Wu PF, Chiang TA, Ko YC, Lee H. Genotoxicity of fumes from heated cooking oils produced in Taiwan. *Environ Res*. 1999;80(2 Pt 1):122–126.
58. Zhong L, Goldberg M, Gao Y, Jin F. Lung cancer and indoor air pollution arising from Chinese-style cooking

131. Mawe, et al. Serotonin signaling in the gut: functions, dysfunctions, and therapeutic targets. *Nat Rev Gastroenterol Hepatol.* 2013;10:473–486.
132. Yano, et al. Indigenous bacteria from the gut microbiota regulate host serotonin biosynthesis. *Cell.* 2015;161(2): 264–276.
133. Mayer, et al. Altered brain-gut Axis in autism: comorbidity or causative mechanisms? *Bioessays.* 2014;36:933–939.
134. Hsiao EY. Gastrointestinal issues in autism spectrum disorder. *Harv Rev Psychiatry.* 2014;22(2):104–111.
135. Ursell, et al. The intestinal metabolome: an intersection between microbiota and host. *Gastroenterology.* 2014; 146:1470–1476.
136. Greenblum S, et al. Extensive strain-level copy-number variation across human gut microbiome species. *Cell.* 2015;160:583–594.
137. Attig L, et al. Nutritional developmental epigenomics: immediate and long-lasting effects. *Proc Nutr Soc.* 2010; 69(2):221–231.
138. Tobi EW, Goeman JJ, Monajemi R, et al. DNA methylation signatures link prenatal famine exposure to growth and metabolism. *Nat Commun.* 2014;5:5592.
139. Galler JR, et al. Infant malnutrition predicts conduct problems in adolescents. *Nutr Neurosci.* 2012;15(4): 186–192.
140. Peter CJ, et al. DNA methylation signatures of early childhood malnutrition associated with impairments in attention and cognition. *Biol Psychiatry.* 2016;80(10): 765–774.
141. Zeevi D, et al. Personalized nutrition by prediction of glycemic responses. *Cell.* 2015;163:1079–1094.
142. Dietary Reference Intakes for Energy, Carbohydrate, Fiber, Fat, Fatty Acids, Cholesterol, Protein, and Amino Acids. *Food and Nutrition Board of the Institute of Medicine.* The National Academy Press; 2005:275 [Chapter 8] www.nap.edu/.

CHAPTER 4

# Obesity Screening in Adolescents

TAMASYN NELSON, DO

## INTRODUCTION

After tripling over three decades, recent data suggest that the prevalence of childhood obesity has plateaued in the past decade. This data comes from the National Health and Nutrition Examination Survey (NHANES), a nationwide survey designed to study trends in the number of children (aged 2–19 years) who are overweight (i.e., with a body mass index [BMI] at or above the 85th percentile but below the 95th percentile) and who are obese (i.e., with a BMI at or above the 95th percentile). The NHANES analysis from 2015 indicates that while the current prevalence of overall childhood obesity is 18.5%, adolescents (ages 12–19 years) have the highest obesity prevalence overall (21%) when compared with older children (ages 6–11 years, 18%) and younger children (ages 2–5 years, 14%).[1,2] Furthermore, although obesity rates have decreased over the past 15 years in younger children, the rate of obesity in adolescents has steadily increased.[3]

Along with increases in the adolescent population, a more critical analysis of childhood obesity data also exposes that childhood obesity disproportionately affects racial and ethnic minority populations. Studies that have analyzed childhood obesity, including race and ethnicity as determinants, have revealed the prevalence of childhood obesity is significantly higher among non-Hispanic black children and adolescents (22%) and Hispanic children and adolescents (26%) than among their non-Hispanic white (14%) and non-Hispanic Asian (11%) peers.[1] The reasons for these differences are complex and not fully understood but include differences in culture, environment, and socioeconomic status (SES).

The increasing prevalence of obesity in adolescents and racial and ethnic minorities remains a challenge despite multiple interventions and programs focused on obesity treatment. Often the best "treatment" comes from taking a preventative approach. This chapter will consist of an overview of the causes and comorbidities of childhood obesity before addressing screening, which can be utilized as a preventative approach in this population.

## CAUSES OF OBESITY IN CHILDREN AND ADOLESCENTS

The causes of childhood obesity are multifactorial and include both genetic and social factors that impact health.

### Genetic Causes

Both epigenetic and genetic factors contribute to the development of obesity. Epigenetics is the study of the heritability of the changes in the expression of genes that are *not* due to changes at the level of the DNA sequence. In other words, epigenetics examines how external factors such as environment, lifestyle choices, and age can impact how genes are expressed in an individual. Genomic imprinting is an epigenetic phenomenon in which DNA methylation occurs without subsequent alteration of the genetic sequence. Normally an individual inherits two copies of every autosomal gene, one from the mother and one from the father. In genomic imprinting, one copy of genes turns off in a parent-of-origin determined manner.[4] Changing the environment in utero and modifying postnatal lifestyle can alter genomic imprinting.[5] Scientists and researchers still have much to discover about the mechanism of action by which epigenetics and genomic imprinting can influence the development of obesity; however, scientists have assembled promising data from a systematic review that has concluded that they have identified the first potential epigenetic markers for obesity and that these markers may be detectable at birth.

Scientists and researchers also do not fully comprehend the extent to which the heritability of genes factors into the potential of a child or adolescent to develop obesity. Through research and testing, they have produced data that shows that an individual's BMI is highly

Adolescent Health Screening: An Update in the Age of Big Data. https://doi.org/10.1016/B978-0-323-66130-0.00004-1

heritable.[3] Additionally, in a meta-analysis of genome-wide association data, scientists found two gene variants associated with fat mass, weight, and obesity risk. These two variants have been identified near the loci of the melanocortin 4 receptor (*MC4R*) gene and near the loci of the fat mass– and obesity-associated (*FTO*) gene. The MC4R binds the $\alpha$-melanocyte stimulating hormone, which plays an important role in appetite control. When there is a mutation in MC4R, individuals have increased hunger and decreased satiety, and as such, researchers have associated this type of mutation with binge eating.[6] Mutations in MC4R are the most common identified genetic defect causing childhood obesity. Despite the progress scientists and researchers have made, identifying additional gene variants associated with obesity remains a difficult process. Even with the identification of multiple gene mutations in an individual, each mutation likely exerts only a small effect on the overall risk of obesity in an individual. For this reason, many scientists and researchers do not view genetics as a main factor contributing to the development of childhood obesity, and instead, focus on the role that social factors play in the development of childhood obesity.

## Social Determinants of Health

Social determinants of health are conditions in the environments in which people are born, live, learn, play, worship, and age that affect a wide range of health, functioning, and quality-of-life outcomes and risks.[7]

### *Socioeconomic status*

SES is a social determinant of health and is defined as the measure of how income, education, and occupation affect an individual's social status. Researchers have found a correlation between low SES and obesity. Several studies have also illuminated a correlation between the presence of limited parental education (used as a proxy for low SES) and obesity.[7,8] Moreover, living in a low-income family corresponds with an increased risk of developing obesity in childhood.

Low-income families have a higher risk of being food insecure or not having access to reliable sources of nutritious food, secondary to financial or other societal restrictions.[9] Food-insecure families more often live in neighborhoods with fewer grocery stores, more fast-food restaurants, and limited access to fresh produce.[10] Additionally, neighborhood stores in food-insecure areas tend to have nutritious foods (fresh produce, lean meats) priced higher than less nutritious, calorie-dense foods (canned fruits and vegetables, packaged foods such as chips and cookies). The cost of food has a more pronounced effect on food-insecure families, which often have less resources to allocate on basic needs such as food.[11] As a result, food-insecure families tend to purchase and eat more of these less nutritious, calorie-dense foods than food-secure families, thus creating the increased risk of obesity in children and adolescents from food-insecure families.

A study of family households with children demonstrated a greater availability of and accessibility to obesogenic foods in food-insecure homes relative to food-secure homes.[12] Of note, the study did not reveal a difference in fruit and vegetable availability among the food-insecure and food-secure homes. The study concluded that the increased availability of nonnutritious foods, and not the presence of nutritious foods, had a greater influence on dietary choices in these food-insecure homes.

### *Race and ethnicity*

When assessing the overall prevalence of obesity in childhood and adolescence, studies have evidenced a significant difference in the rate of obesity between different racial and ethnic groups. While the overall prevalence of obesity is increasing across all adolescents, for groups identifying as non-Hispanic black and Hispanic, the prevalence of obesity has increased among both adolescents and children. When compared with their peers identifying as non-Hispanic white and Asian, the rate of obesity in non-Hispanic blacks and Hispanics is much higher.[2] Some of the observed variation in obesity rates when examining factors such as race and ethnicity may result from differences in habits developed during critical periods of development: the prenatal period, infancy, and early childhood.

A study[13] sought to evaluate whether risk factors beginning in prepregnancy and extending into early childhood could contribute to the racial and ethnic discrepancies observed in childhood and adolescent obesity. A prospective prebirth cohort was followed up for a period of 7 years, and the study uncovered differences when focusing on race and ethnicity with respect to eating behaviors in infancy—notably, whether or not mothers breastfed, timing of the introduction of solid foods—as well as differences in the speed of weight gain in childhood, the quantity of sleep, the presence of television in the bedroom, and the intake of fast food and sugar-sweetened beverages (SSBs).[13] The results indicated that the behaviors associated with an increased likelihood of childhood obesity, such as no breastfeeding, early introduction of solids, insufficient sleep, and higher intake of fast food and sugar-sweetened drinks, tended to exist more often in non-Hispanic black and Hispanic populations.[14] Researchers still have more work to do in understanding what causes these observed differences so that those treating and dealing with childhood obesity can create effective interventions to narrow these noted disparities.

## COMORBIDITIES OF CHILDHOOD AND ADOLESCENT OBESITY

Obesity is a proinflammatory state[15] that leads to many chronic diseases, including heart disease, diabetes, and hypertension. As the prevalence of childhood obesity increases, so do the complications of obesity. Having childhood obesity corresponds with multiple comorbidities that can have damaging short-term and long-term effects on an individual continuing into adulthood. Understanding the scope of these comorbidities is important for providers so that they can share this information with their patients and families as they address prevention and, when necessary, treatment of obesity.

### Cardiovascular

There has been much research conducted to understand what cardiovascular effects can be expected secondary to childhood obesity. Studies have shown that childhood obesity not only increases the risk of developing short-term cardiovascular complications, including hypertension and dyslipidemia, but also increases the risk of long-term complications that extend into adulthood, such as increased cardiometabolic morbidity (ischemic heart disease and stroke) and increased risk of premature mortality.[16–21] To date, a few studies have demonstrated that the presence of these comorbidities in adulthood clearly link to patients having been overweight or obese in adolescence. One study that has been able to demonstrate such a link was the follow-up of the Harvard Growth Study.[19] Researchers carried out the original Harvard Growth Study between 1922 and 1935. During that time, 1800 adolescents aged 13–18 years enrolled in the study had their measurements checked annually until 1935. In 1988, researchers contacted those same individuals to gain information about their medical history. For those who had died, researchers obtained information from their death certificates. The results revealed that those participants who were overweight in adolescence had increased rates of atherosclerosis and coronary artery disease among other comorbidities as adults.

### Endocrinal

Insulin resistance accompanies many of the cardiovascular and metabolic complications of obesity. The presence of insulin resistance and the subsequent development of hyperinsulinemia sets up the potential for developing type 2 diabetes mellitus (T2DM). Additionally, being overweight or obese is the most important risk factor for developing T2DM in children and adolescents.[21,22] Secondary to the increased prevalence of childhood overweight/obesity, T2DM, which was previously known as an adult disease, now represents a significant health concern for children and adolescents.[23] The increased prevalence of T2DM in children and adolescents correlates with their increasing prevalence of overweight and obesity.

### Psychosocial Concerns

As childhood obesity has developed into an increasing concern and public health crisis, those concerned about its increase have made efforts to describe how it affects the quality of life of children and adolescents. In a nationwide study of adolescents that examined self-reported general health, physical health, and emotional health, as well as school and social functioning, found that even when controlling for race, gender, SES, and family structure, significant relationships existed between overweight and obese adolescents and self-reporting of poor general health.[24]

## RISK FACTORS OF OBESITY IN ADOLESCENCE

Adolescence is a crucial developmental period, during which individuals begin to establish tendencies and behaviors that track into adulthood, including behaviors formed around eating habits.[25,26] As such, it is important to understand what factors contribute to unhealthy adolescent eating behaviors in order to better intervene and prevent the progression to obesity.

## LIFE STRESSORS AND THE POTENTIAL EFFECT ON WEIGHT STATUS

Adolescence represents a transitional time in life with respect to an individual's social and emotional sense of self. In transitioning from childhood into adolescence, individuals can encounter increased risk of obesity as a response to stressful life events. That adolescents have a higher sensitivity to stressful events secondary to elevated levels of hypothalamic-pituitary-adrenal activity contributes to this increased risk.[27] Adolescents also do not have fully developed executive functioning, which includes attributes such as decision making, planning, impulse control, and dietary restraint. Such underdevelopment may lead adolescents to cope with life stressors by using food as a coping mechanism, without much thought to how this coping behavior might negatively impact them in adulthood.

Another model of thought of how life stressors affect weight status involves the concept of emotional regulation. Emotional regulation is the ability to cope with negative emotions and maintain a positive effect or suppress a negative effect. Some researchers believe emotional regulation plays a role in mediating between exposure to stress and development of obesity. A small sampling of studies[28–31] have indicated a positive relationship between good emotional regulation skills and the intake of a healthier diet in adolescents.

## PARENTING AND PARENTAL EATING BEHAVIORS

Parental eating behaviors represent another factor influencing adolescents' eating behaviors and choices. Researchers have found that some of this influence can vary based on the gender of the adolescent. For instance, adolescent boys are more likely to eat dairy products if their parents do and adolescent girls are more likely to eat dairy, fruits, and vegetables if their parents do.[32] However, a lack of consensus exists with respect to exactly how parents influence adolescent eating behaviors. Some studies show that adolescents' attitudes toward food, not parenting practices, play the most important role in influencing adolescents' eating behaviors.[26] Yet other studies have demonstrated that more restrictive parenting styles, specifically regarding regulating the consumption of SSBs, may impact adolescents' eating habits, resulting in decreased consumption of SSBs by adolescents.[33] Researchers have advanced adolescent self-efficacy as a potential mediator that can explain how parental eating behaviors influence adolescent eating behaviors. Perceived self-efficacy refers to an individual's belief about his or her ability to accomplish a given outcome. The self-efficacy theory posits that individuals will only attempt to do things they feel confident about achieving and that they will not attempt to do those things they are not confident in achieving.[34] Thus an individual's sense of self-efficacy toward a task increases the more the individual has confidence that he or she will complete the task successfully. The theory credits this tendency to the propensity of people to attempt tasks in which they have confidence they will succeed and avoid tasks in which they believe they may fail. Additionally, individuals who doubt their ability to complete a task successfully not only have lower perceived self-efficacy toward those tasks but also view those tasks as threats, which may increase their resistance toward those tasks. Developing a better understanding of how self-efficacy affects adolescent food choices represents an important step in addressing how assessments of self-efficacy might help with screening for teens at risk for developing obesity.

With regard to adolescent self-efficacy and parenting style, one study[25] found that adolescents whose parents had both a stricter parenting style toward healthy eating behaviors and perceived healthy eating as important for their child were reported to have higher perceived self-efficacy to consume fruits and also actually consumed fruits more than their peers whose parents did not have these characteristics. This study adds to the emerging body of evidence that promoting self-efficacy for healthy eating behaviors represents an important step in helping adolescents to adopt healthier eating behaviors. Given these results, healthcare providers working on preventing and treating adolescent obesity may want to implement self-efficacy assessments to screen for healthy and unhealthy eating behaviors in adolescents as well as assessments examining how parenting styles establish family eating behaviors.

## SCREENING

The US Preventive Services Task Force (USPSTF) recommends screening for obesity using BMI in children and adolescents from 6 to 18 years of age to allow for early detection and treatment of obesity.[35] As more and more evidence emerges that childhood obesity can lead to adult premature mortality and exacerbate adult comorbidities, such screenings for obesity-related risk factors—even before the elevation of a child's or adolescent's BMI—present the best approach to prevention.

In addition to screening for BMI status, risk factors to screen for include the presence of increased food intake and decreased physical activity. To formally screen dietary preferences, healthcare providers can use a food frequency questionnaire (FFQ). FFQs can determine the dietary habits of individuals over a set period. Multiple different versions of FFQs have been developed for various purposes and can contain up to 139 questions (e.g., the NHANES FFQ available at https://epi.grants.cancer.gov/diet/usualintakes/ffq.html?&url=/diet/usualintakes/ffq.html. A study[36] has demonstrated the usefulness of FFQs in assessing adolescent food intake. However, FFQs can take a substantial amount of time to administer, as they require assessment after completion and healthcare providers may not always find this practical depending on the busyness of the office or clinic in which they work.

An international effort, the Adolescence Surveillance System for Obesity Prevention (ASSO), has begun collecting food and lifestyle data in adolescents, with the intent of developing new, reliable dietary surveys (FFQs) that can be used in both the research and clinical settings.[37,38] A meta-analysis[36] noted FFQs in adolescents to be valid and useful, meaning that FFQs (for the most part) accurately measured *actual* adolescent nutrition, could be used to rank adolescents in terms of nutrient and total calorie intake, could be used to provide international comparisons of adolescents in epidemiologic studies, and were adequate to be used in future research. What this study and the overall literature has yet to determine, however, is which specific FFQ survey items might lead to obesity. Obviously, FFQs do not consider emotional, behavioral, or environmental contributors to obesity. In the future, factors such as poverty, single-family households, depression, anxiety, spiritual deficits, social relationship deficits, lack of engagement, etc. might be found associated with obesity and combined with FFQs to provide the primary care provider (PCP) with a list of "leading indicators of obesity." Such a comprehensive screening tool might help healthcare providers intervene long before obesity has had a chance to manifest.

Currently, healthcare providers can get quick and generalizable information by asking their patients for a 24-hour diet history,[39] which consists of an assessment of typical meal patterns and food choices in the course of a day. Consultations between adolescents and dieticians can also help ascertain the adolescent's level of food consumption. As a cursory screening tool, healthcare providers can also assess patterns of eating in adolescents, specifically asking about skipping meals and dependence on packaged snacks as a replacement for meals. As discussed earlier, healthcare providers should also assess the level of physical activity by the adolescent (see chapter 6). However, as we have discussed, this type of general information does not give the PCP specific instructions on which factors might lead to obesity and how to counsel patients who have a habit of, for example, skipping meals (e.g., Will skipping meals lead to obesity? What does the data say about skipping meals? How does the PCP counsel the adolescent patient who eats "too much" of a certain food? Which foods, if consumed excessively, are more likely to lead to obesity? Diet, soft drinks? High consumption of fats? High consumption of carbohydrates?). The PCP is without specific instructions in this realm.

At any rate, although the focus of this chapter in on *screening*, a brief word on *treatment* may help the PCP navigate the waters ahead. Once adolescents have been screened and found to have risk factors, healthcare providers need to address those risk factors through discussion and goal setting to mitigate them and reduce any potential future complications. One method of addressing these issues is motivational interviewing (MI), which is discussed in more detail in the following.

## BEHAVIORAL METHODS FOR ADDRESSING UNCOVERED OBESITY RISK FACTORS (OR FOR COUNSELING FOR ESTABLISHED OBESITY): MOTIVATIONAL INTERVIEWING

Given the prevalence and detrimental effects of childhood obesity, healthcare providers need to equip themselves with as many tools as possible to help address and combat this epidemic. MI, a counseling style that has shown promise in promoting behavior changes in childhood obesity, provides healthcare providers with another useful tool in their toolbox to assist in obesity counseling and treatment.

MI has long shown promise in helping patients explore and resolve their ambivalence toward changing behavior.[40,41]

For healthcare professionals, often trained to consider themselves as experts, allowing for a patient-centered approach can seem difficult. However, when done correctly, MI not only allows for an open dialogue—where the healthcare professional can work with the patient to guide the conversation in the direction of behavior change—but also creates an environment where the patient feels empowered and has increased self-efficacy about making a behavior change. In order to correctly use MI, healthcare professionals must understand the concepts and skills needed to apply MI effectively in a patient encounter, specifically focused in this instance on the prevention of obesity and the future complications associated with it.

### The Motivational Interviewing Spirit

Integral to the effective use of MI is use of the MI spirit. The MI spirit allows for a clinical style that engenders a comfortable environment for a discussion that fosters respect, genuine interest, and partnership. There are four components of MI spirit: compassion, acceptance, partnership, and evocation.[42,43]

*Compassion* refers to the provider's ability to relate to the patient. The provider must empathize with the patient's perspective; this allows the patient to feel understood and respected.

*Acceptance* refers to the acknowledgment that the patient has the autonomy to choose to change a behavior or to continue with the behavior. The patient has the right to change or stay the same, and the provider or professional must respect that right.

*Partnership* refers to creating a collaborative environment in which the patient feels that he or she plays an essential part in the decision-making process. The patient and provider walk hand and hand together toward a decision point. Each have a unique and important contribution to make.

*Evocation* refers to the ability to create an environment where the patient is willing to openly discuss his or her feelings and concerns.

These four components set the stage for the patient-centered approach of MI. Once a healthcare provider understands the spirit of MI, he or she can more effectively use the skills of MI to help patients uncover their motivations for changing or not changing.

## Motivational Interviewing Skills

There are four main skills associated with MI: use of open-ended questions, affirmations, reflections, and summary statements, also known as OARS. Use of these skills facilitates a discussion about behavior change using MI.

### Open-ended Questions

These are questions that a patient cannot answer with a "yes" or "no." Use of open-ended questions can often create a nonjudgmental setting for patients to consider their actions. Open-ended questions can start out broad, "Why did you come to see me today?" and then become narrower as the conversation continues, "Why do you feel frustrated about your weight?"

### Affirmations

These are statements of appreciation for the patient and his or her abilities. Affirmations have no specific structure, but the provider should use them to emphasize a positive action the patient has taken. When used effectively, they can encourage the patient in the direction of making a behavior change, "Your health is really important to you so you have been drinking less soda."

### Reflections

Reflections represent the keystone of MI. Reflections demonstrate to patients that the provider desires to get to know the patient and his or her motivations better. Reflections work to keep the momentum of the conversation flowing. Providers can also use them as a gentle way to challenge patients.[44] Reflections can simply rephrase what the patient has said, or they can show greater complexity by interpreting what the patient has said to the provider. For example, a patient says, "When I weighed less, I used to be able to keep up with my friends when we played football." A simple reflection is, "You can't keep up with your friends anymore when you play together." This exemplifies rephrasing what the patient stated. An example of a more complex reflection—where the provider interprets what the patient said— is, "You worry that your weight is now causing you to spend less time with your friends."

### Summary statements

Summary statements are beneficial in helping patients organize their thoughts. Using summary statements in MI, the provider selectively chooses the statements the patient has made that favor making a change and excludes those that do not favor making a change. Summary statements can be made at any time during the visit when the provider wants to take a moment and capitalize on progress that the patient has made during the conversation.

Using MI providers have an opportunity to gain an insight into what patients think is happening to them and what they feel is most important. Having this insight can make it easier to have a conversation about changing an unhealthy behavior and guide conversation to a point where patients may feel comfortable creating goals to change their behaviors.

## CONCLUSION

Childhood obesity remains a major public health concern, and the national and global trajectories for obesity in children and adolescents remains alarmingly high, despite multiple interventions that have been made in the past two decades. In part due to this, the current generation of children and adolescents may represent the first generation to have a lower life expectancy than their parents.[45] Adolescence is a critical period for establishing healthy lifestyle behaviors. A complex interplay among genetics, social factors, and environmental factors rests behind the development of childhood obesity. As researchers begin to discover the leading indicators of obesity, providers will have to make identifying individuals at risk in the pediatric population a priority so that providers can conduct appropriate screenings that will assist with obesity prevention. Prevention of childhood obesity is of utmost importance, as the complications can exist into adulthood and lead to increased morbidity and mortality.

## REFERENCES


1. Hales C, Carroll M, Fryar C, Ogden C. Prevalence of obesity among adults and youth: United States, 2015–2016. *NCHS Data Brief*. 2017;288. Hyattsville, MD: National Center for Health Statistics.
2. Ogden C, Carroll M, Lawman H, et al. Trends in obesity prevalence among children and adolescents in the United States, 1988–1994 through 2013–2014. *JAMA*. 2016; 315(21):2292. https://doi.org/10.1001/jama.2016.6361.
3. Zylke J, Bauchner H. The unrelenting challenge of obesity. *JAMA*. 2016;315(21):2277. https://doi.org/10.1001/jama.2016.6190.
4. Jirtle R, Jirtle J. What is genomic imprinting? *Genimprint*; 2012. http://www.geneimprint.com/site/what-is-imprinting. Updated March 11, 2019. Accessed March 12, 2019.
5. Herrera B, Keildson S, Lindgren C. Genetics and epigenetics of obesity. *Maturitas*. 2011;69(1):41–49. https://doi.org/10.1016/j.maturitas.2011.02.018.
6. Branson R, Potoczna N, Kral J, Lentes K, Hoehe M, Horber F. Binge eating as a major phenotype of melanocortin 4 receptor gene mutations. *N Engl J Med*. 2003; 348(12):1096–1103. https://doi.org/10.1056/nejmoa021971.
7. Pavela G, Lewis D, Locher J, Allison D. Socioeconomic status, risk of obesity, and the importance of Albert J. Stunkard. *Curr Obes Rep*. 2016;5(1):132–139. https://doi.org/10.1007/s13679-015-0185-4.
8. Shrewsbury V, Wardle J. Socioeconomic status and adiposity in childhood: a systematic review of cross-sectional studies 1990–2005. *Obesity*. 2008;16(2): 275–284. https://doi.org/10.1038/oby.2007.35.
9. Kaiser L, Townsend M. Food insecurity among US children. *Top Clin Nutr*. 2005;20(4):313–320. https://doi.org/10.1097/00008486-200510000-00004.
10. Morland K, Wing S, Diez Roux A, Poole C. Neighborhood characteristics associated with the location of food stores and food service places. *Am J Prev Med*. 2002;22(1):23–29. https://doi.org/10.1016/s0749-3797(01)00403-2.
11. Dachner N, Ricciuto L, Kirkpatrick S, Tarasuk V. Food purchasing and food insecurity among low-income families in Toronto. *Can J Diet Pract Res*. 2010;71(3):e50–e56. https://doi.org/10.3148/71.3.2010.e50.
12. Nackers L, Appelhans B. Food insecurity is linked to a food environment promoting obesity in households with children. *J Nutr Educ Behav*. 2013;45(6):780–784. https://doi.org/10.1016/j.jneb.2013.08.001.
13. Taveras E, Gillman M, Kleinman K, Rich-Edwards J, Rifas-Shiman S. Racial/ethnic differences in early-life risk factors for childhood obesity. *Pediatrics*. 2010;125(4):686–695. https://doi.org/10.1542/peds.2009-2100.
14. Healthy People 2020 [Internet]. *Office of Disease Prevention and Health Promotion*. Washington, DC: U.S. Department of Health and Human Services; Available from: https://www.healthypeople.gov/2020/leading-health-indicators/2020-lhi-topics/Social-Determinants.
15. Wellen K, Hotamisligil G. Inflammation, stress, and diabetes. *J Clin Invest*. 2005;115(5):1111–1119. https://doi.org/10.1172/jci25102.
16. Reilly J. Health consequences of obesity. *Arch Dis Child*. 2003;88(9):748–752. https://doi.org/10.1136/adc.88.9.748.
17. Dietz W. Childhood weight Affects adult morbidity and mortality. *J Nutr*. 1998;128(2):411S–414S. https://doi.org/10.1093/jn/128.2.411s.
18. Dietz W. Health consequences of obesity in youth: childhood predictors of adult disease. *Pediatrics*. 1998;101(Supplement 2):518–525.
19. Must A, Jacques P, Dallal G, Bajema C, Dietz W. Long-term morbidity and mortality of overweight adolescents. *N Engl J Med*. 1992;327(19):1350–1355. https://doi.org/10.1056/nejm199211053271904.
20. Twig G, Yaniv G, Levine H, et al. Body-mass Index in 2.3 million adolescents and cardiovascular death in adulthood. *N Engl J Med*. 2016;374(25):2430–2440. https://doi.org/10.1056/nejmoa1503840.
21. Reilly J, Kelly J. Long-term impact of overweight and obesity in childhood and adolescence on morbidity and premature mortality in adulthood: systematic review. *Int J Obes*. 2010;35(7):891–898. https://doi.org/10.1038/ijo.2010.222.
22. Kapiotis S, Holzer G, Schaller G, et al. A proinflammatory state is detectable in obese children and is accompanied by functional and morphological vascular changes. *Arterioscler Thromb Vasc Biol*. 2006;26(11):2541–2546. https://doi.org/10.1161/01.atv.0000245795.08139.70.
23. Gungor N, Libman I, Arslanian S. *Mechanisms, Manifestations and Management: Type 2 Diabetes Mellitus in Children and Adolescents*. Lippincott, Williams, and Wilkins; 2004: 450–466.
24. Swallen K. Overweight, obesity, and health-related quality of life among adolescents: the national longitudinal study of adolescent health. *Pediatrics*. 2005;115(2):340–347. https://doi.org/10.1542/peds.2004-0678.
25. Pearson N, Ball K, Crawford D. Parental influences on adolescent fruit consumption: the role of adolescent self-efficacy. *Health Educ Res*. 2011;27(1):14–23. https://doi.org/10.1093/her/cyr051.
26. Martens M, Assema P, Brug J. Why do adolescents eat what they eat? Personal and social environmental predictors of fruit, snack and breakfast consumption among 12–14-year-old Dutch students. *Public Health Nutr*. 2005;8(8). https://doi.org/10.1079/phn2005828.
27. Romeo R. The teenage brain. *Current Directions In Psychological Science*. 2013;22(2):140–145. https://doi.org/10.1177/0963721413475445.
28. Aparicio E, Canals J, Arija V, De Henauw S, Michels N. The role of emotion regulation in childhood obesity: implications for prevention and treatment. *Nutr Res Rev*. 2016; 29(01):17–29. https://doi.org/10.1017/s0954422415000153.
29. Wills T, Isasi C, Mendoza D, Ainette M. Self-control constructs related to measures of dietary intake and physical

activity in adolescents. *J Adolesc Health*. 2007;41(6): 551–558. https://doi.org/10.1016/j.jadohealth.2007.06.013.
30. Isasi C, Ostrovsky N, Wills T. The association of emotion regulation with lifestyle behaviors in inner-city adolescents. *Eat Behav*. 2013;14(4):518–521. https://doi.org/10.1016/j.eatbeh.2013.07.009.
31. Riggs N, Chou C, Spruijt-Metz D, Pentz M. Executive cognitive function as a correlate and predictor of child food intake and physical activity. *Child Neuropsychol*. 2010;16(3): 279–292. https://doi.org/10.1080/09297041003601488.
32. Hanson N, Neumark-Sztainer D, Eisenberg M, Story M, Wall M. Associations between parental report of the home food environment and adolescent intakes of fruits, vegetables and dairy foods. *Public Health Nutr*. 2005; 8(1):77–85. https://doi.org/10.1079/phn2005661.
33. van der Horst K, Kremers S, Ferreira I, Singh A, Oenema A, Brug J. Perceived parenting style and practices and the consumption of sugar-sweetened beverages by adolescents. *Health Educ Res*. 2006;22(2):295–304. https://doi.org/10.1093/her/cyl080.
34. Bandura A. *Self Efficacy: The Exercise of Control*. New York: W.H. Freeman; 1997:13–38.
35. Grossman D, Bibbins-Domingo K, Curry S, et al. Screening for obesity in children and adolescents. *JAMA*. 2017; 317(23):2417. https://doi.org/10.1001/jama.2017.6803.
36. Tabacchi G, Filippi A, Amodio E, et al. A meta-analysis of the validity of FFQ targeted to adolescents. *Public Health Nutr*. 2015;19(07):1168–1183. https://doi.org/10.1017/s1368980015002505.
37. Tabacchi G. Asso project: a challenge in the obesity prevention context. *J Sport Sci Law*. 2011;1–3(III):2.
38. Tabacchi G, Bianco A. Methodological aspects in the development of the lifestyle surveillance toolkit in the ASSO project. *J Sport Sci Law IV*. 2011;(4):96–100.
39. Burke B. The dietary history as a tool in research. *J Am Diet Assoc*. 1947;23:1041–1046.
40. Fagot-Campagna A. Emergence of type 2 diabetes mellitus in children: epidemiological evidence. *J Pediatr Endocrinol Metab*. 2000;13(suppl. 6). https://doi.org/10.1515/jpem-2000-s613.
41. Koyuncuoğlu Güngör N. Overweight and obesity in children and adolescents. *J Clin Res Pediatr Endocrinol*. 2014: 129–143. https://doi.org/10.4274/jcrpe.1471.
42. Schwartz R, Hamre R, Dietz W, et al. Office-based motivational interviewing to prevent childhood obesity. *Arch Pediatr Adolesc Med*. 2007;161(5):495. https://doi.org/10.1001/archpedi.161.5.495.
43. Rollnick S, Miller W, Butler C. *Motivational Interviewing in HealthCare: Helping Patients Change Behavior*. 2nd ed. New York: Guilford Press; 2008.
44. Rosengren D. *Building Motivational Interviewing Skills: A Practitioner Workbook*. 1st ed. Guilford Press; 2009:30–88.
45. Rollnick S, Mason P, Butler C. *Health Behavior Change: A Guide for Practitioners*. London, UK: Churchill Livingstone; 1998.

## FURTHER READING

1. Wardle J, Carnell S, Haworth C, Plomin R. Evidence for a strong genetic influence on childhood adiposity despite the force of the obesogenic environment. *Am J Clin Nutr*. 2008;87(2):398–404. https://doi.org/10.1093/ajcn/87.2.398.
2. Thorleifsson G, Walters G, Gudbjartsson D, et al. Genome-wide association yields new sequence variants at seven loci that associate with measures of obesity. *Nat Genet*. 2008; 41(1):18–24. https://doi.org/10.1038/ng.274.
3. Yeo G, Farooqi I, Aminian S, Halsall D, Stanhope R, O'Rahilly S. A frameshift mutation in MC4R associated with dominantly inherited human obesity. *Nat Genet*. 1998;20(2):111–112. https://doi.org/10.1038/2404.
4. Archer E. The childhood obesity epidemic as a result of nongenetic evolution: the maternal resources hypothesis. *Mayo Clin Proc*. 2015;90(1):77–92. https://doi.org/10.1016/j.mayocp.2014.08.006.
5. Sobal J, Stunkard A. Socioeconomic status and obesity: a review of the literature. *Psychol Bull*. 1989;105(2):260–275. https://doi.org/10.1037//0033-2909.105.2.260.
6. Stunkard A, Sorensen T. Obesity and socioeconomic status – a complex relation. *N Engl J Med*. 1993;329(14):1036–1037. https://doi.org/10.1056/nejm199309303291411.
7. Caprio S, Daniels S, Drewnowski A, et al. Influence of race, ethnicity, and culture on childhood obesity: implications for prevention and treatment. *Obesity*. 2008;16(12):2566–2577. https://doi.org/10.1038/oby.2008.398.
8. Darmon N, Drewnowski A. Does social class predict diet quality? *Am J Clin Nutr*. 2008;87(5):1107–1117. https://doi.org/10.1093/ajcn/87.5.1107.
9. Drewnowski A, Specter S. Poverty and obesity: the role of energy density and energy costs. *Am J Clin Nutr*. 2004; 79(1):6–16. https://doi.org/10.1093/ajcn/79.1.6.
10. Fradkin C, Wallander J, Elliott M, Tortolero S, Cuccaro P, Schuster M. Associations between socioeconomic status and obesity in diverse, young adolescents: variation across race/ethnicity and gender. *Health Psychol*. 2015;34(1):1–9. https://doi.org/10.1037/hea0000099.
11. Arslanian S. Type 2 diabetes mellitus in children: pathophysiology and risk factors. *J Pediat Endocrinol Metab*. 2000; 13(suppl. 6). https://doi.org/10.1515/jpem-2000-s612.
12. Boone J, Gordon-Larsen P, Adair L, Popkin B. Screen time and physical activity during adolescence: longitudinal effects on obesity in young adulthood. *Int J Behav Nutr Phys Act*. 2007;4(1):26. https://doi.org/10.1186/1479-5868-4-26.
13. Olshansky S, Passaro D, Hershow R, et al. A potential decline in life expectancy in the United States in the 21st century. *N Engl J Med*. 2005;352(11):1138–1145. https://doi.org/10.1056/nejmsr043743.
14. Golan M, Crow S. Parents are key players in the prevention and treatment of weight-related problems. *Nutr Rev*. 2004; 62(1):39–50. https://doi.org/10.1301/nr.2004.jan.3950.

15. Lien N, Lytle L, Klepp K. Stability in consumption of fruit, vegetables, and sugary foods in a cohort from age 14 to age 21. *Prev Med*. 2001;33(3):217–226. https://doi.org/10.1006/pmed.2001.0874.
16. Pervanidou P, Chrousos G. Metabolic consequences of stress during childhood and adolescence. *Metabolism*. 2012;61(5):611–619. https://doi.org/10.1016/j.metabol.2011.10.005.
17. van Jaarsveld C, Fidler J, Steptoe A, Boniface D, Wardle J. Perceived stress and weight gain in adolescence: a longitudinal analysis. *Obesity*. 2009;17(12):2155–2161. https://doi.org/10.1038/oby.2009.183.
18. Taveras E, Gillman M, Kleinman K, Rich-Edwards J, Rifas-Shiman S. Reducing racial/ethnic disparities in childhood obesity. *JAMA Pediatrics*. 2013;167(8):731. https://doi.org/10.1001/jamapediatrics.2013.85.
19. Welk G, Morrow J, Saint-Maurice P. *Measures Registry User Guide: Individual Physical Activity*. Washington (DC): National Collaborative on Childhood Obesity Research; January 2017. http://nccor.org/tools-mruserguides/wp-content/uploads/2017/.

pathway in the hypothalamus, regulates the length and depth of sleep and is dependent on the timing, duration, and quality of an individual's previous sleep period. It is generally agreed that sleep quality and restfulness are best when the sleep schedules—both the circadian and homeostatic systems—are synchronized to the external light-dark cycle and that individuals should go to bed and wake up at around the same time each day.[14]

A part of both, the homeostatic and circadian processes, melatonin plays an integral role. It is released at its highest rate during nighttime and has two interacting effects on the sleep–wake cycle. It entrains and shifts the circadian rhythm and promotes sleep onset and continuity by increasing the homeostatic drive to sleep.[15] Melatonin secretion in adolescents occurs later in the evening than it does in younger children and adults. Therefore, instead of feeling sleepy in the evening, adolescents actually tend to become more alert and have a difficult time to fall asleep; however, in the morning, when people of other ages are awake and primed for the day, adolescents still have elevated melatonin levels and often feel groggy and sleepy.[16] In their study of individuals between 10 and 13 years of age, Laberge et al. (2001) found evidence of decreasing sleep time, later bedtimes, and a larger gap between weekend and weeknight sleep schedules.[17]

In adolescents, circadian rhythm also adapts more easily to delays than to advances in sleep–wake schedules. This can lead to delayed sleep phase syndrome, in which a person's sleep is delayed by two or more hours beyond the socially acceptable or conventional bedtime, with subsequent sleep loss, disrupted sleep, excessive daytime sleepiness, impaired ability to awaken, and poor school performance.[6] In addition, excessive indoor light exposure (late night computer screens, etc.) can delay melatonin production and subsequently delay the circadian rhythm.[18]

Taken together, all of the above physiologic and habitual factors lead to a tendency for adolescents to want to stay up later and wake later, leaving them susceptible to sleep deficits if an early morning schedule is imposed (as it usually is by school start times, etc.). Such physiologic changes make the adolescent vulnerable to the deleterious effects associated with sleep deficits and sleep disorders as mentioned earlier.

## SLEEP AND AGE

During middle childhood, the average amount of sleep is between 9 and 10 h and there is a gender difference between 4 and 12 years of age with respect to total sleep, with girls sleeping more than boys. In addition, the sleep and wake times shift to nearly 10:00 p.m. and 7:30 a.m., respectively, during this stage. The amount of sleep needed remains the same as children transition to adolescence, but the 10-h average obtained by youth during middle childhood decreases to 7 ½–8 h of sleep per night as individuals approach 16 years of age. In one review,[19] more than a quarter of high school and college students were found to be sleep deprived. With increasing age, the total sleep time and REM sleep decrease, leading eventually to the emergence of the normal adult sleep pattern.[20]

# SECTION TWO: COMMON SLEEP ISSUES IN ADOLESCENCE

There is growing concern regarding adolescents' sleep pattern and the subsequent consequences.

## INSUFFICIENT SLEEP IN ADOLESCENTS

### Introduction

In 2010, the American Medical Association and the American Academy of Sleep Medicine recognized insufficient sleep in adolescents as a serious health risk.[21] The National Sleep Foundation survey reported that 16% of the students in the sixth grade and 75% in 12th grade and above sleep less than 8 h per night.[22] Moreover, Healthy People 2020 aims to reduce sleep loss among adolescents with objective of having students in grades 9 through 12 to get sufficient sleep of ≥8 h.[23]

### Effect of Circadian Rhythm, Electronic Media, and School Start Time

Circadian rhythm disturbance is one of the major factors affecting sleep quality in adolescents. As mentioned earlier, adolescents have a challenge to fall asleep in the early evening and to wake in the early morning.[24] This natural tendency is exacerbated by evening and nighttime screen use and electronic media, social networking, and late sleep and waking time on weekends than on weekdays.[25]

Moreover, poor sleep quality is directly associated with early school start time. The American Academy of Pediatrics recommends middle and high schools delay the start of class to 8:30 a.m. or later to allow school schedules align with the biological circadian rhythms of adolescents, whose sleep–wake cycles begin to shift up to 2 h later at the start of puberty.[26] It was found that delays in school start times resulted in improvement of attendance rates, an increase in the percentage of students continuously enrolled in the same school,[27] increased sleep duration, decreased daytime sleepiness,[28] increased satisfaction with sleep, significant declines in self-reported depressed mood, health center visits for fatigue-related complaints, and first-period tardiness,[29] fewer attention and concentration difficulties, better academic performance,[30] and decreased the average crash rate.[31]

### Effect of Caffeine on Sleep

Effect of caffeine on sleep quality and patterns is complex.[32] Adolescents use caffeine for energy, mood enhancement, and to counteract daytime sleepiness.[33] Adolescents' caffeine intake is associated with shorter sleep duration, sleep-onset and sleep-maintenance insomnia, increased daytime sleepiness,[34] and dose-related decreased slow-wave and REM sleep, both of which are important in learning and memory consolidation.[35] Compared to adults, adolescents experience more caffeine-related tolerance and withdrawal symptoms.[36]

### Consequences of Insufficient Sleep

Insufficient sleep affects almost every system. It has been proved that there is a bidirectional relationship between insufficient sleep and depression, meaning that too much or too little sleep is associated with depression.[37] Chronic sleep loss is also associated with anxiety and risky behaviors such as drinking while driving.[38] Research showed that sleeping less than 8 h at night was found to be associated with a threefold increased risk of suicide attempts and therefore earlier bedtime could potentially be protective against adolescent depression and suicidal ideation.[39]

Many studies showed a clear link between chronic sleep loss and increased risk of obesity, insulin resistance, increased hunger, and decreased satiety.[40] Adolescents with sleep time less than 8 h consume a higher proportion of calories from fats and a higher percentage of daily caloric intake from snacks with increase in the risk of development of type 2 diabetes.[41] Furthermore, the relationship between chronic sleep loss and obesity may be compounded by the presence of obstructive sleep apnea, with poor sleep leading to obesity leading to sleep apnea, which in turn leads to more poor sleep and increased obesity.[42] Chronic sleep loss with subsequent daytime sleepiness is associated with an increased rate of motor vehicle crashes.[43] Attention to proper sleep is vital for the prevention of adolescent motor vehicle crashes.[44]

## INSOMNIA IN ADOLESCENTS

The National Sleep Foundation recommends ≥8 h of sleep for adolescents aged 14–17 years old.[45] Insomnia is defined as difficulty in initiating sleep, maintaining sleep,or waking up earlier than the usual schedule with inability to return to sleep.[46] In adolescence, insomnia may be related to inadequate sleep hygiene, delayed sleep phase, or it can have a psychophysiological origin. Prevalence of insomnia ranges from 15% to 30% among adolescents[47] with higher prevalence in girls aged 11–12 years, which is most likely secondary to hormonal changes.[48]

Insomnia secondary to inadequate sleep hygiene is the most common type in adolescence secondary to irregular sleep schedule between weekdays and the weekend; use of stimulating substances or drugs (licit and illicit); excess caffeine in the late afternoon or at night; and use of electronic devices before going to bed. Social and family pressures, hormonal changes, and the need for belonging to a group also influence sleep quality.[49]

Delayed sleep phase insomnia is another common cause of insomnia in adolescents.[47] It was observed in 3.3% of adolescents aged 16–18 years and resulted in a threefold increased risk for school absenteeism in males and 1.8-fold in females.[50] In psychophysiological insomnia, there is an exaggerated preoccupation with sleep, getting to sleep, and the adverse effects of "not sleeping" on the following day. This type of insomnia occurs through a combination of risk factors (genetic vulnerability, psychiatric comorbidities), triggering factors (stress), and other factors (poor sleep hygiene, caffeine intake).[47]

Sleep deprivation resulting from insomnia has been associated with an eightfold higher risk of depression,[51] 2–3-fold higher risk of ADHD,[52] and more frequent seizures.[53] Moreover, insomnia leads excessive daytime sleepiness and/or hyperactivity, poor academic performance, poor social relationships, and sleep–wake cycle inversion.[54]

## SLEEP DISORDERED BREATHING IN ADOLESCENTS

Sleep-disordered breathing (SDB) refers to the occurrence of repetitive episodes of complete or partial obstruction of the upper airway during sleep, usually in association with loud snoring and daytime sleepiness.[55] Obstructive sleep apnea is the most common type of SDB affecting about 2%–5% of children and adolescents.[56] Risk factors for OSA in adolescents include obesity, African-American race, upper and lower respiratory problems,[57] male gender, and tonsillar hypertrophy.[58]

In adolescents, OSA, with subsequent chronic sleep deprivation, is significantly associated with worse executive function (decision making, attention control, inhibitory control, working memory, cognitive flexibility, planning, etc.), more depression and externalizing symptoms, daytime sleepiness,[59] greater risk of metabolic syndrome including dyslipidemia, insulin resistance, obesity, and hypertension,[60] and higher risk for cardiovascular morbidities such as systemic hypertension,[61] left ventricular hypertrophy,[62] pulmonary hypertension, and right ventricular dysfunction[63] secondary to increases in sympathetic activity and reactivity,[64] endothelial dysfunction,[65] and OSA-induced inflammatory response with increased level of C-reactive protein.[66]

## CIRCADIAN RHYTHM DISORDERS IN ADOLESCENTS

Circadian rhythm sleep disorders are persistent or recurrent patterns of sleep disturbance due to misalignment of the circadian clock in relation to environmental cues and the terrestrial light–dark cycle. In adolescents, they are associated with insomnia, daytime sleepiness, increased daytime irritability, poor school performance, and psychiatric disorders. Delayed sleep phase and advanced sleep phase disorders are the most common circadian rhythm disorders. Biological, physiologic, and genetic factors play an important role in pathogenesis of circadian rhythm disorders.[67] Similarly, individuals who live in extreme latitudes and are exposed to extended periods of light may also be at increased risk.[68] Polymorphisms in circadian clock genes have been identified in familial delayed and advanced sleep phase syndromes.[69]

Delayed sleep phase syndrome (DSPD) is commonly found in teenagers and young adults.[70] It is characterized by sleep onset and wake times that are typically delayed 3–6 h relative to conventional sleep–wake times. The amount and quality of sleep are not affected but delayed resulting in social and often psychological difficulties.[71] DSPD prevalence is 7%–16% among adolescents and young adults, and represents 10% of individuals diagnosed with chronic insomnia disorder. When forced out of bed at conventional wake-up times, adolescents with DSPD continually experience short sleep duration and feel permanently jet lagged. Adolescents may present to a general practitioner with a history of taking "hours" to get to sleep and being extremely difficult to wake in the morning for school, university, or work. They may also describe himself or herself as a "night owl." The disorder could be misdiagnosed as psychophysiological insomnia. Depression and anxiety are commonly associated with DSPD.[72]

On the other hand, advanced sleep phase syndrome is characterized by involuntary bedtimes and awake times that are more than 3 h earlier than societal means. Advanced sleep phase disorder is uncommon in adolescence, although it may manifest secondary to anxiety and depression. Sleep onset occurs early in the evening (6–9 p.m.), despite efforts to achieve a later bedtime. Sleep quality is typically normal but duration is often curtailed because of early morning waking (2–5 a.m.). Staying in bed until the desired waking time will fragment sleep, and it may be misdiagnosed as an irregular sleep–wake pattern.[67]

## PARASOMNIAS IN ADOLESCENTS

Parasomnias are undesirable events that can result from arousals during REM or non-REM (NREM) sleep.[73] Sleepwalking, confusional arousals, and sleep terrors occur from arousals during stages N2 and N3 NREM sleep mainly during the first third of the night.[74] Ohayon et al. (1999) estimated that the prevalence of sleep terrors, sleepwalking, and confusional arousals were 2.2%, 2%, and 4.2%, respectively, among adolescents and adults of 15–24 years old. The prevalence significantly decreased after age 25, and no sex differences were observed.[75] A detailed history, sleep diaries, and comprehensive physical and neurological exams are required for diagnosis.[76] (see section on screening later).

REM sleep behavior disorder, sleep paralysis, sleep hallucinations, and nightmares result from arousals during REM sleep. REM sleep behavior disorder is characterized by complex movements during REM sleep.[77] Conditions that may mimic REM sleep behavior disorder include nocturnal seizures; sleepwalking, sleep terrors; hypnogenic paroxysmal dystonia, nocturnal frontal lobe epilepsy, and obstructive sleep apnea with agitated arousals; nocturnal psychogenic dissociative disorders; and malingering. Medications such as tricyclic antidepressants, SSIRS, and SNIRS may cause REM sleep behavior disorder.[78]

**Sleep paralysis**, which usually begins in childhood or adolescence, occurs during the transition between sleep and wakefulness.[79] It occurs in episodes that may last for few minutes and may be associated with hallucinations. Consciousness is usually preserved. Fatigue, stress, irregular schedules, shift work, sleeping, alcohol and caffeine use, and sleep deprivation may predispose individuals to sleep paralysis.[80] Genetic factors may also play a role in sleep paralysis.[81] Panic disorder, anxiety, bipolar disorder, posttraumatic stress disorder, and depression are associated with sleep paralysis.[82] Atonic seizures, cataplexy, hypokalemic periodic paralysis, anxiolytic withdrawal and abuse, and psychosis may mimic sleep paralysis.[81]

**Sleep related hallucinations** can occur at sleep onset (hypnagogic hallucinations) or on awakening (hypnopompic hallucinations). They are usually visual, but they can also include tactile, auditory, or kinetic phenomena and may be associated with episodes of sleep paralysis.[73]

**Nightmares** usually occur during REM sleep in the second half of the night and are most common between ages of 3 and 6 years.[83] Those with nightmares in childhood tend to have nightmares as adolescents and adults.[84]

**Other parasomnias** include nocturnal enuresis, sleep dissociative disorder, sleep-related eating disorder, exploding head syndrome, and catathrenia. In adolescence, only 1%–3% have nocturnal enuresis.[85] Polyuria, sudden involuntary detrusor contraction, and decreased arousability secondary to obstructive sleep apnea are the most common causes of nocturnal enuresis.[86] Sleep-related dissociative disorders can emerge during transition from wakefulness to sleep or within several minutes after awakening from stages 1 or 2 NREM sleep or REM sleep. They are commonly associated with childhood traumatic events and include dissociative fugue, dissociative identity disorder, and dissociative disorder not otherwise specified. The age of onset can range from childhood to middle adulthood.[73] In exploding head syndrome, patients have terrifying loud noise that may be accompanied by myoclonic jerks or the perception of a flash of light. EEG is usually normal.[87] Patients with sleep-related eating disorder experience a partial arousal from sleep, often 2–3 h after sleep onset with subsequent out-of-control eating. Majority of cases begin in adolescence or early adulthood.[88] Catathrenia, or nocturnal groaning, can occur in NREM sleep and REM sleep. The onset of catathrenia may begin during childhood or adolescence.[89] Each of these parasomnias is associated with chronic sleep loss and thus adolescents experiencing parasomnias are susceptible to all consequences of chronic sleep loss noted earlier, that is, depression, poor school performance, daytime sleepiness, etc.

## SECTION THREE: SCREENING FOR SLEEP DISORDERS IN ADOLESCENTS

Although adolescents spend one-third to one-half of their life sleeping, sleep disorders are often overlooked by primary care providers.[90] It is estimated that sleep disorders in adolescents are highly prevalent, with prevalence rates ranging from 25% to 40%. In addition, adolescent sleep disorders are more common in those with other medical, psychiatric, or neurological disorders.[91]

The assessment of sleep disorders in adolescents is performed by subjective and, when needed, objective tools. Subjective assessment relies on sleep history, sleep diaries, and sleep questionnaires—structured queries that explore the most relevant sleep-related behaviors. Objective tools such as polysomnography, actigraphy, multiple sleep latency test, and multiple wakefulness test are used to diagnose specific sleep disorders such as obstructive sleep apnea, narcolepsy, and hypersomnolence. This section covers the most common screening tools that could be used by primary care providers to screen adolescents for sleep disorders as well as an overview of the objective studies that are commonly used by Sleep Medicine Specialist to diagnose specific sleep disorders.

## SECTION THREE A: SUBJECTIVE ASSESSMENT OF SLEEP

### SLEEP HISTORY

A comprehensive sleep history is the most important subjective tool to screen for sleep disorders in adolescents. Review of sleep schedule and sleep–wake cycle is an essential element and includes bedtime, wake time, and naptimes with differences across weekdays and weekends or holidays.[92] Evening activities, such as television viewing, computer use, studying, and bedtime routines, should be evaluated as well. Bedtime difficulties, including bedtime stalling, bedtime refusal, bedtime fears, and inability to fall asleep independently, should be addressed. Sleep history should address the time to fall asleep, behaviors during the night, and the number and duration of nighttime awakenings.[93] Abnormal events during sleep, such as night terrors, confusional arousals, respiratory disturbances, seizures, and enuresis should be assessed as well.[94]

Furthermore, the bedroom environment should be considered as a potential contributor to sleep difficulties, including room temperature, noise, and comfort level. Daytime behaviors including wake time and daytime sleepiness, naps, meals, medications, and caffeine intake should be detailed in the sleep history.[95] Moreover, daytime functioning including school performance, psychological functioning, social functioning and family functioning should be assessed. It is important to address family issues such as financial or marital difficulties that can also contribute to adolescent sleep difficulties.[96]

## SLEEP DIARIES

Sleep diary is another important tool that is used to collect information from adolescents about their daily sleep behaviors and pre-bedtime practices. These diaries contain nightly recordings of specific sleep-related information, including the time at which the adolescent goes to bed, the time and frequency of night awakenings, the time at which the adolescent wakes in the morning, and the times of daytime naps. Diaries may also include parents' report on antecedents, behaviors, and consequences surrounding bedtime. Sleep diary helps to identify the type of sleep problems and different factors that may influence sleep, and monitor change over the course of an intervention. Moreover, in comparison to sleep questionnaires, sleep diaries provide information at multiple time points over a period of time, and do not require adolescents to retrospectively recall information confounded by memory and other preceding factors. The number of diary entries needed to ensure validity remains unclear; however, a minimum of 14 days has been proposed. Sleep diaries may be perceived as laborious and vulnerable to reporter bias, however, when completed consistently, sleep diaries provide valuable information to help identify sleep patterns and contributing factors, and track treatment progress of sleep disturbances.[97]

Sleep diaries have been in clinical use for decades. The Pittsburgh Sleep Diary, which is one of the oldest sleep diaries, contains 23 questions with 6point scale.[98] The Consensus Sleep Diary that contains 23 questions on 5-point scale was developed because of collaborations with insomnia experts and potential users.[97] Other commonly used sleep diaries include National Sleep Foundation (15 questions with 3-point scale), Get Self Help Sleep Diary (14 questions with 11-point scale), National Heart, Lung, and Blood Institute (12 questions with 3–4-point scale), NPS (National Prescribing Service) MedicineWise Sleep Diary (11 questions with 3-point scale), and Loughborough Sleep Research Center (8 questions with 5-point scale).[99] Electronic sleep diaries are also available as mobile apps.[100]

## SLEEP QUESTIONNAIRES

The following are the most commonly used sleep questionnaires that can be used in clinical practice to screen for sleep disorders in adolescents.

### Questionnaires Assessing Sleep Initiation and Maintenance

#### *Adolescent sleep–wake scale*

The Adolescent Sleep–Wake Scale (ASWS), which is a 28-item questionnaire, is one of the best known and most widely used measures of sleep quality in adolescents. The tool is comprised of five behavioral domains of sleep quality: (1) going to bed (5 items), (2) falling asleep (6 items), (3) maintaining sleep (6 items), (4) reinitiating sleep (6 items), and (5) returning to wakefulness (5 items). Respondents should report the frequency of various sleep problems within the past month using a 6-point scale with anchors "always" and "never." Five subscale scores corresponding to each behavioral dimension and a total sleep quality score can be yielded with higher scores reflecting better sleep quality.[101]

Because of its validity, the ASWS has been proven valid to assess sleep quality in community adolescents, and in adolescents with medial or psychiatric problems, with a lower score indicating poor sleep initiation or poor sleep maintenance. Poor sleep initiation or sleep maintenance in turn may indicate poor sleep habits, suboptimal adolescent psychologic health, and may forewarn of future learning and behavioral issues.[102]

### Questionnaires Assessing Daytime Sleepiness

#### *Cleveland adolescent sleepiness questionnaire*

Cleveland adolescent sleepiness questionnaire (CASQ), which is a brief, 16-item, self-completed instrument, measures excessive daytime sleepiness in adolescents of 11–17 years old. It tests two domains: degree of sleepiness (11 questions testing sleepiness in school, at home, and while in transit) and degree of alertness (5 questions testing alertness in school).[103]

#### *Epworth sleepiness scale*

The Epworth sleepiness scale (ESS) measures daytime sleepiness and consists of eight items (situations) where individuals assess how likely they would fall asleep.

A sum of responses is calculated for a total score ranging from 0 to 24 with a total score ≥10 represents excessive daytime sleepiness.[104] To investigate the daytime sleepiness and hyperactivity secondary to obstructive sleep apnea in adolescents, the ESS was modified by Melendres et al. (2004) to make it more appropriate for use with adolescents. Results supported the validity of the modified ESS where adolescents with sleep disordered breathing scored higher on the ESS than controls.[105] Moore et al. (2009) demonstrated that the ESS scores correlated with self-reports of anxiety and general health status.[106] However, no psychometrics for the ESS in adolescents or children have been established.

#### Pediatric daytime sleepiness scale

Pediatric daytime sleepiness scale (PDSS) is a brief 8-item scale that assesses subjective daytime sleepiness in adolescents in a variety of settings over the course of the day that impacts on academic performance. The PDSS was developed and tested in a population of 442 middle school students (11–15 years) to examine the relationship of daytime sleepiness and academic outcomes. Those with scores >26 had poor academic performance.[107] In a cross-sectional survey of 2884 students of 11–15 years old from seven schools in four cities of Argentina, Perez-Chada et al. (2007) found that frequent snorers had higher mean PDSS scores than occasional or nonsnorers (18 ± 5, 15.7 ± 6 and 15.5 ± 6, respectively; $P < .001$).[108]

### Questionnaires Assessing Sleep Hygiene

#### Adolescent sleep hygiene scale

Sleep hygiene is a multidimensional behavioral practice that is essential for good sleep quality, adequate sleep duration, and full daytime alertness.[109] The Adolescent Sleep Hygiene Scale (ASHS) is a self-reported 33-item questionnaire that assesses eight sleep hygiene domains that may inhibit or facilitate sleep in adolescents. These domains are physiological (five items, e.g., evening caffeine consumption, going to bed with stomachache or feeling hungry); behavioral (seven items, e.g., using bed for things other than sleep such as talking on the telephone, watching TV, playing video games, doing homework); cognitive (six items) and emotional (three items, e.g., thinking about things that need to be done at bedtime, going to bed feeling upset); sleep environment (four items, e.g., falling asleep with the lights on); sleep stability (four items, e.g., different bedtime/wake time pattern on weekdays and weekends); substance use (two items, e.g., evening alcohol use); daytime sleep (one item, e.g., napping); and having a bedtime routine (one item, e.g., bathing, brushing teeth, reading). Eight subscale scores corresponding to each domain and a total sleep quality score can be yielded with higher scores reflecting better success on each of these dimensions of sleep hygiene.[101] It was rated as "approaching well-established" by Lewandowski et al. (2011).[110]

### Multidimensional Questionnaires

#### BEARS questionnaire

The BEARS questionnaire was developed to address the most common sleep issues in children and adolescents in the 2–18-year-old range. It incorporates five basic sleep domains that reflect the most common presenting sleep complaints in children and adolescents: bedtime problems including difficulty going to bed and falling asleep, excessive daytime sleepiness, awakenings during the night, regularity of sleep/wake cycles (bedtime, wake time), and snoring.[111] In their study of 8862 children and adolescents in the age range between 9 and 17 years in 24 schools in Bogotá, Colombia, Ramirez-Velez et al. (2017) found that BEARS questionnaire is a valid tool to screen adolescents for sleep disorders in primary care.[112] Although BEARS is a quick, simple, and inexpensive screener for pediatricians, it does not ask information about excessive leg movements or other movements in sleep and may miss children who have periodic limb movement disorder, restless leg syndrome, or other parasomnias that are fairly common sleep disorders in children, some of which may cause or exacerbate some behavior problems in children.

#### Pediatric sleep questionnaire

The pediatric sleep questionnaire (PSQ), which is also known as Sleep-Related Breathing Disorders scale, is a 22-item questionnaire that is developed and validated at the University of Michigan as a research tool to identify children and adolescents of 2–18 years old at risk for sleep-related breathing disorders.[113] It includes items intended to measure childhood sleep-related breathing disorder with subscores for snoring, sleepiness, and behavior. The scales within the questionnaire include a 9-item breathing subscale, a 2-item sleepiness subscale, a 6-item behavior subscale, and a 5-item other subscale; the latter includes questions pertaining to weight, rate of growth since birth, nocturnal enuresis, ability to awaken in the morning, and feeling unrefreshed in the morning. The PSQ scale showed a sensitivity of 81% and a specificity of 87%. Instrument performance did not vary with participant age (2–18 years). The PSQ scale showed good internal consistency and test–retest reliability. In a study of 105 participants, the PSQ predicted polysomnographic

3. Zepelin H, Siegel JM, Tobler I. Mammalian sleep. In: Kryger MH, Roth T, Dement WC, eds. *Principles and Practice of Sleep Medicine*. 4th ed. Philadelphia: Elsevier/Saunders; 2005:91–100.
4. Westerman D. *The Concise Sleep Medicine Handbook*. 2nd ed. Atlanta (GA): Independent Publishing Platform; 2013:1–10.
5. Dement WC, Vaughn C. *The Promise of Sleep*. New York: Dell Publishing; 1999.
6. Dahl RE, Lewin DS. Pathways to adolescent health: sleep regulation and behavior. *J Adolesc Health*. 2002;31: 175–184.
7. Carskadon M, Dement W. Normal human sleep: an overview. In: Kryger MH, Roth T, Dement WC, eds. *Principles and Practice of Sleep Medicine*. 4th ed. Philadelphia: Elsevier Saunders; 2005:13–23.
8. Crick F, Mitchison G. The function of dream sleep. *Nature*. 1983;304(5922):111–114.
9. Smith C, Lapp L. Increases in number of REMS and REM density in humans following an intensive learning period. *Sleep*. 1991;14(4):325–330.
10. Borberly AA. A two process model of sleep regulation. *Hum Neurobiol*. 1982;1:195–204.
11. Carskadon MA. Sleep in adolescents: the perfect storm. *Pediatr Clin North Am*. 2011;58:637–647. https://doi.org/10.1016/j.pcl.2011.03.003.
12. Rosenburg RS. Aging and circadian rhythms. In: *Encyclopedia of Sleep and Dreaming*. Vol. 1. New York, NY: Macmillan Publishing Company; 1993:12–14.
13. Shanahan T, Czeisler C. Physiological effects of light on the human circadian pacemaker. *Semin Perinatol*. 2000; 24:299–320.
14. Basheer R, Strecker RE, Thakkar MM, et al. Adenosine and sleep-wake regulation. *Prog Neurobiol*. 2004;73:379–396.
15. Grivas TB, Savvidou OD. Melatonin the "light of night" in human biology and adolescent idiopathic scoliosis. *Scoliosis*. 2007;2:6. https://doi.org/10.1186/1748-7161-2-6.
16. Arendt J. Melatonin and human rhythms. *Chronobiol Int*. 2006;23(1–2):21–37. https://doi.org/10.1080/07420520500464361.
17. Laberge L, Petit D, Simard C, Vitaro F, Tremblay RE, Montplaisir J. Development of sleep patterns in early adolescence. *J Sleep Res*. 2001;10:59–67.
18. Hagenauer MH, Perryman JI, Lee TM, Carskadon MA. Adolescent changes in the homeostatic and circadian regulation of sleep. *Dev Neurosci*. 2009;31:276–284.
19. Mercer PW, Merritt SL, Cowell JM. Differences in reported sleep need among adolescents. *J Adolesc Health*. 1998; 23(5):259–263.
20. Karacan I, Anch M, Thornby JI, et al. Longitudinal sleep patterns during pubertal growth: four-year follow up. *Pediatr Res*. 1975;9(11):842–846.
21. American Medical Association, American Academy of Sleep Medicine. *Resolution 503: Insufficient Sleep in Adolescents*. Chicago, IL: American Medical Association, American Academy of Sleep Medicine; 2010.
22. National Sleep Foundation. *2006 Teens and Sleep. Sleep in America Polls*. Washington, DC: National Sleep Foundation; 2006. Available at: www.sleepfoundation.org/article/sleep-america-polls/2006-teens-and-sleep.
23. Sleep Health. *Healthy People 2020 Topics and Objectives*. Available at: www.healthypeople.gov/2020/topics objectives2020/overview.aspx?topicid=38.
24. Cain N, Gradisar M. Electronic media use and sleep in school-aged children and adolescents: a review. *Sleep Med*. 2010;11(8):735–742.
25. Crowley SJ, Carskadon MA. Modifications to weekend recovery sleep delay circadian phase in older adolescents. *Chronobiol Int*. 2010;27(7):1469–1492.
26. American Academy of Pediatrics, Adolescent Sleep Working Group, Committee on Adolescence, Council on School Health. School start times for adolescents. *Pediatrics*. 2014;134(3).
27. Wahlstrom K. Changing times: findings from the first longitudinal study of later high school start times. *NASSP Bull*. 2002;86(633):3–21.
28. Dexter D, Bijwadia J, Schilling D, Applebaugh G. Sleep, sleepiness and school start times: a preliminary study. *WMJ*. 2003;102(1):44–46.
29. Owens JA, Belon K, Moss P. Impact of delaying school start time on adolescent sleep, mood, and behavior. *Arch Pediatr Adolesc Med*. 2010;164(7):608–614.
30. Wolfson AR, Spaulding NL, Dandrow C, Baroni EM. Middle school start times: the importance of a good night's sleep for young adolescents. *Behav Sleep Med*. 2007; 5(3):194–209.
31. Vorona RD, Szklo-Coxe M, Wu A, Dubik M, Zhao Y, Ware JC. Dissimilar teen crash rates in two neighboring southeastern Virginia cities with different high school start times. *J Clin Sleep Med*. 2011;7(2):145–151.
32. Kristjansson AL, Sigfusdottir ID, Allegrante JP, James JE. Adolescent caffeine consumption, daytime sleepiness and anger. *J Caffeine Res*. 2011;1(1):75–82.
33. O'Dea JA. Consumption of nutritional supplements among adolescents: usage and perceived benefits. *Health Educ Res*. 2003;18(1):98–107.
34. Bryant Ludden A, Wolfson AR. Understanding adolescent caffeine use: connecting use patterns with expectancies, reasons, and sleep. *Health Educ Behav*. 2010;37(3): 330–342.
35. Gromov I, Gromov D. Sleep and substance use and abuse in adolescents. *Child Adolesc Psychiatr Clin N Am*. 2009; 18(4):929–946.
36. Strain EC, Griffiths RR. Caffeine Dependence: fact or fiction? *J R Soc Med*. 1995;88(8):437–440.
37. Chen MC, Burley HW, Gotlib IH. Reduced sleep quality in healthy girls at risk for depression. *J Sleep Res*. 2012; 21(1):68–72.
38. Catrett CD, Gaultney JF. Possible insomnia predicts some risky behaviors among adolescents when controlling for depressive symptoms. *J Genet Psychol*. 2009;170(4): 287–309.
39. An H, Ahn JH, Bhang SY. The association of psychosocial and familial factors with adolescent suicidal ideation: a population-based study. *Psychiatry Res*. 2010;177(3): 318–322.

40. Leproult R, Van Cauter E. Role of sleep and sleep loss in hormonal release and metabolism. *Endocr Dev*. 2010;17: 11–21.
41. Weiss A, Xu F, Storfer-Isser A, Thomas A, Ievers-Landis CE, Redline S. The association of sleep duration with adolescents' fat and carbohydrate consumption. *Sleep*. 2010;33(9):1201–1209.
42. Kang KT, Chou CH, Weng WC, Lee PL, Hsu WC. Associations between adenotonsillar hypertrophy, age, and obesity in children with obstructive sleep apnea. *PLoS One*. 2013;8(10). e78666.
43. Pizza F, Contardi S, Antognini AB, et al. Sleep quality and motor vehicle crashes in adolescents. *J Clin Sleep Med*. 2010;6(1):41–45.
44. Smith-Coggins R, Howard SK, Mac DT, et al. Improving alertness and performance in emergency department physicians and nurses: the use of planned naps. *Ann Emerg Med*. 2006;48(5):596–604, 604.e1–e3.
45. Hirschkowitz M, Whiton K, Albert SA, et al. The National Sleep Foundation's sleep time duration recommendations: methodology and results summary. *Sleep Health*. 2015;1:40–43.
46. Bruni O, Angriman M. L'insonnia in eta evolutiva. *Medico Bam-Bino*. 2015;34:224–233.
47. Owens JA, Mindell JA. Pediatric insomnia. *Pediatr Clin North Am*. 2011;58:555–569.
48. Calhoun SL, Fernandez-Mendoza J, Vgontzas AN, Liao D, Bixler EO. Prevalence of insomnia symptoms in a general population sample of young children and preadolescents: gender effects. *Sleep Med*. 2014;15:91–95.
49. Fossum IN, Nordnes LT, Storemark SS, Bjorvatn B, Pallesen S. The association between use of electronic media in bed before going to sleep and insomnia symptoms, daytime sleepiness, morning-ness, and chronotype. *Behav Sleep Med*. 2014;12:343–357.
50. Sivertsen B, Pallesen S, Stormark KM, Bøe T, Lundervold AJ, Hysing M. Delayed sleep phase syndrome in adolescents: prevalence and correlates in a large population based study. *BMC Public Health*. 2013;13:1163.
51. Sivertsen B, Harvey AG, Lundervold AJ, Hysing M. Sleep problems and depression in adolescence: results from a large population-based study of Norwegian adolescents aged 16–18years. *Eur Child Adolesc Psychiatry*. 2014;23: 681–689.
52. Corkum P, Davidson F, MacPherson M. A Framework for the assessment and treatment of sleep problems in children with attention-deficit/hyperactivity disorder. *Pediatr Clin North Am*. 2011;58:667–683.
53. Pereira AM, Bruni O, Ferri R, Palmini A, Nunes ML. The impact of epilepsy on sleep architecture during childhood. *Epilepsia*. 2012;53:1519–1525.
54. Merikanto I, Lahti T, Puusniekka R, Partonen T. Late bedtimes weaken school performance and predispose adolescents to health hazards. *Sleep Med*. 2013;14: 1105–1111.
55. Phillipson EA. Sleep apnea–a major public health problem. *N Engl J Med*. 1993;328:1271–1273.
56. Lumeng JC, Chervin RD. Epidemiology of pediatric obstructive sleep apnea. *Proc Am Thorac Soc*. 2008;5(2): 242–252.
57. Redline S, Tishler PV, Schluchter M, Aylor J, Clark G, Graham G. Risk factors for sleep-disordered breathing in children associations with obesity, race, and respiratory problems. *Am J Respir Crit Care Med*. May 1999; 159(5 Pt 1):1527–1532.
58. Baker M, Scott B, Johnson RF, Mitchell RB. Predictors of obstructive sleep apnea severity in adolescents. *JAMA Otolaryngol Head Neck Surg*. 2017;143(5):494–499. https://doi.org/10.1001/jamaoto.2016.4130.
59. Xanthopoulos MS, Gallagher PR, Berkowitz RI, Radcliffe J, Bradford R, Marcus CL. Neurobehavioral functioning in adolescents with and without obesity and obstructive sleep apnea. *Sleep*. 2015;38(3): 401–410. https://doi.org/10.5665/sleep.4498.
60. Patinkin ZW, Feinn R, Santos M. Metabolic consequences of obstructive sleep apnea in adolescents with obesity: a systematic literature review and meta-analysis. *Child Obes*. 2017;13(2):102–110. https://doi.org/10.1089/chi.2016.0248.
61. Kohyama J, Ohinata JS, Hasegawa T. Blood pressure in sleep disordered breathing. *Arch Dis Child*. 2003;88:139–142.
62. Amin RS, Kimball TR, Bean JA, et al. Left ventricular hypertrophy and abnormal ventricular geometry in children and adolescents with obstructive sleep apnea. *Am J Respir Crit Care Med*. 2002;165:1395–1399.
63. Shiomi T, Guilleminault C, Stoohs R, Schnittger I. Obstructed breathing in children during sleep monitored by echocardiography. *Acta Paediatr*. 1993;82:863–871.
64. O'Brien LM, Gozal D. Autonomic dysfunction in children with sleep-disordered breathing. *Sleep*. 2005;28:747–752.
65. O'Brien LM, Serpero LD, Tauman R, Gozal D. Plasma adhesion molecules in children with sleep-disordered breathing. *Chest*. 2006;129:947–953.
66. Tauman R, Ivanenko A, O'Brien LM, Gozal D. Plasma C-reactive protein levels among children with sleep-disordered breathing. *Pediatrics*. 2004;113:e564–e569.
67. Reid KJ, Zee PC. Circadian disorders of the sleep-wake cycle. In: Kryger MH, Roth T, Dement WC, eds. *Principles and Practice of Sleep Medicine*. 4th ed. Philadelphia: Elsevier/Saunders; 2005:691–701.
68. Czeisler CA, Richardson GS, Zimmerman JC, et al. Entrainment of human circadian rhythms by light-dark cycles: a reassessment. *Photochem Photobiol*. 1981;34(2): 239–247.
69. Pereira DS, Tufik S, Louzada FM, et al. Association of the length polymorphism in the human Per3 gene with the delayed sleep-phase syndrome: does latitude have an influence upon it? *Sleep*. 2005;28(1):29–32.
70. Wyatt J, Stepanki E, Kirby J. Circadian phase in delayed sleep phase syndrome: predictors and temporal stability across multiple assessments. Sleep 2006;29:1075–1080.
71. Weitzman ED, Czeisler CA, Coleman RM, et al. Delayed sleep phase syndrome. A chronobiological disorder with sleep-onset insomnia. *Arch Gen Psychiatry*. 1981; 38(7):737–746.

72. Lewy AJ. Circadian misalignment in mood disturbances. *Curr Psychiatry Rep*. 2009;11:459–465.
73. American Academy of Sleep Medicine. *International Classification of Sleep Disorders*. 3rd ed. Darien, IL: American Academy of Sleep Medicine; 2014.
74. Broughton R. NREM arousal parasomnias. In: Kryger MH, RT, Dement WC, eds. *Principles and Practice of Sleep Medicine*. 3rd ed. Philadelphia: W.B. Saunders Co; 2000:693–706.
75. Ohayon MM, Guilleminault C, Priest RG. Night terrors, sleepwalking, and confusional arousals in the general population: their frequency and relationship to other sleep and mental disorders. *J Clin Psychiatry*. 1999;60: 268–276.
76. Mindell JA, Owens J. *Sleepwalking and Sleep Terrors. A Clinical Guide to Pediatric Sleep*. Philadelphia: Lipincott Williams &Wilkins; 2003:88–96.
77. Schenck CH, Bundlie SR, Ettinger MG, Mahowald MW. Chronic behavioral disorders of human REM sleep: a new category of parasomnia. *Sleep*. 1986;9:293–308.
78. Chokroverty SHW, Walters AS. An approach to the patient with movement disorders during sleep and classification. In: Chokroverty SHW, Walters AS, eds. *Sleep and Movement Disorders*. Philadelphia: Butterworth-Heinemann; 2003:201–218.
79. Ohayon MM, Zulley J, Guilleminault C, Smirne S. Prevalence and pathologic associations of sleep paralysis in the general population. *Neurology*. 1999;52:1194–1200.
80. Montagna P. Sleep-related non epileptic motor disorders. *J Neurol*. 2004;251:781–794.
81. Dahlitz M, Parkes JD. Sleep paralysis. *Lancet*. 1993;341: 406–407.
82. Paradis CM, Friedman S. Sleep paralysis in African Americans with panic disorder. *Transcult Psychiatry*. 2005;42: 123–134.
83. Levin R, Fireman G. Nightmare prevalence, nightmare distress, and self-reported psychological disturbance. *Sleep*. 2002;25:205–212.
84. Nielsen TA, Laberge L, Paquet J, et al. Development of disturbing dreams during adolescence and their relation to anxiety symptoms. *Sleep*. 2000;23:727–736.
85. Bader G, Neveus T, Kruse S, Sillen U. Sleep of primary enuretic children and controls. *Sleep*. 2002;25:579–583.
86. Umlauf MG, Chasens ER. Sleep disordered breathing and nocturnal polyuria: nocturia and enuresis. *Sleep Med Rev*. 2003;7:403–411.
87. Sachs C, Svanborg E. The exploding head syndrome: polysomnographic recordings and therapeutic suggestions. *Sleep*. 1991;14:263–266.
88. Winkelman JW. Clinical and polysomnographic features of sleep related eating disorder. *J Clin Psychiatry*. 1998;59: 14–19.
89. Vetrugno R, Provini F, Plazzi G, et al. Catathrenia (nocturnal groaning): a new type of parasomnia. *Neurology*. 2001;56:681–683.
90. Meissner HH, Riemer A, Santiago SM, et al. Failure of physician documentation of sleep complaints in hospitalized patients. *West J Med*. 1998;169:146–149.
91. Meltzer LJ, Johnson C, Crosette J, Ramos M, Mindell JA. Prevalence of diagnosed sleep disorders in pediatric primary care practices. *Pediatrics*. 2010;125(6): e1410–e1418. https://doi.org/10.1542/peds.2009-2725.
92. Ohayon MM, Roberts RE, Zulley J, Smirne S, Priest RG. Prevalence and patterns of problematic sleep among older adolescents. *J Am Acad Child Adolesc Psychiatry*. 2000;39:1549–1556.
93. Short MA, Gradisar M, Gill J, Camfferman D. Identifying adolescent sleep problems. *PLoS One*. 2013;8(9). https://doi.org/10.1371/journal.pone.0075301. e75301.
94. Wolfson AR, Carskadon MA. Sleep schedules and daytime functioning in adolescents. *Child Dev*. 1998;69(4): 875–887.
95. Link SC, Ancoli-lsrael S. Sleep and the teenager. *Sleep Res*. 1995;24a:184.
96. Blum D, Kahn A, Mozin MJ, Rebuffat E, Sottiaux M, Van de Merckt C. Relation between chronic insomnia and school failure in preadolescents. *Sleep Res*. 1990;19:194.
97. Carney CE, Buysse DJ, Ancoli-Israel S, et al. *Sleep*. 2012; 35(2):287–302.
98. Monk TH, Reynolds CF, Kupfer DJ, et al. The Pittsburgh sleep diary. *J Sleep Res*. 1994;3(2):111–120. https://doi.org/10.1111/j.1365-2869.1994.tb00114.x.
99. Ibáñez V, Silva J, Cauli O. A survey on sleep questionnaires and diaries. *Sleep Medicine*. 2018;42:90–96. https://doi.org/10.1016/j.sleep.2017.08.026.
100. Tonetti L, Mingozzi R, Natale V. Comparison between paper and electronic sleep diary. *Biol Rhythm Res*. 2016; 47(5):743–753. https://doi.org/10.1080/09291016.2016.1191689.
101. LeBourgeois MK, Giannotti F, Cortesi F, Wolfson AR, Harsh J. The relationship between reported sleep quality and sleep hygiene in Italian and American adolescents. *Pediatrics*. 2005;115(suppl. 1):257–265.
102. LeBourgeois MK, Avis K, Mixon M, Olmi J, Harsh J. Snoring, sleep quality, and sleepiness across attention-deficit/hyperactivity disorder subtypes. *Sleep*. 2004;27(3): 520–525.
103. Spilsbury JC, Drotar D, Rosen CL, Redline S. The Cleveland adolescent sleepiness questionnaire: a new measure to assess excessive daytime sleepiness in adolescents. *J Clin Sleep Med*. 2007;3(6):603–612.
104. Johns M. A new method for measuring daytime sleepiness: the epworth daytime sleepiness scale. *Sleep*. 1991; 14:540–545.
105. Melendres CS, Lutz JM, Rubin ED, Marcus CL. Daytime sleepiness and hyperactivity in children with suspected sleep-disordered breathing. *Pediatrics*. 2004;114: 768–775.
106. Moore M, Kirchner L, Drotar D, et al. Relationships among sleepiness, sleep time, and psychological functioning in adolescents. *J Pediatr Psychol*. 2009;34: 117–183.
107. Drake C, Nickel C, Burduvali E, Roth T, Jefferson C, Pietro B. The Pediatric Daytime Sleepiness Scale (PDSS): sleep habits and school outcomes in middle-school children. *Sleep*. 2003;26(4):455–458.

108. Perez-Chada D, Perez-Lloret S, Videla AJ, et al. Sleep disordered breathing and daytime sleepiness are associated with poor academic performance in teenagers. A study using the pediatric daytime sleepiness scale (PDSS). *Sleep*. 2007;30(12):1698–1703. https://doi.org/10.1093/sleep/30.12.1698.
109. Malone SK. Early to bed, early to rise?: an exploration of adolescent sleep hygiene practices. *J Sch Nurs*. 2011;27: 348–354.
110. Lewandowski AS, Toliver-Sokol M, Palermo TM. Evidence-based review of subjective pediatric sleep measures. *J. Pediatr Psychol*. 2011;36:780–793.
111. Mindell JA, Owens JA. *A Clinical Guide to Pediatric Sleep: Diagnosis and Management of Sleep Problems*. Philadelphia: Lippincott Williams & Wilkins; 2003.
112. Ramírez-Vélez, Robinson H-Z, Libardo, Correa-Bautista, Enrique J, Cárdenas-Calderón, Giovanni E. *Reliability and Validity of the BEARS Sleep Disorder Questionnaire in Children and Adolescent Students Fr*. Retos, [S.l.], N. 34; 2017:89–93. ISSN:1988-2041 https://recyt.fecyt.es/index.php/retos/article/view/58585.
113. Chervin RD, Hedger K, Dillon JE, Pituch KJ. Pediatric sleep questionnaire (PSQ): validity and reliability of scales for sleep-disordered breathing, snoring, sleepiness, and behavioral problems. *Sleep Med*. 2000;1(1):21–32.
114. Chervin RD, Weatherly RA, Garetz SL, et al. Pediatric sleep questionnaire: prediction of sleep apnea and outcomes. *Arch Otolaryngol Head Neck Surg*. 2007; 133(3):216–222.
115. Duarte J, Nelas P, Chaves C, Ferreira M, Coutinho E, Cunha M. Sleep-wake patterns and their influence on school performance in Portuguese adolescents. *Aten Primaria*. 2014;46:160–164.
116. Wolfson AR, Carskadon MA, Acebo C, et al. Evidence for the validity of a sleep habits survey for adolescents. *Sleep*. 2003;2:213–216.
117. O'Brien EM, Mindell JA. Sleep and risk-taking behavior in adolescents. *Behav Sleep Med*. 2005;3(3):113–133.
118. Acebo C, Carskadon MA. Influence of irregular sleep patterns on waking behavior. In: Carskadon MA, ed. *Adolescent Sleep Patterns: Biological, Social, and Psychological Influences*. New York, NY, US: Cambridge University Press; 2002:220–235.
119. Bruni O, Ottavianio S, Guidetti V, et al. The sleep disturbance scale for children (SDSC): construction and validation of an instrument to evaluate sleep disturbances in childhood and adolescence. *J Sleep Rrs*. 1996;5:251–261.
120. Romeo DM, Bruni O, Brogna C, et al. Application of the sleep disturbance scale for children (SDSC) in preschool age. *Eur J Paediatr Neurol*. 2013;17(4):374–382.
121. Carotenuto M, Bruni O, Santoro N, Del Giudice EM, Perrone L, Pascotto A. Waist circumference predicts the occurrence of sleep-disordered breathing in obese children and adolescents: a questionnaire-based study. *Sleep Med*. 2006;7(4):357–361.
122. Hartshorne TS, Heussler HS, Dailor AN, Williams GL, Papadopoulos D, Brandt KK. Sleep disturbances in CHARGE syndrome: types and relationships with behavior and caregiver well-being. *Dev Med Child Neurol*. 2009;51(2):143–150.
123. Haynes PL. The role of behavioral sleep medicine in the assessment and treatment of sleep disordered breathing. *Clin Psychol Rev*. 2005;25:673–705.
124. Pandi-Perumal SR, Spence DW, BaHammam AS. Polysomnography: an overview. In: Pagel J, Pandi-Perumal S, eds. *Primary Care Sleep Medicine*. New York: Springer; 2014.
125. Robertson B, Marshall B, Carno MA. *Polysomnography for the Sleep Technologist*. St. Louis: Elsevier; 2014.
126. American Academy of Sleep Medicine. *ICSD-3, International Classification of Sleep Disorders: Diagnostic and Coding Manual*. 3rd ed. 2014.
127. Cruz SD, Littner MR, Zeidler MR. Home sleep testing for the diagnosis of obstructive sleep apnea-indications and limitations. *Semin Respir Crit Care Med*. 2014;35(5): 552–559. https://doi.org/10.1055/s-0034-1390066.
128. Kapoor M, Greenough G. Home sleep tests for obstructive sleep apnea (OSA). *J Am Board Fam Med*. 2015; 28(4):504–509. https://doi.org/10.3122/jabfm.2015.04.140266.
129. Carskadon MA, Dement WC. Sleepiness and sleep state on a 90-minute schedule. *Psychophysics*. 1977;14:127–133.
130. Carskadon MA. Guidelines for the multiple sleep latency test (MSLT): a standard measure of sleepiness. *Sleep*. 1986; 9(4):519–524. https://doi.org/10.1093/sleep/9.4.519.
131. Meira L, Van Zeller M, Eusébio E, Santa Clara E, Viana P, Drummond M. Maintenance of wakefulness test in clinical practice. *ERJ Open Res*. 2017;3:P5. https://doi.org/10.1183/23120541.sleepandbreathing-2017.P5.
132. Morgenthaler T, Alessi C, Friedman L, et al. Practice parameters for the use of actigraphy in the assessment of sleep and sleep disorders. *Sleep*. 2007;30:519–529.
133. Sadeh A. Assessment of intervention for infant night waking: parental reports and activity-based home monitoring. *J Consult Clin Psychol*. 1994;62:63–68.
134. Malow B, Adkins KW, McGrew SG, et al. Melatonin for sleep in children with autism: a controlled trial examining dose, tolerability, and outcomes. *J Autism Dev Disord*. 2012;42:1729–1737.
135. Acebo C, Sadeh A, Seifer R, et al. Estimating sleep patterns with activity monitoring in children and adolescents: how many nights are necessary for reliable measures? *Sleep*. 1999;22:95–103.
136. Berger AM, Wielgus KK, Young-McCaughan S, Fischer P, Farr L, Lee KA. Methodological challenges when using actigraphy in research. *J. Pain Symptom Manag*. 2008;36: 191–199.
137. Quante M, Kaplan ER, Cailler M, et al. Actigraphy-based sleep estimation in adolescents and adults: a comparison with polysomnography using two scoring algorithms. *Nat Sci Sleep*. 2018;10:13–20. https://doi.org/10.2147/NSS.S151085.
138. Carskadon MA, Wolfson AR, Acebo C, Tzischinsky O, Seifer R. Adolescent sleep patterns, circadian timing, and sleepiness at a transition to early school days. *Sleep*. 1998;21:871–881.

139. Lemke MR, Mieth B, Pleuse S, Spath C. Motor behavior in depression: applications and limitations of actigraphic analyses. *Psychiatr Prax*. 2001;28:219–225.
140. Armitage R, Hoffmann R, Emslie G, Rintelman J, Moore J, Lewis K. Rest-activity cycles in childhood and adolescent depression. *J Am Acad Child Adolesc Psychiatry*. 2004;43:761–769.
141. Teixeira LR, Fischer FM, de Andrade MM, Louzada FM, Nagai R. Sleep patterns of day-working, evening high-schooled adolescents of Sao Paulo, Brazil. *Chronobiol Int*. 2004;21:239–252.

CHAPTER 6

# Adolescent Exercise Screening

ZACHARY M. HOOD, MD • VINCENT MORELLI, MD

## COMMON TERMINOLOGY AND DEFINITIONS

Before delving into the topic of adolescent exercise screening, it is important to take a moment to be clear and precise with our terminology, as the discussion that follows relies partly on linguistic distinction. Despite the predominant colloquial usage, *physical activity* and *exercise* are not interchangeable terms.[1] *Physical activity* is a broad term defined as bodily movement produced by the contraction of skeletal muscle that increases energy expenditure above the basal level. *Exercise* is a form of physical activity that is planned, structured, repetitive, and purposeful, with a focus on improving or maintaining one or more components of physical fitness. *Physical fitness*, then, can be considered as the ability to accomplish daily tasks with vigor and alertness, without undue fatigue, and with ample energy to enjoy leisure time pursuits and meet unforeseen emergencies.[1] The scope of physical fitness includes cardiorespiratory and skeletal muscular endurance, skeletal muscular strength and power, speed, flexibility, agility, balance, reaction time, and body composition.[2]

Providing further refinement, the *metabolic equivalent of task* (MET) is a widely accepted physiological measure used to quantify physical activity.[3] METs are units used to estimate the metabolic cost (i.e., oxygen consumption) of physical activity, with one MET unit accepted to be the resting metabolic rate (~3.5 mL O2/kg/min). *Moderate-intensity physical activity* (MPA) includes those activities performed at an intensity of three to six METs and *vigorous-intensity physical activity* (VPA) includes those activities performed at an intensity >6 METs. Table 6.1 lists various ways of achieving MPA.[3]

## IMPORTANCE OF PHYSICAL ACTIVITY ON ADOLESCENT DEVELOPMENT

It should come as no surprise that physical activity and exercise have numerous benefits. Evidence clearly demonstrates long-term adaptations to exercise training include effects upon the musculoskeletal, metabolic, cardiovascular, and respiratory systems, with beneficial effects on cardiovascular disease and all-cause mortality.[4] Although the beneficial effects appear to be dose-dependent (to a certain degree), current evidence indicates engaging in as few as one or two 75-min sessions of exercise per week decreases all-cause, cardiovascular, and cancer-related mortality compared to sedentary individuals.[5] It is, therefore, imperative to promote physical activity to patients, as inactivity increases the relative risk of coronary artery disease, stroke, hypertension, and osteoporosis by 45%, 60%, 30%, and 59%, respectively.[6] Table 6.2 highlights some of the ways in which physical activity and exercise favorably impact multiple systems and health outcomes.[1] The evidence also suggests that the benefits of physical activity on reducing mortality may plateau after a certain activity level,[5] and doses above 100 min/day of MPA in healthy individuals do not appear to be associated with additional reductions in mortality rates.[5]

Among children and adolescents, however, these benefits usually are not the motivating factors for physical activity. Rather, their motivation for physical activity often relates to one or more of the following[7]:

1. Improving physical fitness, performance, body composition, and body image
2. Alleviating boredom
3. Socializing

Regardless of the motivations, physical activity during adolescence can have profound and lasting effects. Recently, two systematic reviews[8,9] have identified many benefits of regular physical activity in school-aged children, as highlighted in Table 6.3.

To appreciate the impact of physical activity during adolescence and the challenges of caring for adolescent patients, a brief review of normal development follows. Adolescence is the developmental stage (roughly between 10 and 19 years of age) mediated by hormonal, genetic, and environmental factors leading to physical,

Adolescent Health Screening: An Update in the Age of Big Data. https://doi.org/10.1016/B978-0-323-66130-0.00006-5

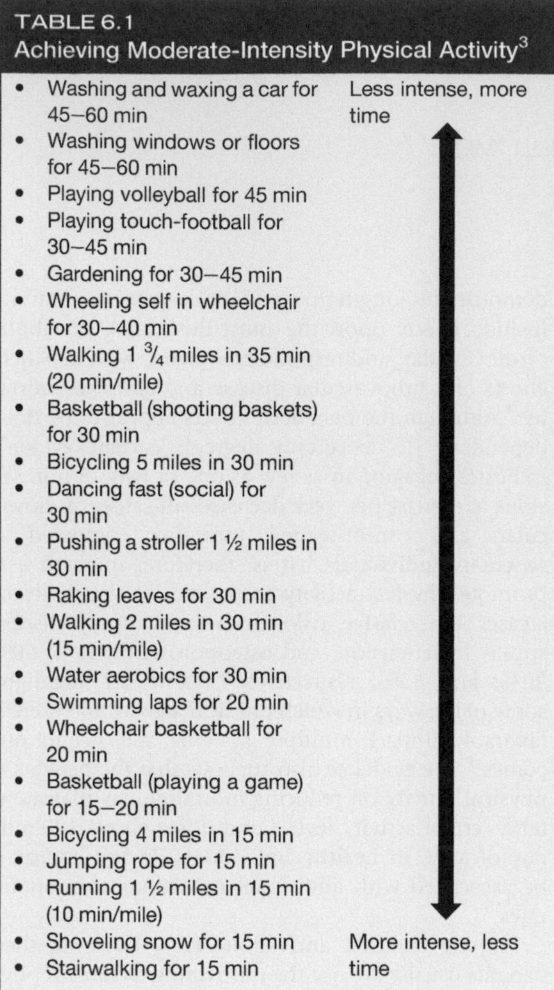

**TABLE 6.1**
**Achieving Moderate-Intensity Physical Activity[3]**

|  |  |
|---|---|
| Washing and waxing a car for 45–60 min | Less intense, more time |
| Washing windows or floors for 45–60 min | ↑ |
| Playing volleyball for 45 min | |
| Playing touch-football for 30–45 min | |
| Gardening for 30–45 min | |
| Wheeling self in wheelchair for 30–40 min | |
| Walking 1 3/4 miles in 35 min (20 min/mile) | |
| Basketball (shooting baskets) for 30 min | |
| Bicycling 5 miles in 30 min | |
| Dancing fast (social) for 30 min | |
| Pushing a stroller 1 ½ miles in 30 min | |
| Raking leaves for 30 min | |
| Walking 2 miles in 30 min (15 min/mile) | |
| Water aerobics for 30 min | |
| Swimming laps for 20 min | |
| Wheelchair basketball for 20 min | |
| Basketball (playing a game) for 15–20 min | |
| Bicycling 4 miles in 15 min | |
| Jumping rope for 15 min | |
| Running 1 ½ miles in 15 min (10 min/mile) | ↓ |
| Shoveling snow for 15 min | More intense, less time |
| Stairwalking for 15 min | |

**TABLE 6.2**
**Benefits of Exercise on Multiple Systems and Health Outcomes[1]**

- Reduces risk of dying prematurely
- Reduces risk of dying from heart disease
- Reduces risk of stroke
- Reduces risk of developing diabetes
- Reduces risk of developing high blood pressure
- Helps reduce blood pressure in people who already have high blood pressure
- Reduces risk of developing colon cancer
- Reduces feelings of depression and anxiety
- Helps control weight
- Helps build and maintain healthy bones, muscles, and joints
- Helps older adults become stronger and better able to move about without falling
- Promotes psychological well-being

**TABLE 6.3**
**Benefits of Regular Physical Activity in School-Aged Children[8,9]**

- Reduced adiposity in overweight youth[10–12]
- Reduced blood pressure in youth with mild essential hypertension[10,13,14]
- Reduced cholesterol and/or triglyceride levels in youth with high cholesterol or obesity[15]
- Improved bone health[16–18]
- Improved aerobic fitness[19,20]
- Improved muscular strength and endurance[19]
- Improved psychosocial well-being[21–24]
- Improved cognitive performance/academic achievement[25,26]

sexual, and psychosocial maturation. The normal child-to-adolescent transition is mediated by neuroendocrine changes. Gonadotropin-releasing hormone (GnRH) is activated and leads to an increased secretion of gonadotrophs (follicle-stimulating hormone (FSH) and luteinizing hormone (LH) from the pituitary). The increased secretion of FSH and LH, in turn, promotes the production of androgens and estrogens from the ovaries and testes. At the same time, the triggers that stimulate GnRH secretion also incite corticotropin-releasing hormone secretion from the hypothalamus, which then stimulates the anterior pituitary to secrete adrenocorticotropic hormone, which acts on the adrenal glands to increase the secretion of the adrenal androgens, dehydroepiandrosterone and androstenedione. The elevated levels of estrogen and gonadal and adrenal androgens begin to initiate sexual development and simultaneously stimulate an increase in the release of growth hormone from the pituitary. Together, these well-orchestrated changes lead to an increase in physical stature, the development of secondary sexual characteristics, and the ultimate transition into adulthood.[27–30]

Neurologically, as a child transitions from adolescence to adulthood, the amount of gray matter (neurons) decreases, as selective elimination of redundant pathways (i.e., "pruning") takes place. Conversely, the amount of cortical white matter (myelin-coated axons) increases, as more and more cell-to-cell connections are formalized.[31] These connections continue to form through early adulthood and are important in learning, imagination, memory, and physical memory. Importantly, any arrest in white matter growth during this time could lead to potential interconnectivity deficits and impaired learning. One specific area of importance when looking at white matter development is the prefrontal cortex, the seat of impulse control, decision making, delayed gratification, and goal-directed behavior. White matter connections formed in this area are not complete until a person reaches their mid-20s.[32–34] Additionally, the adolescent brain has a relative lack of mood modulating and behavioral control neurotransmitters (e.g., serotonin) and an excess in excitatory neurotransmitters (e.g., glutamate, dopamine), resulting in a propensity for excitability amid a general lack of impulse control and executive function.

An awareness of the normal neuroendocrine changes that occur during adolescence is critical for parents, teachers, and policy makers, as any factors that further delay or impede maturation in these areas could be expected to compound these deficits and lead to further learning and behavioral problems and risky behaviors.[35] Several prospective studies have looked at the effects on academic and cognitive performance in low-income adolescents, a population known to be particularly at risk and associated with lower levels of physical activity.[36] One study[37] examining attention span and reading comprehension in low-income adolescents found that aerobic exercise improved both attention span and reading comprehension to a greater degree in low-income students than their higher-income counterparts. The study recommended that "schools serving low-income adolescents should consider implementing brief sessions of aerobic exercise during the school day." Another study[38] examining fitness and cognitive performance in 83,000 children in the New York Public School system found that, although all children improved academic performance with increased fitness, the effect was most pronounced in impoverished youths, especially boys.

Regular physical activity has been shown to enhance neurogenesis via increased levels of brain-derived neurotropic factor[39,40] and serotonin.[41] This enhanced neurogenesis may account for the structural advantages seen in the brains of fit children. In other words, the physically fit children have been shown to have larger hippocampal volumes (memory storage and association area)[41] and larger basal ganglia volumes (areas important in task completion). Cognitively, exercise has been shown to improve attention span[42] and mental processing speed.[43] Exercise has been shown to enhance learning, especially with challenging subjects,[44] and to strengthen multitasking ability,[45] resulting in higher test scores.[46–48] Fit children also have superior relational or associative memory (able to associate dissimilar bits of information), an area important in learning and imagination. In all, physically fit children have an increased ability to focus, learn, process, and shut out distractions and conflicting impulses.[49,50]

Childhood habits are proven to carry forward strongly into adulthood.[51–53] As such, instilling a habit of activity during adolescence can profoundly impact and enhance mental health and school performance, fostering long-term socioeconomic gain and health in adults who have carried forward a habit of activity from childhood.[54,55]

## GUIDELINES ANDEMOGRAPHICS: EXPECTATION VERSUS REALITY

### Expectation

In 1997, the Centers for Disease Control and Prevention (CDC) suggested a multifaceted approach to promote physical activity among young people.[56] These guidelines recommended that healthcare providers, schools, the community, and the fitness industry cooperate to provide safe environments and facilities for developmentally appropriate physical activity, as well as appropriate instruction, supervision, and role models for youth. Curiously, although physical activity guidelines for adults have been updated several times since 1997,[57,58] recommendations specific to children and adolescents have remained consistent: at least 60 min per day of moderate-to-vigorous physical activity (MVPA) for school-aged children.[8,58,59] The World Health Organization (WHO) and the American College of Sports Medicine (ACSM) recommend the same,[60,61] and the American Academy of Pediatrics (AAP)/Bright Futures, the American Academy of Family Physicians (AAFP), and the US Preventive Services Task Force (USPSTF) concur.[8,62,63] The CDC specifies that aerobic activity should make up most of a child's 60 or more minutes of daily MVPA (with VPA on at least 3 days per week), with regular contribution from muscle strengthening (e.g., gymnastics, push-ups) and bone strengthening (e.g., running, jumping rope) on at least 3 days per week as part of the 60 or more minutes per day.[59]

### Reality

In the United States, only 42% of children and 8% of adolescents meet these modest recommendations,[64,65] with underserved children (Black and Hispanic children) exhibiting the lowest levels of physical activity. The lowest levels of physical activity are seen in children with poorly educated mothers, those living in high-crime neighborhoods, those from low-income families, those with few adult role models, those in schools lacking sufficient PE classes, and those living in communities with low community-based physical activity opportunities.[66,67] In addition, as children age from 9 to 15 years, the time spent in MVPA drops significantly (from a daily average of 181 min at age 9–124 min at age 11[68]), again with the greatest declines seen in children of low-income families (and girls).[68] Longitudinal data from the Study of Early Child Care and Youth Development (2000–2006) indicate that virtually all 9-year-old children met the CDC guideline for MVPA, engaging in an average of approximately 3 h of MVPA per day (as measured by an accelerometer).[68] However, by age 15, MVPA declined to an average of 50 min/day on weekdays and 37 min/day on weekends, with only 32% and 18% of 15-year-olds meeting the CDC guidelines for MVPA on weekdays and weekends, respectively. According to the 2010 National Youth Physical Activity and Nutrition Survey, only 15% of high school students participate in ≥60 min of aerobic physical activity per day.[69] Contributing to the problem is the fact that in 2014 only 3.6% of elementary schools, 3.4% of middle schools, and 4.0% of high schools nationwide required daily PE for all students,[70] thus disregarding the recommendations of the nation's Healthy People 2020 goals (Table 6.4).[71]

**TABLE 6.4**
**Healthy People 2020 Objectives for Preventing Chronic Diseases of Adulthood[71]**

| |
|---|
| *Increase the proportion of adults who engage in aerobic physical activity of at least MPA for more than 300 min/week, or more than 150 min/week of VPA, or an equivalent combination*<br>• Goal of 10% improvement from 28.4% of adults that currently (2008) meet the guideline<br>• Latest data (2016) suggest surpassing the goal (35.9%) |
| *Increase the proportion of adolescents who meet current Federal physical activity guidelines of aerobic physical activity*<br>• Goal of 10% improvement from 28.7% of adolescents that currently (2011) meet the guideline<br>• Latest data (2015) suggest decline to 27.1% |
| *Increase the proportion of adolescents who participate in daily school physical education*<br>• Goal of 10% improvement from 33.3% of adolescents that currently (2009) participate in daily school physical education<br>• Latest data (2015) suggest decline to 29.8% |

Reduced physical activity levels in adolescence predict reduced physical activity levels in adulthood, with potential long-term health implications.[72] Worldwide, one out of five adults is physically inactive.[62,73] Inactivity is particularly prevalent in more developed countries and among women, older persons, and those with lower incomes. Meanwhile, the time spent in sedentary behaviors (e.g., screen time) is increasing.[74,75] In the United States, many Americans do not meet national guidelines for being physically active. In a sample of children and adults from the National Health and Nutrition Examination Survey (NHANES) 2003 to 2004, activity monitoring found that 55% of waking hours were spent in sedentary behaviors,[76] and subsequent NHANES data in 2005–2006 indicate that the percentage of sedentary time is increasing (58%), while time spent in light activity is decreasing.[76] It is important to note that national prevalence data are often based on self-report measures of questionable validity, and when more objective measures are used (e.g., heart rate monitor, accelerometer), estimates of the proportion of youth meeting the guidelines drop dramatically.[77] Unsurprisingly, it is estimated that one-third of children and adolescents in the United States are overweight or obese,[78] and, if this trend continues, over 40% will be obese by 2036.[79]

## THE IMPACT OF INACTIVITY

As alluded to earlier, it is well established that physical activity in childhood helps in disease prevention, promotes mental health and well-being,[58,80,81] enhances social skills,[82] and improves academic achievement.[83,84] These benefits are seen regardless of a child's socioeconomic background. The transition from childhood to adolescence is particularly crucial in promoting healthy habits because it is during this time that children gain more dietary decision-making power, more freedom as to how they spend their leisure time, and are more likely to initiate unhealthy behaviors such as skipping breakfast, dropping out of organized sports, or increasing screen time.[85–87] Importantly, both medical and psychological maladies, begun in childhood, often persist into adulthood,[88–90] making childhood a critical time for proper healthful habit formation.[51–53]

In the United States and other developed countries, these considerations are even more significant in underserved communities, where there is a significant tie between obesity and lower socioeconomic status. Childhood obesity is clearly associated with medical conditions such as diabetes, hypertension, and heart disease. Overweight children are also subject to psychological stressors such as discrimination, lowered self-esteem, depression, loneliness, and nervousness.[91]

Obesity also has a racial bias. In the United States, Black and Hispanic children have a rate of obesity twice that of White/non-Hispanic children,[92] and although overweight and obesity have increased in *all* children over the last 30 years, the increase has been significantly greater in Black children and Hispanic children.[93,94] For example, while White children have experienced a threefold increase in overweight and obesity between 1971 and 2002, Black children experienced a fivefold increase over the same period. It is also significant to note that obesity tracking into adulthood is especially high among minorities.[95] For a more in-depth discussion of obesity and obesity screening, see the Obesity Chapter in this publication.

Inactivity is associated with worse health outcomes. Large prospective cohort studies from several countries around the world have found that sedentary behavior is associated with a variety of poor health outcomes, including increased mortality.[74,96–99] One study calculated the attributable risk for premature mortality and estimated that physical inactivity worldwide causes 9% of premature mortality, accounting for 5.3 million deaths worldwide in 2008.[100] Prolonged sitting and/or sedentary time has also been associated with an increased risk for diabetes, cardiovascular disease, and cancer,[101,102] and is an independent risk factor for mortality[101–106] according to emerging evidence. A 2016 meta-analysis of 16 studies involving over one million individuals confirmed the risks associated with prolonged sitting (over 8 hours daily) and found higher mortality rates among individuals in the lower quartiles of physical activity as compared to the referent group (i.e., those sitting <4 h/day and in the most active quartile of >35.5 MET-hours per week; approximately 60–75 min per day).[106]

## THE PROBLEM

Despite the above compelling data and medical intuition, clinicians do not routinely screen patients (adolescents or otherwise) for physical inactivity or provide adequate counseling. In developed countries, studies suggest only 13%–34% of primary care patients report receiving advice on physical activity from their primary care clinician.[107–109] Lack of training, experience, or validated screening tools about how best to identify those at risk (not to mention a lack of consensus about how best to proceed once a patient has been identified) makes exercise intervention logistically and psychologically challenging.

The first step in solving a problem is often by recognizing that there is a problem. More specifically, that usually requires clearly defining, naming, and articulating the problem. By doing so, awareness can be raised expeditiously and steps can be taken toward improvement. To that end, there has been progress. Recently, a new phrase in the literature has emerged with the hopes of raising awareness among patients, parents, policy makers, and physicians, with the goal of beginning the process of improvement. Exercise deficit disorder (EDD) is a term used to describe a condition characterized by reduced levels of MVPA that are inconsistent with long-term health, well-being, and public health recommendations.[110] From this platform and understanding, progress is possible.

## PROPOSALS

### Screening General Principles

Before continuing our discussion, please review the general principles of screening tests in the introductory chapter.

### Extant Adolescent Screening Guidelines

Among the adolescent population, screening is routinely performed for many conditions despite a lack of evidence supporting the beneficial effects and/or quantifying the potential benefits and harms for many of these conditions (Table 6.5[111]). However, this lack of evidence does not necessarily indicate that screening is not beneficial, only that it has not yet been adequately investigated. Consequently, when deciding whether screening should be performed, the potential benefits and harms of screening must be considered, with an understanding that the balance between risk and benefit varies (upon the condition, the clinical circumstances of the child and family, the availability of resources, and the values that the patients or patients' caregivers place on the potential benefits and harms).[112] For many conditions, screening is regulated by local, state, or federal policies, in addition to several professional groups (CDC, AAP, AAFP, USPSTF, to name a few). See Table 6.5 for adolescent screening recommendations from the USPSTF.[111]

On average, an estimated 70% of adolescents have a preventive health visit every 4 years[113,114] and most youth visit their primary care physician (PCP) at least once per year. As such, PCPs are well positioned to deliver important health advice and promote physical activity to adolescents by

TABLE 6.5
USPSTF Recommendations for Screening and Counseling in Adolescents (2018)[111]

| | |
|---|---|
| **CANCER** | |
| • Cervical | Start screening every 3 years at the age of 21 years. |
| • Testicular | Not recommended |
| • Skin | Counsel patients with fair skin about minimizing exposure to UV radiation |
| **CARDIOVASCULAR** | |
| • Blood Pressure | Insufficient evidence for adolescents. Start screening at the age of 18 years. |
| • Lipids | Insufficient evidence |
| **DEVELOPMENT AND BEHAVIOR, INJURY PREVENTION, MENTAL HEALTH, AND SUBSTANCE ABUSE** | |
| • Alcohol Misuse | Insufficient evidence for adolescents. Start screening at 18 years old. |
| • Child Maltreatment | Insufficient evidence |
| • Depression | Screen ages 12–18 years. Insufficient evidence for 11 years or younger. |
| • Illicit Drug Use | Insufficient evidence |
| • Motor Vehicle Occupant Restraints | Refer to CDC guidelines |
| • Suicide Risk | Insufficient evidence |
| • Tobacco Use | Screen to provide interventions (education, counseling) to prevent initiation |
| • Youth Violence | Refer to CDC guidelines |
| **METABOLIC, NUTRITION, ENDOCRINE** | |
| • Celiac | Insufficient evidence |
| • Obesity | Screen with body mass index and offer behavioral interventions if indicated |
| **MUSCULOSKELETAL** | |
| • Scoliosis | Insufficient evidence |
| **OBSTETRIC AND GYNECOLOGIC CONDITIONS** | |
| • Asymptomatic Bacteriuria | Screen pregnant women at 12–16 weeks gestation |
| • Bacterial Vaginosis | Not recommended for low risk, asymptomatic women. Insufficient evidence for high risk, asymptomatic women |
| • Gestational Diabetes Mellitus | Screen pregnant women at 24 weeks gestation |
| • Hepatitis B | Screen pregnant women at first prenatal visit |
| • HIV | Screen all pregnant women |
| • Iron Deficiency Anemia | Insufficient evidence |
| • Lead levels | Not recommended routinely in asymptomatic pregnant women |
| • Syphilis | Screen pregnant women early |
| **INFECTIOUS DISEASES** | |
| • Chlamydia and Gonorrhea | Screen sexually active women of age 24 years and younger. Insufficient evidence for men. |
| • Genital Herpes | Not recommended for asymptomatic adolescents |
| • Hepatitis B | Screen adolescents at high risk |
| • HIV | Screen adolescents and adults aged 15–65 years |
| • Immunizations | Refer to CDC guidelines |
| • Sexually Transmitted Infections | Intensive behavioral counseling for all sexually active adolescents |
| • Syphilis | Screen at risk adolescents |

1. Encouraging daily physical activity in all children and youth
2. Helping parents determine the readiness of their child to participate in organized sports or strength-training programs
3. Performing preparticipation physical evaluations
4. Identifying contraindications and limitations to participation and defining modifications to participation and training
5. Providing education and anticipatory guidance regarding nutrition, hydration, ergogenic aids, or performance-enhancing drugs (e.g., anabolic steroids)
6. Educating families on how to select experienced and qualified fitness or strength and conditioning specialists

However, expectation does not match reality in most primary care settings. Although medical practitioners often perform health screenings related to vision, hearing, and body mass index, patient interactions are typically void of any meaningful assessment of physical activity, making the well-child visit a missed opportunity to evaluate each child's daily exercise habits and impart guidance. This gap in adherence to indicated clinical services is especially pronounced during adolescent preventive visits,[115] with physicians often failing to discuss risks or offer anticipatory guidance[115,116] for reasons including limited evidence for behavior counseling with adolescents, lack of physician confidence in behavior counseling skills, lack of feedback to physicians about how often they provide recommended services, and physicians' perceived lack of interest from adolescents.[116] Influencing behavior change is difficult in patients of all ages, but adolescents pose special challenges, as the period is characterized by dramatic physical, cognitive, and emotional transformation. Taking time to assess the cognitive and emotional abilities of the patient, and the role their caregivers play in making decisions, is challenging but crucial.

## Screening for Adolescent Exercise

To guide physical activity counseling, accurate and reproducible screening measures are needed. A study[117] published in JAMA in 2001 sought to develop a reliable and valid physical activity screening measure for use with adolescents in primary care settings. Three studies were conducted to evaluate the test–retest reliability and concurrent validity of six single-item and three composite measures of physical activity, with accelerometer (a step counting/speed monitoring device) data serving as the criterion standard for tests of validity. To pass muster for the clinical setting, a screening tool must be accurate and reproducible, be brief enough to be practical, and yield clinically useful scores. The purpose of the screening tool is not to comprehensively assess individuals' physical activity habits, but rather to identify individuals not meeting the guidelines (i.e., those with EDD, see later) who could benefit from counseling.

Study 1 sought to examine the test–retest reliability of nine measures of physical activity, indicating temporal stability of the measure or how constant scores remain from one testing occasion to another.[118] Subjects were recruited from two high schools and two middle schools in San Diego, CA and Pittsburgh, PA and completed six single-item self-report measures of physical activity, from which three composite measures of physical activity were derived. Data analysis consisted of one-way model intraclass correlation coefficients (ICCs) for evaluating reliability at the item level and computed K statistics to evaluate the measures' reliability for classifying subjects as meeting or not meeting current recommended activity guidelines.[119] Scores from the nine measures of physical activity are summarized in Table 6.6.

The VPA and 60-min MPA composite measures had the strongest reliabilities (ICC = 0.76 and 0.79, respectively), but only the 60-min MPA composite measure reached the criterion to be considered "substantial"[120] (K = 61%).

Study 2 examined the concurrent validity of the physical activity measures. Historically, the greatest obstacle to validate physical activity assessments has been the lack of an adequate criterion standard.[121] However, recently developed electronic accelerometers (e.g., The Computer Science and Applications (CSA) accelerometers) have been validated for youth[122,123] and offer the advantage of storing minute-by-minute activity levels, allowing detailed data on frequency and intensity of physical activity to be compared with self-reports. Subjects wore a CSA (Computer Science and Applications) accelerometer on their right hip for 7 days and were instructed to wear the monitor continuously, except when sleeping, showering, or swimming. At the end of the week, subjects completed the self-report measures. Validity correlations were significant for the VPA and the 60-min MPA measures, but not for the 30-min MPA measures. The 60-min MPA composite out-performed all other measures and significantly correlated with minutes of MVPA assessed by the CSA monitor.

Finally, in Study 3, based on the findings of Studies 1 and 2, the researchers modified the measure into a 60-min MVPA measure to assess participation in physical

TABLE 6.6
Descriptive Statistics and Test–Retest Reliability for Physical Activity Measures[a,117]

| Intensity | Duration | Reference Period | No. of Items | Mean (SD) | ICC | κ, % |
|---|---|---|---|---|---|---|
| Vigorous | 20-min bout | Typical week | 1 | 4.1 (2.0) | 0.67 | 49 |
| | | Past 7 days | 1 | 4.1 (2.1) | 0.66 | 47 |
| | | Composite | 2 | 4.1 (1.8) | 0.76 | 54 |
| Moderate | Accumulate 30 min | Typical week | 1 | 4.1 (2.1) | 0.55 | 45 |
| | | Past 7 days | 1 | 3.9 (2.1) | 0.64 | 47 |
| | | Composite | 2 | 4.0 (1.8) | 0.71 | 59 |
| | Accumulate 60 min | Typical week | 1 | 2.4 (2.1) | 0.65 | 50 |
| | | Past 7 days | 1 | 2.4 (2.2) | 0.72 | 56 |
| | | Composite | 2 | 2.4 (1.9) | 0.79 | 61 |

[a] $N = 250$, ICC indicates intraclass correlation coefficient.

activity more broadly and without specification on intensity levels. This refined 60-min MVPA measure was incorporated into the PACE+ (Patient-Centered Assessment and Counseling for Exercise Plus Nutrition) physical activity computer-based intervention[124] and evaluated for reliability and validity as in the previous studies. The 60-min MVPA measure proved reliable (ICC = 0.77), substantial ($K = 61\%$), and valid (correlation coefficient $r = 0.40$; $P < .001$), with values comparable to those reported previously in the literature.[125]

In all, the 60-min MVPA composite is a reasonable method for assessing participation in overall physical activity and for assessing achievement of current guidelines. Researchers found the 60-min MVPA Screening Measure (Fig. 6.1) to be brief and easy to score, yielding clinically meaningful scores that estimate adolescent physical activity and correlate significantly with an objective measure of physical activity.

Another effort to address physical inactivity was colaunched by the ACSM and American Medical

**PACE+ Adolescent Physical Activity Measure**

**Physical activity** is any activity that increases your heart rate and makes you get out of breath some of the time.

**Physical activity** can be done in sports, playing with friends, or walking to school.

Some examples of **physical activity** are running, brisk walking, rollerblading, biking, dancing, skateboarding, swimming, soccer, basketball, football, and surfing.

Add up all the time you spend in physical activity each day (don't include your physical education or gym class).

**P1** Over the past 7 d, on how many days were you physically active for a total of at least 60 min per day?

○ 0 days ○ 1 ○ 2 ○ 3 ○ 4 ○ 5 ○ 6 ○ 7 days

**P2** Over a typical or usual week, on how many days are you physically active for a total of at least 60 min per day?

○ 0 days ○ 1 ○ 2 ○ 3 ○ 4 ○ 5 ○ 6 ○ 7 days

Scoring: (P1 + P2)/2 < 5 indicates not meeting physical activity guidelines.

FIG. 6.1 Sixty-minute measure for moderate-to-vigorous physical activity: PACE+ (Patient-Centered Assessment and Counseling for Exercise Plus Nutrition).

Association (AMA) in 2007. *Exercise is Medicine* (EIM) is a nonprofit initiative that calls for physical activity to be included as a standard part of medical treatment and the patient care process.[126] EIM urges healthcare providers to assess the physical activity levels of their patients at every visit, provide physically inactive patients with brief counseling, and to "write" a basic exercise prescription. Before leaving the clinic setting, inactive patients should also receive a referral to available physical activity resources in the local community to assist them in becoming more physically active. The *Exercise is Medicine* ***Solution*** is the practical implementation of EIM in a health system[127] and is designed as a simple, brief four-step process that can be completed in the clinic setting in under 5 min by the entire healthcare team (Table 6.7).

Although the initial scope of EIM was aimed primarily toward adults, this approach can create a framework for inquiring about physical activity during pediatric visits as well. Recently, a committee has been established to adapt and promote the EIM initiative for use in pediatric populations as a strategy for increasing the physical activity levels of children and adolescents, with a focus on creating and validating a pediatric Physical Activity Vital Sign (PAVS), promoting advanced training for pediatric healthcare providers, and developing materials for the promotion of EIM to pediatric healthcare providers.[128]

A study[138] published in *Pediatric Cardiology* in 2015 from Poland sought to develop a reference system for use in screening the cardiorespiratory fitness of 6–12-year-old children. Among other parameters, physical fitness can be correlated with the postexercise heart rate, an indicator of cardiorespiratory fitness.[139,140] With this premise, 14,501 children from primary schools in Gdansk, Poland participated in a 3-min *Kasch Pulse Recovery Test* (KPR Test), first described in 1961 by Kasch[141] and later utilized by various organizations, including the YMCA,[140] in epidemiologic studies,[142,143] and in health training programs[144] and emergency personnel field testing,[145] as a means to easily screen and classify cardiorespiratory fitness of individuals. In this study, the KPR test consisted of climbing a 0.305-m step at a rate of 24 steps up and down per minute while continuously monitoring heart rate electronically. Postexercise heart rates (i.e., the values recorded 1 min after completion of the test) were recorded and included in the final analysis. The reference range for the classification of cardiorespiratory fitness was developed from the age-specific percentile distribution of postexercise heart rate in 6–9-year-old and 10–12-year-old children (Fig. 6.2).

The presented age- and gender-specific reference range for postexercise heart rate, determined after the KPR Test, enables assessment and monitoring of submaximal exercise-induced changes in the cardiovascular system and, consequently, the physical fitness of a given individual. The KPR Test is easy to perform and well tolerated by school-aged children and, if validated by future studies in other adolescent age groups, potentially represents a useful clinical method of assessing an adolescent's fitness.

TABLE 6.7
Exercise is Medicine Solution[126,127]

| Exercise is Medicine Solution |
|---|
| **Assessment** |
| • Systematic assessment of every patient's physical activity levels[129] |
| • The Physical Activity Vital Sign (PAVS) is an evidence- and practice-based tool for assessing patient physical activity levels that has been successfully integrated into several Kaiser Permanente health locations[130–132] |
| **Exercise Prescription** |
| • Provide eligible patients (i.e., patients who are not completing 150 min of MVPA in a week) with a basic physical activity prescription[133] |
| **Physical Activity Counseling** |
| • In addition to giving a physical activity prescription, healthcare providers may also wish to provide their patients with brief physical activity counseling |
| • Several physical activity counseling models have been shown to be effective in increasing patient physical activity levels, including the "5As,"[134,135] motivational interviewing,[136] and the use of the transtheoretical model[137] |
| **Physical Activity Referral** |
| • Ensuring that all eligible patients receive a physical activity referral to supportive resources to assist them in engaging in greater physical activity levels |
| • Patients may be referred to existing physical activity resources within a health system (i.e., wellness programs, physical therapy), self-directed programs (i.e., walking programs, smartphone apps), or community-based resources |

| Cardiorespiratory fitness | Boys (6–9 years) | Boys (10–12 years) | Girls (6–9 years) | Girls (10–12 years) |
|---|---|---|---|---|
| Excellent ($HR_{mean\ post\text{-}ex}$ < 5th %tile) | <95 | <93 | <100 | <102 |
| Very good ($HR_{mean\ post\text{-}ex}$ ≤ 25th %tile) | 95–106 | 93–105 | 100–113 | 102–116 |
| Good ($HR_{mean\ post\text{-}ex}$ ≤ 50th %tile) | 107–115 | 106–116 | 114–123 | 117–128 |
| Sufficient ($HR_{mean\ post\text{-}ex}$ ≤ 75th %tile) | 116–126 | 117–128 | 124–134 | 129–141 |
| Poor ($HR_{mean\ post\text{-}ex}$ ≤ 95th %tile) | 127–142 | 129–147 | 135–152 | 142–157 |
| Very poor ($HR_{mean\ post\text{-}ex}$ > 95th %tile) | >142 | >147 | >152 | >157 |

**FIG. 6.2** Classification for ranges of reference values of mean postexercise heart rates of 6–12-year-old children.

## Exercise Deficit Disorder

Preventive medicine in pediatrics suggests that positive health-related habits initiated early in life provide the basis for lifelong well-being.[146] Unfortunately, 80.3% of 13–15-year-old adolescents do not meet the recommended 60 min of MVPA[147] and there is currently no comprehensive strategy for encouraging children to eat a healthy diet and engage in regular exercise.[148] Although physicians are expected to intervene, most physicians lack formal training in exercise science and lack experience in prescribing exercise to patients.[149] Exercise deficit disorder is defined as reduced levels of moderate-to-vigorous physical activity that are inconsistent with long-term health and well-being.[110] The evaluation and management of EDD can be summarized into the following principle objectives:

1. Early identification of physically inactive children by PCPs
2. Exercise prescription followed by intervention via consultation and treatment by a specialist trained in pediatric exercise science and youth fitness
3. Evidence-based training protocols that target motor skill deficiency and muscle weakness

To assist and encourage physicians in the diagnosis and treatment of children with EDD, Faigenbaum et al. propose integrating exercise assessment into primary care practice, and, when appropriate, referral to a pediatric exercise specialist[150] (several organizations offer certification courses to become an exercise specialist, including the American College of Sports Medicine (www.acsm.org) and the American Council on Exercise (www.acefitness.org). The timely identification of children with EDD is essential in preventing resistance to intervention. Additionally, it is critical that physicians recognize that all inactive children (regardless of body weight, shape, or physical ability) are at risk to diseases related to a sedentary lifestyle. Early intervention is essential because the window of opportunity to establish healthy lifestyle behaviors is narrow and begins to close coincident with the decline in physical activity that can occur in late childhood.[151] As such, physicians require a screening mechanism that is efficient, sensitive, and logistically feasible in a busy clinical environment. Fig. 6.3[150] provides a theoretical treatment algorithm for physicians identifying and treating children with EDD.

## SUMMARY

Adolescence is a sensitive period of life, characterized by dynamic changes in physiological and psychological development, as well as the establishment of healthy and unhealthy behaviors. Sedentary lifestyle and poor nutrition will challenge children who are genetically predisposed to the metabolic disease.[152] The U.S. population is plagued by physical inactivity, lack of cardiorespiratory fitness, and sedentary lifestyles. There is a linear relationship between physical activity and health status, with those maintaining an active lifestyle generally being healthier and living longer.[153] Meanwhile, sedentary individuals suffer greater morbidity and premature mortality, with some estimates attributing roughly 50% of deaths to unhealthy lifestyle behaviors, such as poor quality diet, cigarette smoking, and physical inactivity.[154]

Although this chapter focuses on *screening*, we briefly mentioned *treatment* for EDD to help the PCP properly refer or counsel patients. If the PCP chooses to refer, they should refer to a pediatric exercise specialist or a Sports Medicine Physician versed in the best methods to address EDD. Best counseling methods include cognitive and behavioral intervention (e.g., cognitive reframing of exercise, motivational interviewing) and short follow-up (e.g., weekly) initially to reinforce new habits and address any potential barriers.

Physical activity, like smoking, is a learned behavior that is influenced by one's family, friends, and environment.[155] As a result, children who are not exposed to an environment with opportunities to enhance motor skill proficiency (e.g., catching, kicking, hopping)

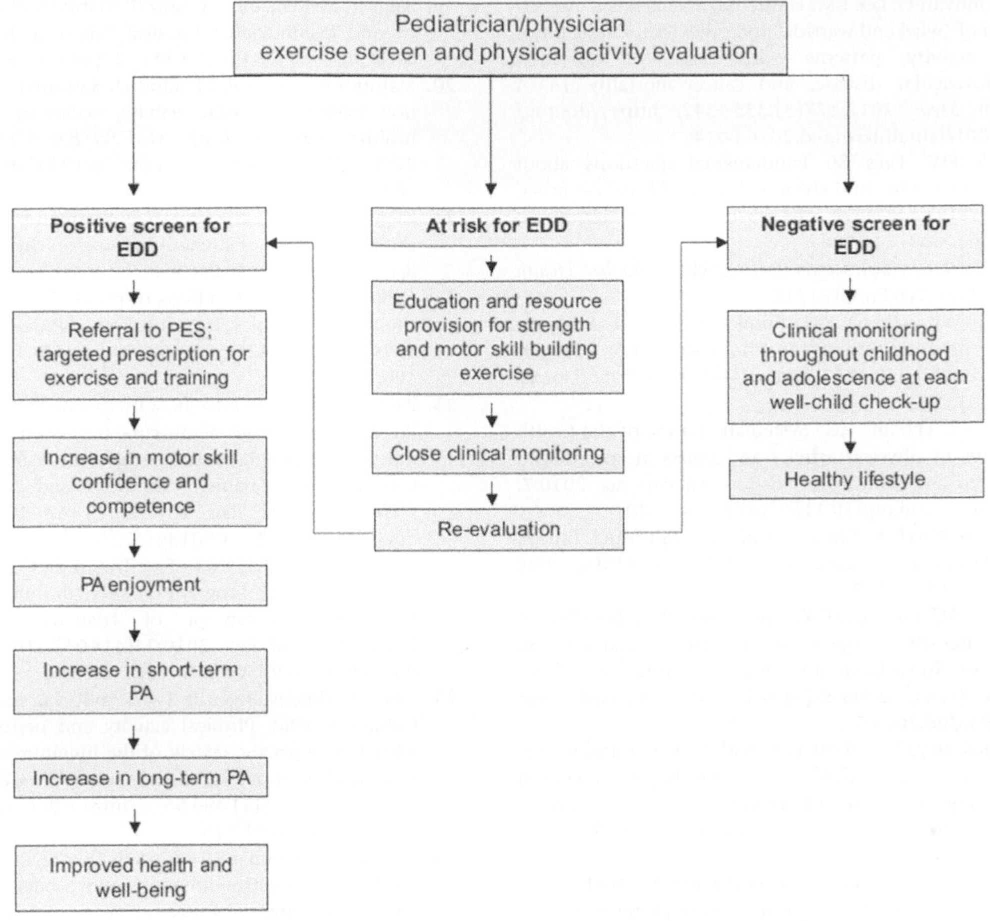


**Abbreviations:** EDD, exercise-deficit disorder; PA, physical activity; PES, pediatric exercise specialist.

**FIG. 6.3** Physician detection-and-intervention algorithm for EDD in children.

tend to be less active during adolescence, increasing the possibility of a sedentary lifestyle during adulthood.[156–158] The construct of physical inactivity or EDD is unique, in that there are no clinical markers or laboratory tests to aid in diagnosis. Recently, Sallis[159] suggested that healthcare providers should obtain an "exercise vital sign" on every adult patient they see. Perhaps more importantly, for reasons presented throughout this chapter, and in concert with obtaining an "exercise vital sign" in adults, pediatric healthcare providers should screen all youth with a "play history" to identify those not meeting the current recommendations for 60 min or more of MVPA each day and, once identified, adolescents with EDD should be managed with the same intensity and resolve as would a young patient with hypertension or dyslipidemia.

## REFERENCES

1. US Department of Health and Human Services. *2008 Physical Activity Guidelines for Americans*. Hyattsville, MD: US Department of Health and Human Services; 2008.
2. U.S. Department of Health and Human Services. *Physical Activity and Health: A Report of the Surgeon General*. U.S. Department of Health and Human Services, Centers for Disease Control and Prevention, National Center for Chronic Disease Prevention and Health.
3. Pate RR, Pratt M, Blair SN, et al. Physical activity and public health. A recommendation from the Centers for disease control and prevention and the American college of sports medicine. *JAMA*. 1995;273(5):402–407.
4. Kodama S, Saito K, Tanaka S, et al. Cardiorespiratory fitness as a quantitative predictor of all-cause mortality and cardiovascular events in healthy men and women: a meta-analysis. *JAMA*. 2009;301(19):2024–2035. https://doi.org/10.1001/jama.2009.681.

5. O'Donovan G, Lee I-M, Hamer M, Stamatakis E. Association of "weekend warrior" and other leisure time physical activity patterns with risks for all-cause, cardiovascular disease, and cancer mortality. *JAMA Intern Med*. 2017;177(3):335–342. https://doi.org/10.1001/jamainternmed.2016.8014.
6. Booth FW, Lees SJ. Fundamental questions about genes, inactivity, and chronic diseases. *Physiol Genomics*. 2007;28(2):146–157. https://doi.org/10.1152/physiolgenomics.00174.2006.
7. McKeag DB. Adolescents and exercise. *J Adolesc Health Care*. 1986;7(6 Suppl):121S–129S.
8. Strong WB, Malina RM, Blimkie CJR, et al. Evidence based physical activity for school-age youth. *J Pediatr*. 2005;146(6):732–737. https://doi.org/10.1016/j.jpeds.2005.01.055.
9. Janssen I, Leblanc AG. Systematic review of the health benefits of physical activity and fitness in school-aged children and youth. *Int J Behav Nutr Phys Act*. 2010;7:40. https://doi.org/10.1186/1479-5868-7-40.
10. Gutin B, Basch C, Shea S, et al. Blood pressure, fitness, and fatness in 5- and 6-year-old children. *JAMA*. 1990;264(9):1123–1127.
11. Benson AC, Torode ME, Fiatarone Singh MA. The effect of high-intensity progressive resistance training on adiposity in children: a randomized controlled trial. *Int J Obes (Lond)*. 2008;32(6):1016–1027. https://doi.org/10.1038/ijo.2008.5.
12. Watts K, Beye P, Siafarikas A, et al. Exercise training normalizes vascular dysfunction and improves central adiposity in obese adolescents. *J Am Coll Cardiol*. 2004;43(10):1823–1827. https://doi.org/10.1016/j.jacc.2004.01.032.
13. Hansen HS, Froberg K, Hyldebrandt N, Nielsen JR. A controlled study of eight months of physical training and reduction of blood pressure in children: the Odense schoolchild study. *BMJ*. 1991;303(6804):682–685.
14. Shea S, Basch CE, Gutin B, et al. The rate of increase in blood pressure in children 5 years of age is related to changes in aerobic fitness and body mass index. *Pediatrics*. 1994;94(4 Pt 1):465–470.
15. Sung RYT, Yu CW, Chang SKY, Mo SW, Woo KS, Lam CWK. Effects of dietary intervention and strength training on blood lipid level in obese children. *Arch Dis Child*. 2002;86(6):407–410.
16. Rubin K, Schirduan V, Gendreau P, Sarfarazi M, Mendola R, Dalsky G. Predictors of axial and peripheral bone mineral density in healthy children and adolescents, with special attention to the role of puberty. *J Pediatr*. 1993;123(6):863–870.
17. Janz KF, Gilmore JM, Burns TL, et al. Physical activity augments bone mineral accrual in young children: the Iowa bone development study. *J Pediatr*. 2006;148(6):793–799. https://doi.org/10.1016/j.jpeds.2006.01.045.
18. Sardinha LB, Baptista F, Ekelund U. Objectively measured physical activity and bone strength in 9-year-old boys and girls. *Pediatrics*. 2008;122(3):e728–e736. https://doi.org/10.1542/peds.2007-2573.
19. Sallis JF, McKenzie TL, Alcaraz JE. Habitual physical activity and health-related physical fitness in fourth-grade children. *Am J Dis Child*. 1993;147(8):890–896.
20. Marques A, Santos R, Ekelund U, Sardinha LB. Association between physical activity, sedentary time, and healthy fitness in youth. *Med Sci Sports Exerc*. 2015;47(3):575–580. https://doi.org/10.1249/MSS.0000000000000426.
21. Faigenbaum A, Zaichkowsky LD, Westcott WL, et al. Psychological effects of strength training on children. *J Sport Behav*. 1997;20(2):164–175.
22. Calfas KJ, Taylor WC. Effects of physical activity on psychological variables in adolescents. *Pediatr Exerc Sci*. 1994;6(4):406–423. https://doi.org/10.1123/pes.6.4.406.
23. Padilla-Moledo C, Ruiz JR, Ortega FB, Mora J, Castro-Pinero J. Associations of muscular fitness with psychological positive health, health complaints, and health risk behaviors in Spanish children and adolescents. *J Strength Cond Res*. 2012;26(1):167–173. https://doi.org/10.1519/JSC.0b013e31821c2433.
24. Velez A, Golem DL, Arent SM. The impact of a 12-week resistance training program on strength, body composition, and self-concept of Hispanic adolescents. *J Strength Cond Res*. 2010;24(4):1065–1073. https://doi.org/10.1519/JSC.0b013e3181cc230a.
25. Singh A, Uijtdewilligen L, Twisk JWR, van Mechelen W, Chinapaw MJM. Physical activity and performance at school: a systematic review of the literature including a methodological quality assessment. *Arch Pediatr Adolesc Med*. 2012;166(1):49–55. https://doi.org/10.1001/archpediatrics.2011.716.
26. Donnelly JE, Hillman CH, Castelli D, et al. Physical activity, fitness, cognitive function, and academic achievement in children: a systematic review. *Med Sci Sports Exerc*. 2016;48(6):1197–1222. https://doi.org/10.1249/MSS.0000000000000901.
27. Chulani VL, Gordon LP. Adolescent growth and development. *Prim Care*. 2014;41(3):465–487. https://doi.org/10.1016/j.pop.2014.05.002.
28. Colvin CW, Abdullatif H. Anatomy of female puberty: the clinical relevance of developmental changes in the reproductive system. *Clin Anat*. 2013;26(1):115–129. https://doi.org/10.1002/ca.22164.
29. Tena-Sempere M. Ghrelin, the gonadal axis and the onset of puberty. *Endocr Dev*. 2013;25:69–82. https://doi.org/10.1159/000346055.
30. Lee Y, Styne D. Influences on the onset and tempo of puberty in human beings and implications for adolescent psychological development. *Horm Behav*. 2013;64(2):250–261. https://doi.org/10.1016/j.yhbeh.2013.03.014.
31. Gogtay N, Giedd JN, Lusk L, et al. Dynamic mapping of human cortical development during childhood through early adulthood. *Proc Natl Acad Sci U S A*. 2004;101(21):8174–8179. http://www.pnas.org/content/101/21/8174.abstract.
32. Casey BJ, Thomas KM, Welsh TF, et al. Dissociation of response conflict, attentional selection, and expectancy

with functional magnetic resonance imaging. *Proc Natl Acad Sci.* 2000;97(15):8728–8733. http://www.pnas.org/content/97/15/8728.abstract.

33. Casey BJ, Tottenham N, Fossella J. Clinical, imaging, lesion, and genetic approaches toward a model of cognitive control. *Dev Psychobiol.* 2002;40(3):237–254.
34. Casey BJ, Tottenham N, Liston C, Durston S. Imaging the developing brain: what have we learned about cognitive development? *Trends Cogn Sci.* 2005;9(3):104–110. https://doi.org/10.1016/j.tics.2005.01.011.
35. Hare TA, Tottenham N, Galvan A, Voss HU, Glover GH, Casey BJ. Biological substrates of emotional reactivity and regulation in adolescence during an emotional go-nogo task. *Biol Psychiatry.* 2008;63(10):927–934. https://doi.org/10.1016/j.biopsych.2008.03.015.
36. Sallis JF, Zakarian JM, Hovell MF, Hofstetter CR. Ethnic, socioeconomic, and sex differences in physical activity among adolescents. *J Clin Epidemiol.* 1996;49(2):125–134.
37. Tine M. Acute aerobic exercise: an intervention for the selective visual attention and reading comprehension of low-income adolescents. *Front Psychol.* 2014;5:575. https://doi.org/10.3389/fpsyg.2014.00575.
38. Bezold CP, Konty KJ, Day SE, et al. The effects of changes in physical fitness on academic performance among New York City youth. *J Adolesc Heal.* 2014;55(6):774–781. https://doi.org/10.1016/j.jadohealth.2014.06.006.
39. Cotman CW, Berchtold NC, Christie L-A. Exercise builds brain health: key roles of growth factor cascades and inflammation. *Trends Neurosci.* 2007;30(9):464–472. https://doi.org/10.1016/j.tins.2007.06.011.
40. Phillips C, Baktir MA, Srivatsan M, Salehi A. Neuroprotective effects of physical activity on the brain: a closer look at trophic factor signaling. *Front Cell Neurosci.* 2014;8:170. https://doi.org/10.3389/fncel.2014.00170.
41. Klempin F, Beis D, Mosienko V, Kempermann G, Bader M, Alenina N. Serotonin is required for exercise-induced adult hippocampal neurogenesis. *J Neurosci.* 2013;33(19):8270–8275. http://www.jneurosci.org/content/33/19/8270.abstract.
42. Hillman CH, Buck SM, Themanson JR, Pontifex MB, Castelli DM. Aerobic fitness and cognitive development: event-related brain potential and task performance indices of executive control in preadolescent children. *Dev Psychol.* 2009;45(1):114–129. https://doi.org/10.1037/a0014437.
43. Hillman CH, Castelli DM, Buck SM. Aerobic fitness and neurocognitive function in healthy preadolescent children. *Med Sci Sports Exerc.* 2005;37(11):1967–1974.
44. Raine LB, Lee HK, Saliba BJ, Chaddock-Heyman L, Hillman CH, Kramer AF. The influence of childhood aerobic fitness on learning and memory. *PLoS One.* 2013;8(9). https://doi.org/10.1371/journal.pone.0072666.e72666.
45. Chaddock L, Neider MB, Lutz A, Hillman CH, Kramer AF. Role of childhood aerobic fitness in successful street crossing. *Med Sci Sports Exerc.* 2012;44(4):749–753. https://doi.org/10.1249/MSS.0b013e31823a90cb.
46. Castelli DM, Hillman CH, Buck SM, Erwin HE. Physical fitness and academic achievement in third- and fifth-grade students. *J Sport Exerc Psychol.* 2007;29(2):239–252.
47. Donnelly JE, Greene JL, Gibson CA, et al. Physical activity across the curriculum (PAAC): a randomized controlled trial to promote physical activity and diminish overweight and obesity in elementary school children. *Prev Med (Baltim).* 2009;49(4):336–341. https://doi.org/10.1016/j.ypmed.2009.07.022.
48. Etnier JL, Nowell PM, Landers DM, Sibley BA. A meta-regression to examine the relationship between aerobic fitness and cognitive performance. *Brain Res Rev.* 2006;52(1):119–130. https://doi.org/10.1016/j.brainresrev.2006.01.002.
49. Chaddock L, Erickson KI, Prakash RS, et al. Basal ganglia volume is associated with aerobic fitness in preadolescent children. *Dev Neurosci.* 2010;32(3):249–256. https://www.karger.com/DOI/10.1159/000316648.
50. Chaddock L, Erickson KI, Prakash RS, et al. A functional MRI investigation of the association between childhood aerobic fitness and neurocognitive control. *Biol Psychol.* 2012;89(1):260–268. https://doi.org/10.1016/j.biopsycho.2011.10.017.
51. Tripodi A, Severi S, Midili S, Corradini B. Community projects in Modena (Italy): promote regular physical activity and healthy nutrition habits since childhood. *Int J Pediatr Obes.* 2011;6(Suppl. 2):54–56. https://doi.org/10.3109/17477166.2011.613675.
52. Velde S, Twisk J, Brug J. Tracking of fruit and vegetable consumption from adolescence into adulthood and its longitudinal association with overweight. *Br J Nutr.* 2007;98(02):431–438. https://doi.org/10.1017/S0007114507721451.
53. Cleland V, Dwyer T, Venn A, Cleland V, Dwyer T, Venn A. Which domains of childhood physical activity predict physical activity in adulthood? A 20-year prospective tracking study. *Br J Sports Med.* 2012;46(8):595–602. *Br J Sports Med.* 2012;46(8):595–602 http://bjsm.bmj.com/content/46/8/595.abstract.
54. Koivusilta LK, Nupponen H, Rimpelä AH, Koivusilta LK, Nupponen H, Rimpelä AH. Adolescent physical activity predicts high education and socio-economic position in adulthood. *Eur J Public Health.* 2012;22:203–209. https://doi.org/10.1093/eurpub/ckr037. *Eur J Public Health.* 2012;22(2):203–209.
55. Aarnio M, Winter T, Kujala U, Kaprio J. Associations of health related behavior, social relationships, and health status with persistent physical activity and inactivity: a study of Finnish adolescent twins. *Br J Sport Med.* 2002;36(5):360–364. https://doi.org/10.1136/bjsm.36.5.360.
56. Guidelines for school and community programs to promote lifelong physical activity among young people. Centers for Disease Control and Prevention. *MMWR Recomm Reports Morb Mortal Wkly Report Recomm Reports.* 1997;46(RR-6):1–36.
57. Haskell WL, Lee I-M, Pate RR, et al. Physical activity and public health: updated recommendation for adults from

the American College of Sports Medicine and the American Heart Association. *Med Sci Sports Exerc*. 2007; 39(8):1423–1434. https://doi.org/10.1249/mss.0b013e3180616b27.

58. Physical Activity Guidelines Advisory Committee. *Physical Activity Guidelines Advisory Committee Report, 2008*. Washington, DC: U.S. Department of Health and Human Services; 2008.
59. https://www.cdc.gov/physicalactivity/basics/children/index.htm.
60. Fact Sheet Physical Activity. *Global Recommendations on Physical Activity for Health*. Available at: http://www.euro.who.int/__data/assets/pdf_file/0005/288041/WHO-Fact-Sheet-PA-2015.pdf.
61. *ACSM, AHA Support Federal Physical Activity Guidelines*. https://www.acsm.org/about-acsm/media-room/acsm-in-the-news/2011/08/01/acsmaha-support-federal-physical-activity-guidelines.
62. Guthold R, Stevens GA, Riley LM, Bull FC. Worldwide trends in insufficient physical activity from 2001 to 2016: a pooled analysis of 358 population-based surveys with 1.9 million participants. *Lancet Glob Heal*. 2018; 6(10):e1077–e1086. https://doi.org/10.1016/S2214-109X(18)30357-7.
63. Healthy People 2020. *Physical Activity and Fitness*. Available from: http://www.healthypeople.gov/2020/topicsobjectives2020/overview.aspx?topicid=33.
64. Whitt-Glover MC, Taylor WC, Floyd MF, Yore MM, Yancey AK, Matthews CE. Disparities in physical activity and sedentary behaviors among US children and adolescents: prevalence, correlates, and intervention implications. *J Public Health Policy*. 2009;30(Suppl 1): S309–S334. https://doi.org/10.1057/jphp.2008.46.
65. Troiano RP, Berrigan D, Dodd KW, Masse LC, Tilert T, McDowell M. Physical activity in the United States measured by accelerometer. *Med Sci Sports Exerc*. 2008; 40(1):181–188. https://doi.org/10.1249/mss.0b013e31815a51b3.
66. Gordon-Larsen P, McMurray RG, Popkin BM. Adolescent physical activity and inactivity vary by ethnicity: the national longitudinal study of adolescent health. *J Pediatr*. 1999;135(3):301–306. https://doi.org/10.1016/S0022-3476(99)70124-1.
67. Gordon-Larsen P, McMurray RG, Popkin BM. Determinants of adolescent physical activity and inactivity patterns. *Pediatrics*. 2000;105(6):E83.
68. Nader P, Bradley R, Houts R, McRitchie S, O'brien M. Moderate-to-vigorous physical activity from ages 9 to 15 years. *J Am Med Assoc*. 2008;300(3):295–305. https://doi.org/10.1001/jama.300.3.295.
69. Physical activity levels of high school students — United States, 2010. *MMWR Morb Mortal Wkly Rep*. 2011;60(23): 773–777.
70. US DHHS, Centers for Disease Control and Prevention. *Results from the School Health Policy and Practices Study 2014*. Available at: www.cdc.gov/healthyyouth/data/shpps/pdf/shpps-508-final_101315.pdf.
71. Centers for Disease Control and Prevention. *Healthy People 2020*. Available at: http://www.cdc.gov/nchs/healthy_people/hp2020.htm.
72. Baranowski T, Cullen KW, Basen-Engquist K, et al. Transitions out of high school: time of increased cancer risk? *Prev Med (Baltim)*. 1997;26(5 Pt 1):694–703. https://doi.org/10.1006/pmed.1997.0193.
73. Dumith SC, Hallal PC, Reis RS, Kohl 3rd HW. Worldwide prevalence of physical inactivity and its association with human development index in 76 countries. *Prev Med (Baltim)*. 2011;53(1–2):24–28. https://doi.org/10.1016/j.ypmed.2011.02.017.
74. Owen N, Sparling PB, Healy GN, Dunstan DW, Matthews CE. Sedentary behavior: emerging evidence for a new health risk. *Mayo Clin Proc*. 2010;85(12): 1138–1141. https://doi.org/10.4065/mcp.2010.0444.
75. Rey-Lopez JP, Vicente-Rodriguez G, Ortega FB, et al. Sedentary patterns and media availability in European adolescents: the HELENA study. *Prev Med (Baltim)*. 2010;51(1):50–55. https://doi.org/10.1016/j.ypmed.2010.03.013.
76. Matthews CE, Chen KY, Freedson PS, et al. Amount of time spent in sedentary behaviors in the United States, 2003–2004. *Am J Epidemiol*. 2008;167(7):875–881. https://doi.org/10.1093/aje/kwm390.
77. Armstrong N, Balding J, Gentle P, Kirby B. Patterns of physical activity among 11 to 16 year old British children. *Br Med J*. 1990;301(6745):203–205. http://www.bmj.com/content/301/6745/203.abstract.
78. Ogden CL, Carroll MD, Kit BK, et al. Prevalence of obesity and trends in body mass index among US children and adolescents, 1999–2010. *JAMA*. 2012;307(5):483–490.
79. Kopelman PG. Obesity as a medical problem. *Nature*. 2000;404:635–643.
80. Biddle SJH, Fox K, Boutcher SH, et al. The way forward for physical activity and the promotion of psychological well-being. In: Biddle SJH, Fox K, Boutcher SH, eds. *Physical Activity and Psychological Well-Being*. London: Routledge; 2000:154–168.
81. Hills AP, Andersen LB, Byrne NM. Physical activity and obesity in children. *Br J Sports Med*. 2011;45(11): 866–870.
82. Mahoney JL, Cairns BD, Farmer TW. Promoting interpersonal competence and educational success through extracurricular activity participation. *Journal of Educational Psychology*. 2003;95:409–418.
83. Centers for Disease Control and Prevention. *The Association between School Based Physical Activity, Including Physical Education, and Academic Performance*. Atlanta, GA: U.S. Department of Health and Human Services; 2010. Available at: www.cdc.gov/healthyy.
84. Singh A, Uijtdewilligen L, Twisk JW, et al. Physical activity and performance at school: a systematic review of the literature including a methodological quality assessment. *Arch Pediatr Adolesc Med*. 2012;166:49–55.
85. Demory-Luce D, Morales M, Nicklas T, et al. Changes in food group consumption patterns from childhood to

young adulthood: the Bogalusa Heart Study. *J Am Diet Assoc.* 2004;104:1684–1691.

86. Kimm SY, Glynn NW, Obarzanek E, et al. Relation between the changes in physical activity and body-mass index during adolescence: a multicentre longitudinal study. *Lancet.* 2005;366:301–307.
87. Windle M, Grunbaum JA, Elliott M, et al. Healthy passages – a multilevel, multimethod longitudinal study of adolescent health. *Am J Prev Med.* 2004;27:164–172.
88. Dietz WH. Health consequences of obesity in youth: childhood predictors of adult disease. *Pediatrics.* 1998; 101:518–525.
89. Daniels SR. The consequences of childhood overweight and obesity. *Future Child.* 2006;16:47–67.
90. Juonala M, Magnussen CG, Berenson GS, et al. Childhood adiposity, adult adiposity, and cardiovascular risk factors. *N Engl J Med.* 2011;365:1876–1885.
91. Strauss RS. Childhood obesity and self-esteem. *Pediatrics.* 2000;105:e15.
92. Ogden CL, Flegal KM, Carroll MD, et al. Prevalence and trends in overweight among US children and adolescents, 1999–2000. *JAMA.* 2002;288:1728–1732.
93. Freedman DS, Khan LK, Serdula MK, et al. Racial and ethnic differences in secular trends for childhood BMI, weight, and height. *Obesity (Silver Spring).* 2006;14: 301–308.
94. Wang Y, Beydoun MA. The obesity epidemic in the United States—gender, age, socioeconomic, racial/ethnic, and geographic characteristics: a systematic review and meta-regression analysis. *Epidemiol Rev.* 2007;29:6–28.
95. Freedman DS, Kettle Khan L, Serdula MK, et al. Racial differences in the tracking of childhood BMI to adulthood. *Obes Res.* 2005;13:928–935.
96. Proper KI, Singh AS, van Mechelen W, Chinapaw MJM. Sedentary behaviors and health outcomes among adults: a systematic review of prospective studies. *Am J Prev Med.* 2011;40(2):174–182. https://doi.org/10.1016/j.amepre.2010.10.015.
97. Pavey TG, Peeters GG, Brown WJ. Sitting-time and 9-year all-cause mortality in older women. *Br J Sports Med.* 2015; 49(2):95–99. https://doi.org/10.1136/bjsports-2012-091676.
98. Leon-Munoz LM, Martinez-Gomez D, Balboa-Castillo T, Lopez-Garcia E, Guallar-Castillon P, Rodriguez-Artalejo F. Continued sedentariness, change in sitting time, and mortality in older adults. *Med Sci Sports Exerc.* 2013;45(8):1501–1507. https://doi.org/10.1249/MSS.0b013e3182897e87.
99. Matthews CE, Cohen SS, Fowke JH, et al. Physical activity, sedentary behavior, and cause-specific mortality in black and white adults in the Southern Community Cohort Study. *Am J Epidemiol.* 2014;180(4):394–405. https://doi.org/10.1093/aje/kwu142.
100. Lee I-M, Shiroma EJ, Lobelo F, Puska P, Blair SN, Katzmarzyk PT. Effect of physical inactivity on major non-communicable diseases worldwide: an analysis of burden of disease and life expectancy. *Lancet (London, England).* 2012;380(9838):219–229. https://doi.org/10.1016/S0140-6736(12)61031-9.
101. van der Ploeg HP, Chey T, Korda RJ, Banks E, Bauman A. Sitting time and all-cause mortality risk in 222 497 Australian adults. *Arch Intern Med.* 2012;172(6): 494–500. https://doi.org/10.1001/archinternmed.2011.2174.
102. Biswas A, Oh PI, Faulkner GE, et al. Sedentary time and its association with risk for disease incidence, mortality, and hospitalization in adults: a systematic review and meta-analysis. *Ann Intern Med.* 2015;162(2):123–132. https://doi.org/10.7326/M14-1651.
103. Diaz KM, Howard VJ, Hutto B, et al. Patterns of sedentary behavior and mortality in U.S. Middle-aged and older adults: a national cohort study. *Ann Intern Med.* 2017; 167(7):465–475. https://doi.org/10.7326/M17-0212.
104. Gennuso KP, Gangnon RE, Matthews CE, Thraen-Borowski KM, Colbert LH. Sedentary behavior, physical activity, and markers of health in older adults. *Med Sci Sports Exerc.* 2013;45(8):1493–1500. https://doi.org/10.1249/MSS.0b013e318288a1e5.
105. Chau JY, Grunseit A, Midthjell K, et al. Sedentary behaviour and risk of mortality from all-causes and cardiometabolic diseases in adults: evidence from the HUNT3 population cohort. *Br J Sports Med.* 2015;49(11): 737–742. https://doi.org/10.1136/bjsports-2012-091974.
106. Ekelund U, Steene-Johannessen J, Brown WJ, et al. Does physical activity attenuate, or even eliminate, the detrimental association of sitting time with mortality? A harmonised meta-analysis of data from more than 1 million men and women. *Lancet (London, England).* 2016;388(10051):1302–1310. https://doi.org/10.1016/S0140-6736(16)30370-1.
107. Wee CC, McCarthy EP, Davis RB, Phillips RS. Physician counseling about exercise. *JAMA.* 1999;282(16): 1583–1588.
108. Eakin E, Brown W, Schofield G, Mummery K, Reeves M. General practitioner advice on physical activity–who gets it? *Am J Health Promot.* 2007;21(4):225–228. https://doi.org/10.4278/0890-1171-21.4.225.
109. Croteau K, Schofield G, McLean G. Physical activity advice in the primary care setting: results of a population study in New Zealand. *Aust N Z J Public Health.* 2006; 30(3):262–267.
110. Faigenbaum AD, Stracciolini A, Myer GD. Exercise deficit disorder in youth: a hidden truth. *Acta Paediatr.* 2011; 100(11):1423–1425. https://doi.org/10.1111/j.1651-2227.2011.02461.x.
111. https://www.uspreventiveservicestaskforce.org/BrowseRec/Index/browse-recommendations.
112. Barratt A, Irwig L, Glasziou P, et al. Users' guides to the medical literature: XVII. How to use guidelines and recommendations about screening. Evidence-Based Medicine Working Group. *JAMA.* 1999;281(21):2029–2034.
113. Kang M, Cannon B, Remond L, Quine S. 'Is it normal to feel these questions ...?': a content analysis of the health

concerns of adolescent girls writing to a magazine. *Fam Pract.* 2009;26(3):196–203.
114. Nordin JD, Solberg LI, Parker ED. Adolescent primary care visit patterns. *Ann Fam Med.* 2010;8(6):511–516.
115. Mangione-Smith R, DeCristofaro AH, Setodji CM, et al. The quality of ambulatory care delivered to children in the United States. *N Engl J Med.* 2007;357(15): 1515–1523.
116. Whitlock EP, Orleans CT, Pender N, Allan J. Evaluating primary care behavioral counseling interventions: an evidence-based approach. *Am J Prev Med.* 2002;22(4): 267–284.
117. P JJ, S JF, Long B. A physical activity screening measure for use with adolescents in primary care. *Arch Pediatr Adolesc Med.* 2001;155(5):554–559. https://doi.org/10.1001/archpedi.155.5.554.
118. DeVellis RF. *Scale Development: Theory and Applications*. In: *Applied Social Research Method Series*. Vol. 26. London: England Sage Publications; 1991.
119. Fleiss JL. *Statistical Methods for Rates and Proportions*. 2nd ed. New York, NY: John Wiley & Sons; 1981:212–236.
120. Landis JR, Koch GG. The measurement of observer agreement for categorical data. *Biometrics.* 1977;33(1): 159–174.
121. Montoye HJ. *Measuring Physical Activity and Energy Expenditure.* Champaign, IL: Human Kinetics; 1996.
122. Janz KF. Validation of the CSA accelerometer for assessing children's physical activity. *Med Sci Sports Exerc.* 1994;26: 369–375.
123. Trost SG, Ward DS, Moorehead SM, Watson PD, Riner W, Burke JR. Validity of the computer science and applications (CSA) activity monitor in children. *Med Sci Sports Exerc.* 1998;30:629–633.
124. Prochaska JJ, Zabinski MF, Calfas KJ, Sallis JF, Patrick K. PACE+: interactive communication technology for behavior change in clinical settings. *Am J Prev Med.* 2000;19(2):127–131.
125. Sallis JF, Saelens BE. Assessment of physical activity by self-report: status, limitations, and future directions. *Res Q Exerc Sport.* 2000;71(Suppl 2):1–14. https://doi.org/10.1080/02701367.2000.11082780.
126. Lobelo F, Stoutenberg M, Hutber A. The exercise is medicine global health initiative: a 2014 update. *Br J Sports Med.* 2014;48(22):1627–1633. https://doi.org/10.1136/bjsports-2013-093080.
127. Sallis R, Franklin B, Joy L, Ross R, Sabgir D, Stone J. Strategies for promoting physical activity in clinical practice. *Prog Cardiovasc Dis.* 2015;57(4):375–386. https://doi.org/10.1016/j.pcad.2014.10.003.
128. https://www.exerciseismedicine.org/support_page.php/pediatrics/.
129. Sallis RE, Matuszak JM, Baggish AL, et al. Call to action on making physical activity assessment and prescription a medical standard of care. *Curr Sports Med Rep.* 2016; 15(3):207–214. https://doi.org/10.1249/JSR.0000000000000249.
130. Coleman KJ, Ngor E, Reynolds K, et al. Initial validation of an exercise "vital sign" in electronic medical records. *Med Sci Sports Exerc.* 2012;44(11):2071–2076. https://doi.org/10.1249/MSS.0b013e3182630ec1.
131. Young DR, Coleman KJ, Ngor E, Reynolds K, Sidell M, Sallis RE. Associations between physical activity and cardiometabolic risk factors assessed in a Southern California health care system, 2010–2012. *Prev Chronic Dis.* 2014;11:E219. https://doi.org/10.5888/pcd11.140196.
132. Ball TJ, Joy EA, Gren LH, Shaw JM. Concurrent validity of a self-reported physical activity "vital sign" questionnaire with adult primary care patients. *Prev Chronic Dis.* 2016; 13:E16. https://doi.org/10.5888/pcd13.150228.
133. https://www.exerciseismedicine.org/support_page.php/health-care-providers5/.
134. Carroll JK, Fiscella K, Epstein RM, Sanders MR, Williams GC. A 5A's communication intervention to promote physical activity in underserved populations. *BMC Health Serv Res.* 2012;12:374. https://doi.org/10.1186/1472-6963-12-374.
135. Carroll JK, Antognoli E, Flocke SA. Evaluation of physical activity counseling in primary care using direct observation of the 5As. *Ann Fam Med.* 2011;9(5):416–422. https://doi.org/10.1370/afm.1299.
136. O'Halloran PD, Blackstock F, Shields N, et al. Motivational interviewing to increase physical activity in people with chronic health conditions: a systematic review and meta-analysis. *Clin Rehabil.* 2014;28(12):1159–1171. https://doi.org/10.1177/0269215514536210.
137. Stonerock GL, Blumenthal JA. Role of counseling to promote adherence in healthy lifestyle medicine: strategies to improve exercise adherence and enhance physical activity. *Prog Cardiovasc Dis.* 2017;59(5):455–462. https://doi.org/10.1016/j.pcad.2016.09.003.
138. Jankowski M, Niedzielska A, Brzezinski M, Drabik J. Cardiorespiratory fitness in children: a simple screening test for population studies. *Pediatr Cardiol.* 2015;36: 27–32. https://doi.org/10.1007/s00246-014-0960-0.
139. Cole CR, Blackstone EH, Pashkow FJ, Snader CE, Lauer MS. Heart-rate recovery immediately after exercise as a predictor of mortality. *N Engl J Med.* 1999;341(18): 1351–1357. https://doi.org/10.1056/NEJM199910283411804.
140. Golding LA, Myers CR, Sinning WE. *Y's Way to Physical Fitness: The Complete Guide to Fitness Testing and Instruction.* Champaign: Human Kinetics Publishers; 1989.
141. Kasch FW. A comparison of the exercise tolerance of post-rheumatic and normal boys. *J Assoc Phys Mental Rehabil.* 1961;15:35–40.
142. Beunen G, Malina RM, Ostyn M, Renson R, Simons J, Van Gerven D. Fatness, growth and motor fitness of Belgian boys 12 through 20 years of age. *Hum Biol.* 1983;55(3): 599–613.
143. Johnston FE. Somatic and motor development of Belgian secondary schoolboys. By M. Ostyn, J. Simons,

G. Beunen, R. Renson, and D. Van Gerven. Leuven (Louvain), Belgium: Leuven University Press. 1980. 158 pp., figures, tables. 990 bf ($23.60) (paper). *Am J Phys Anthropol.* 2018;58(4):464. https://doi.org/10.1002/ajpa.1330580417.
144. McArdle WD, Katch FI, Katch VL. *Exercise Physiology: Energy, Nutrition, and Human Performance.* New York: Lippincott, Williams and Wilkins; 2001.
145. Davis JA, Wilmore JH. Validation of a bench stepping test for cardiorespiratory fitness classification of emergency service personnel. *J Occup Med.* 1979;21(10):671–673.
146. Rowland TW. *Exercise and Children's Health.* Champaign, IL, England: Human Kinetics Publishers; 1990.
147. Hallal PC, Andersen LB, Bull FC, Guthold R, Haskell W, Ekelund U. Global physical activity levels: surveillance progress, pitfalls, and prospects. *Lancet (London, England).* 2012;380(9838):247–257. https://doi.org/10.1016/S0140-6736(12)60646-1.
148. Ludwig DS. Childhood obesity–the shape of things to come. *N Engl J Med.* 2007;357(23):2325–2327. https://doi.org/10.1056/NEJMp0706538.
149. Jaques R, Loosemore M. Sports and exercise medicine in undergraduate training. *Lancet (London, England).* 2012; 380(9836):4–5. https://doi.org/10.1016/S0140-6736(12)60992-1.
150. Stracciolini A, Myer GD, Faigenbaum AD. Exercise-deficit disorder in children: are we ready to make this diagnosis? *Phys Sportsmed.* 2013;41(1):94–101. https://doi.org/10.3810/psm.2013.02.2003.
151. Nader PR, Bradley RH, Houts RM. Data error in study of moderate-to-vigorous physical activity from ages 9 to 15 years. *JAMA.* 2009;301(20):2094–2095. https://doi.org/10.1001/jama.2009.701.
152. Sothern MS, Gordon ST. Prevention of obesity in young children: a critical challenge for medical professionals. *Clin Pediatr (Phila).* 2003;42(2):101–111. https://doi.org/10.1177/000992280304200202.
153. Lee IM, Hsieh CC, Paffenbarger RSJ. Exercise intensity and longevity in men. The Harvard alumni health study. *JAMA.* 1995;273(15):1179–1184.
154. Mokdad AH, Marks JS, Stroup DF, Gerberding JL. Actual causes of death in the United States, 2000. *JAMA.* 2004; 291(10):1238–1245. https://doi.org/10.1001/jama.291.10.1238.
155. National Association of Sport and Physical Education and American Heart Association. *Shape of the Nation Report: Status of Physical Education in the USA.* Reston (VA): National Association of Sport and Physical Education; 2010.
156. Barnett LM, Van Beurden E, Morgan PJ, Brooks LO, Beard JR. Does childhood motor skill proficiency predict adolescent fitness? *Med Sci Sports Exerc.* 2008;40(12):2137–2144. https://doi.org/10.1249/MSS.0b013e31818160d3.
157. Barnett LM, van Beurden E, Morgan PJ, Brooks LO, Beard JR. Childhood motor skill proficiency as a predictor of adolescent physical activity. *J Adolesc Health.* 2009; 44(3):252–259. https://doi.org/10.1016/j.jadohealth.2008.07.004.
158. Stodden D, Langendorfer S, Roberton MA. The association between motor skill competence and physical fitness in young adults. *Res Q Exerc Sport.* 2009;80(2):223–229. https://doi.org/10.1080/02701367.2009.10599556.
159. Sallis R. Developing healthcare systems to support exercise: exercise as the fifth vital sign. *Br J Sports Med.* 2011;45(6):473–474. https://doi.org/10.1136/bjsm.2010.083469.

CHAPTER 7

# ACES: Screening for Adverse Childhood Experiences

HEATHER O'HARA, MD, MSPH • VINCENT MORELLI, MD

*It is easier to build strong children than to repair broken men.*[1]

FREDRICK DOUGLAS, 1855.

Adverse childhood experiences (ACEs) are associated with a multitude of nonnormative traumatic events that affect the development and epigenetics of a child.[1a–c] The Chapter on Resilience provides that, "psychological trauma is an intense emotional experience that overwhelms a person's ability to cope. It may be a single event or repetitive ongoing insults such as child abuse, neglect or poverty." (See Chapter on Resilience in this publication). Adverse outcomes including obesity, poor lifestyle choices (i.e., physical inactivity, substance abuse, and smoking), cardiovascular disease, diabetes, mental illness, and even some cancers (Table 7.1) are associated with these traumatic incidents. There is a graded relationship to developing these adverse outcomes in accordance with the number, frequency, and type of trauma experienced during the early developmental periods of life.[2] The 1998 ACE study by Felitti and Anda focused on childhood exposure to three areas of abuse, two categories of neglect, and five types of household dysfunction (Table 7.2). This study has triggered a movement into how healthcare, community, and even families interact to improve the development and outcomes of the next generation (See section on 15)[2a–b].

Understanding the basic tenets of ACEs is the foundation to fully implement a process that can lessen the likelihood, or possibly eliminate the effects, of traumatic events through all stages of development (Fig. 7.1) to improve the emotional and physical well-being of the adolescent[2c].

Although ACE is a relatively new term, a 1989 study suggested the connection between early childhood adversities and mental health.[3] This study followed over 3000 9–11-year-old children in the mid-1960s from the Isle of Wight for 25 years to assess for psychiatric conditions and educational disturbances. Children who were from a low social status, experienced stressful early life events, or family discord had a higher incidence of adverse psychological outcomes.[3] The findings from this study and many others before the sentinel ACE study initiated the interest into the communal effort required to raise healthy, productive, and integral members of society giving credence to the African proverb, "it takes a village to raise a child."

In 1998, Felitti through his keen recognition of the pattern of sexual abuse in his obese patients sparked the development of the current ACE questionnaire and his subsequent study that has provided a foundation for understanding how early trauma increases the risk of adverse health outcomes. This study not only unveiled the connections of these traumatic experiences to adverse life outcomes, but also illuminated the commonality of these nonnormative experiences. Of the over 17,000 participants, more than one in five reported having experienced either physical or sexual abuse, and growing up in a home that included marital discord, mental illness, and/or a substance use disorder (Fig. 7.2) was also very prominent.[3a] Considering the commonality of these experiences in this study, it is extremely disturbing as children should not have to endure these atrocities, however the increased risk of adverse outcomes due to the number and frequency of these events is even more alarming (Fig. 7.3). Multiple studies have shown that participants who experienced one or more ACE categories when compared to those who had no ACEs have an increased risk of behavioral and mental health problems noting an amplification of risk with each additional ACE category.[2,4,5] A 2018 study that incorporated teachers' assessments of children from 10 elementary schools in Spokane, WA found that 13% of their students had three or more ACEs. When compared to students with no known ACEs, this group was found to have three to six times the rate of academic failure, poor health, severe attendance problems, and behavior problems.[6]

Adolescent Health Screening: An Update in the Age of Big Data. https://doi.org/10.1016/B978-0-323-66130-0.00007-7

TABLE 7.1
Adverse Outcomes Associated With Adverse Childhood Experiences (

| Adolescent Pregnancy | Fetal Death | Poor Work Performance |
|---|---|---|
| Alcoholism and alcohol abuse | Financial stress | Multiple sexual partners |
| Cancer | Health-related quality of life | Risk for intimate partner violence |
| Chronic obstructive pulmonary disease | Illicit drug use | Risk for sexual violence |
| Depression | Ischemic heart disease | Sexually transmitted diseases |
| Diabetes | Liver disease | Smoking |
| Early initiation of sexual activity | Obesity | Suicide attempts |
| Early initiation of smoking | Poor academic achievement | Unintended pregnancies |

TABLE 7.2
Content Covered in the Adverse Childhood Experience Questionnaire

| Abuse | Neglect | Household Dysfunction |
|---|---|---|
| Physical | Emotional | Divorce or separation |
| Sexual | Physical | Mother treated violently |
| Psychological | | Substance abuse |
| | | Mentally ill or suicidal |
| | | Imprisonment |

The studies that have explored the level of ACE categories within discrete cohorts suggests that more children than not fall victim to these events. Despite the common occurrence of these experiences, the risk of adverse outcomes based on the number of ACEs is not 100% correlated. Resilience, in terms of a material, is the ability for something to maintain its elasticity, it will bend, but it will not break and it will resume its shape (Merriam-Webster). Numerous studies support the ability for many faced with various adversities or traumas to be resilient and successful.[7–10] The experience will not overwhelm them to the point that recovery is not possible. It is therefore important to recognize that what one person perceives as a traumatic event may not be the same for another person[10a].

The tools available to effectively screen for ACEs (Table 7.3) and provide community resources (Table 7.4) based on need offer a mechanism to assist those affected at various levels of life interactions. Screening in healthcare, school, church, or community center settings could enable the appropriate assessment, follow-up, and resilience building necessary to influence change on a greater scale. Several entities have different versions of the original ACE questionnaire (see appendix) that were specific to certain age ranges or groups. The Centers for Disease Control and Prevention (CDC) provides access to two publicly available screening tools, The Family Health History Questionnaire (FHH) and the Health Appraisal Questionnaire (HA). These tools collect a wide range of past and current health and environmental information. The areas covered by the FHH include categories covering child abuse, physical abuse, or sexual abuse, as well as exposure to various forms of household dysfunction such as criminal behavior, violent treatment of a mother or stepmother, mental illness, or substance abuse. Coupling this survey with the HA, which collects information about current health concerns from perceived to diagnosed conditions related to obesity, mental illness, cardiovascular disease, diabetes, alcohol and drug use, and sexual activity can serve as a comprehensive approach to understanding the patient holistically. These two screening tools served as the foundation to Felitti's 1998 study correlating childhood exposures and adverse outcomes (Felitti, 1998).

Since 1984, the CDC has collected various information on chronic health conditions, injury, use of preventive health services, and access to care through the Behavioral Risk Factor Surveillance System (BRFSS). In 2008, questions related to several of the ACE categories, or simply the ACE module, were included in the BRFSS data collection. Arkansas, Louisiana, New Mexico, Tennessee, and Washington were the first five states to use the ACE module in 2009, with Pennsylvania and Wisconsin added in 2010. By 2014, 32 states plus the

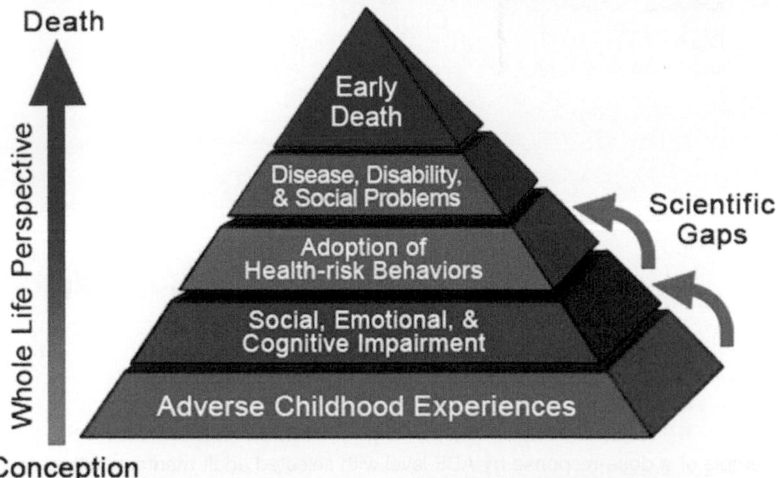


FIG. 7.1 ACE as the foundation for development. Substance Abuse and Mental Health Services Administration (SAMHSA), Center for the Application of Prevention Technologies, Practicing Effective Prevention, Prevention and Behavioral Health, Adverse Childhood Experiences.

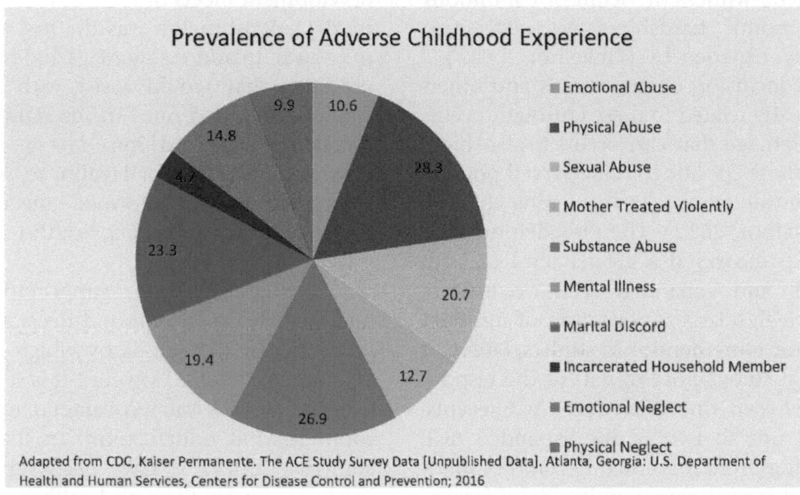


FIG. 7.2 Categories of adverse childhood exposures (CDC, 2016). (Adapted from CDC, Kaiser Permanente. The ACE Study Survey Data [Unpublished Data]. Atlanta, Georgia: U.S. Department of Health and Human Services, Centers for Disease Control and Prevention; 2016.)

District of Columbia included the module at least once during the annual BRFSS surveying cycles.[11] The conclusion from these surveys supported the initial findings from the 1998 study, with again having one in five respondents experiencing at least one ACE and around one in eight experiencing four or more ACEs.[11] These findings along with the other data collected through the BRFSS survey further confirm the poor outcomes linked to these exposures[12,13,13a]. However, despite the far-reaching ability of the BRFSS data collection to understand the common occurrences of select ACE events, the participants were not representative of minority populations [14].

The sentinel ACE study covered a large cohort of participants, with a predominant composition of White, non-Hispanic, middle-class, and 55–65-year-old respondents. Considering this and other studies that mainly reported findings from a similar demographic, several subsequent studies included additional questions related to likely experiences of urban, low

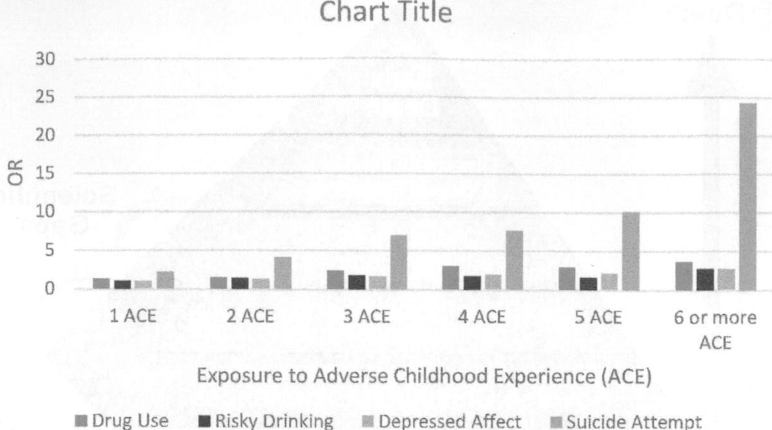


**FIG. 7.3** Example of a dose-response by ACE level with selected adult mental health outcomes. (Adapted from Merrick MT et al. Unpacking the impact of adverse childhood experiences on adult mental health. 2017)

socioeconomic populations and surveyed these respective areas. The various expanded ACE surveys included the death of a parent, witness or victim of community violence, socioeconomic hardship, peer adversities, and discriminatory experiences (Finkelhor, 2012).[14] Findings from the inclusion of these areas and others present the complexity related to these traumatic events and the lifelong damage that can occur. It also highlights some areas more specific to underserved populations that need consideration when screening children or adults[14,15](Finkelhor, 2012). The Philadelphia ACE Survey (PHLACES) uncovered a greater level of both conventional ACE and expanded ACE occurrences within its sample with a larger proportion of minority respondents than the aforementioned studies. Different from the 1998 ACE study, close to half of the respondents reported between one and three ACE events, and half affirmed one to two of the expanded ACE events [14]. The findings from this and other studies solidify the need for inclusion across a multitude of factors. The differences in environment including access to food and healthcare, socioeconomic status, gender, and race warrant the understanding that experiences with nonnormative traumatic events are more expansive than the original 10 areas provided by Felitti and Anda.

The American Academy of Pediatrics recognizes the lifelong adverse effects of physical, environmental, and household trauma and recommends developing innovative evidence-based strategies that will decrease or eliminate these negative outcomes.[16] The recommendations go further to support training all physicians, regardless of specialty or level of practice, about the interconnection of childhood traumas with adverse health outcomes and unhealthy social practices. Several states and clinics have adopted various methods to ensure that a multidisciplinary approach to caring for and supporting child development meets or exceeds these recommendations. In 2011, Washington was the first state to enact a law to commit to addressing ACEs and recognized two organizations that would assist with implementing TIC (trauma informed care) in the state. In 2014, Vermont successfully adopted into law a state-led healthcare program, Blueprint for Health, to study the impact of incorporating ACE-informed medical practices into the community and other health teams within its purview [16a].

Although there is clear support to increase awareness and facilitate action around decreasing or eliminating ACEs, the best methods by which to do so are, as of yet, undetermined. However, it is safe to say that whatever the algorithmic recommendation, there has to be room for individualization. In that vein, several resources (Table 7.5) have been successful at multiple levels of contact through healthcare, community, government, and religious entities.

One such method of approaching the scourge of ACEs is that of TIC. SAMHSA recommends the use of a trauma-informed approach that outlines the following:

1. *Realizes* the widespread impact of trauma and understands potential paths for recovery;
2. *Recognizes* the signs and symptoms of trauma in clients, families, staff, and others involved with the system;
3. *Responds* by fully integrating knowledge about trauma into policies, procedures, and practices; and
4. Seeks to actively resist *retraumatization.*

TABLE 7.3
Available Screening Tools

| Title | Group | Setting | Access |
|---|---|---|---|
| ACE Questionnaire | Adults | Healthcare/Judicial/Community | https://acestoohigh.com/got-your-ace-score/—Felitti and Anda |
| ACE Family History | Adults | Healthcare/Judicial/Community | https://www.cdc.gov/violenceprevention/acestudy/about.html—CDC, Felitti and Anda |
| ACE Health Questionnaire | Adults | Healthcare/Judicial/Community | https://www.cdc.gov/violenceprevention/acestudy/about.html—CDC, Felitti and Anda |
| Center for Youth Wellness | Child/Teen | Healthcare | https://centerforyouthwellness.org/cyw-aceq/—Nadine Burke Harris, MD |
| Bright Future™ Intake Form | Child/Teen | Healthcare | https://www.brightfutures.org/mentalhealth/pdf/professionals/ped_intake_form.pdf |
| Child Stress Disorders Checklist—Short Form | Child/Teen | Healthcare/Judicial/Community | https://www.nctsn.org/treatments-and-practices/screening-and-assessments/trauma-screening—Glenn Saxe, MD NCTSN[a] |
| Elsie Allen Health Center Survey | Child/Teen | Healthcare/Judicial/Community | https://acestoohigh.files.wordpress.com/2015/10/acesquestions.pdf |
| Maltreatment and Abuse Chronology of Exposure Scale (MACE) | Child/Teen/Adult | Healthcare/Judicial/Community | https://www.ncbi.nlm.nih.gov/pmc/articles/PMC4340880/#pone.0117423.s011 |
| Philadelphia Urban ACE Study | Adult | Healthcare/Judicial/Community | http://www.instituteforsafefamilies.org/sites/default/files/isfFiles/Philadelphia%20Urban%20ACE%20Report%202013.pdf |
| Whole Child Assessment | Child/Teen | Healthcare/Judicial/Community | https://www.acesconnection.com/g/resource-center/fileSendAction/fcType/0/fcOid/445474934934941772/filePointer/468559927008283106/fodoid/468559927008283100/WholeChildAssessmentEnglishJune2017.pdf |
| Childhood Trauma Questionnaire | Child/Teen/Adult | Healthcare/Judicial/Community | http://www.midss.org/sites/default/files/trauma.pdf—Pennebaker and Sussman |
| Juvenile Victimization Toolkit | Child/Teen/Adult | Healthcare/Judicial/Community | http://www.unh.edu/ccrc/jvq/available_versions.html—Hamby et al. 2017[16b] |
| Traumatic Antecedents Questionnaire | Child/Teen/Adult | Healthcare/Judicial/Community | http://www.traumacenter.org/products/pdf_files/Traumatic%20Antecedents%20Questionnaire-Final%20Version%202016.pdf—van der Kolk et al., 2016 |

[a] NCTSN—National Child Traumatic Stress Network.

The expectation through the implementation of this generalizable approach is that the providers will be able to better care for those that have experienced traumatic events because they themselves operate in an environment that understands the impact trauma can have on people. Several programs and studies support the concept of instituting a trauma-informed approach that requires the providers are trained to recognize and engage in inquiries that utilize the thought of "What happened to you?" as opposed to "What's wrong with you?" The premise of understanding ACE-related adversities in someone sets the stage for a more trusting relationship whether in a healthcare, judicial, religious, or community setting[17,18] (Leitch, 2017). This understanding is evident through the provider, the policies and procedures of the system, and the readiness to

**TABLE 7.4**
**Common Community Resources**

| | |
|---|---|
| https://www.childwelfare.gov | Schools |
| https://www.bbbs.org/ | Libraries |
| https://www.thehotline.org/ | Local Health Departments |
| https://www.womenshelters.org/ | Health Clinics |
| https://www.nctsn.org/resources/building-community-resilience-children-and-families | Community Centers |
| Food Pantries | Churches |

**TABLE 7.5**
**Intervention Resources**

| | |
|---|---|
| Baltimore: A Trauma and Resilience Informed City for Children and Families | http://fittcenter.umaryland.edu/Portals/0/OverallTraumaResilientInformedCityBaltimoreBSCreport.FINAL.pdf |
| Center on the Developing Child | https://developingchild.harvard.edu/ |
| Washington Family Policy Council Research Findings | https://www.ncbi.nlm.nih.gov/pmc/articles/PMC3483862/pdf/wpic40_325.pdf |
| Substance Abuse Mental Health Services Administration | https://www.samhsa.gov/capt/practicing-effective-prevention/prevention-behavioral-health/adverse-childhood-experiences |
| Arizona State University PBS | http://www.asset.asu.edu/strongkids/ |
| Strengthening Families | https://cssp.org/our-work/project/strengthening-families/ |
| RWJF ACEs | https://www.rwjf.org/en/library/collections/aces.html |
| Theory of Liberation | https://rysecenter.org/our-approach/ |
| ACEs Response Toolkit | https://www.iowaaces360.org/resiliency-toolkit.html |
| Building Community Resilience Collaborative | https://publichealth.gwu.edu/departments/redstone-center/resilient-communities |

provide the care needed to address the effects of ACEs in individuals and families. It is a whole systems approach that can foster not only healing, but also resilience building (Leitch, 2017).

Although the TIC approach is a widely adaptable framework, other models do exist. The development of the Building Community Resilience (BCR) model occurred through the guidance of key stakeholders with various roles under the child health systems (i.e., healthcare providers, school-based agency leaders, and those that work directly with child health systems) across 10 US urban centers. The premise of this model focuses on the shared responsibility of the larger community, the need to work together and understand the impact trauma has at an individual and community level, and ensure the resources are available to be resilient.[19] The model encompasses four components (adapted from Ref. [19]):

1. Shared understanding of childhood adversity
2. Assess system readiness to respond and build supports
3. Create a cross-sector community-based network
4. Engage parents, families, and community residents

Test sites for this model include Cincinnati, OH, Dallas, TX, the State of Oregon, Washington, DC, and the Alive and Well Communities in Missouri and Kansas.

Another approach to addressing ACEs is available through the Prevention Institute, a national organization with a long-standing history of working to improve communities through a public health perspective. Their initiative, Urban Networks to Increase Thriving Youths (UNITY), promotes the development of a framework to ameliorate the effects of ACEs through sociocultural (people), economic (opportunities), and built environment (place) interventions. It defines the symptoms of community trauma as issues brought on by limited employment and intergenerational poverty, dilapidated surroundings, the use of unhealthy building materials, disrupted social relations, and social tolerance for violence among others. Individual and community level trauma can be supported through methods that support these areas. The focus of the framework includes rebuilding relationships, promoting activities to support the uplifting of the community in safe public spaces, training, and encouraging the use of nonviolent conflict resolution along with building trust that serves to heal the community, as well as promoting economic empowerment and workforce development.[20] It is a common belief that people resort to unsafe behaviors such as crime out of necessity; creating a community that can address these needs is an underlying theme to mitigating traumatic experiences.

The ability for these approaches and many others to be successful is inclusive of one central theme, the need for everyone to be informed, trained, and ready to participate in these efforts. Utilizing multidisciplinary interventions early can be successful in mitigating both the acute and long-term sequelae of ACE events [1,20a–b].

The responsibility of screening and the linkage of services from that screening means that healthcare, political, judicial, religious, community, governmental, and nongovernmental systems bear this burden along with the individuals and communities that are suffering. Although there are several resources available to help in this process of training, increasing awareness, and implementing programs that would be beneficial, the available evidence of which method best treats/mitigates the effects of trauma has yet to be determined. However, the understanding of the relationship between adverse childhood experiences and the protective factors that support the growth and development of an afflicted person and community is clear.[19,21–25] While there is no easy path to eliminating adverse childhood experiences, there are tools and resources available to assist with decreasing the acute and chronic outcomes from these exposures. Action is required now to advance this process so that the past, current, and future generations can thrive.

## REFERENCES


1. https://drandrewrowland.wordpress.com/2014/04/25/it-is-easier-to-build-strong-children-than-to-repair-broken-men-frederick-douglass-1817-1895/; Accessed 13.10.2018.

1a. Kundakovic M, Champagne FA. Early-Life Experience, Epigenetics, and the Developing Brain. *Neuropsychopharmacology*. 2015;40(1):141–153.

1b. Kaufman J, Montalvo-Ortiz JL, Holbrook H, O'Loughlin K, Orr C, Kearney C, et al. Adverse Childhood Experiences, Epigenetic Measures, and Obesity in Youth. *J Pediatr*. 2018;202:150–156.e3.

1c. Shonkoff JP, Garner AS, Committee on Psychosocial Aspects of Child and Family Health, Committee on Early Childhood, Adoption, and Dependent Care, Section on Developmental and Behavioral Pediatrics. The lifelong effects of early childhood adversity and toxic stress. *Pediatrics*. 2012;129(1):e232–e246.

2. Felitti VJ, Anda RF, Nordenberg D, et al. Relationship of childhood abuse and household dysfunction to many of the leading causes of death in adults. The Adverse Childhood Experiences (ACE) Study. *Am J Prev Med*. 1998;14(4): 245–258.

2a. Hall J, Porter L, Longhi D, Becker-Green J, Dreyfus S. Reducing Adverse Childhood Experiences (ACE) by Building Community Capacity: a Summary of Washington Family Policy Council Research Findings. *J Prev Interv Community*. 2012;40:325–334.

2b. Leitch L. Action steps using ACEs and trauma-informed care: a resilience model. *Health Justice*. 2017;5:5. Accessed 14.10.2018.

2c. Balistreri KS, Alvira-Hammond M. Adverse childhood experiences, family functioning, adolescent health, and emotional well-being. *Public Health*. 2016 Mar;132: 72–78.

3. Rutter M. Isle of Wight revisited: twenty-five years of child psychiatric epidemiology. *J Am Acad Child Adolesc Psychiatry*. 1989;28(5):633–653.

3a. Gilbert LK, Breiding MJ, Merrick MT, et al. Childhood adversity and adult chronic disease: an update from ten states and the District of Columbia, 2010. *Am J Prev Med*. 2015;48(3):345–349.

4. Schilling EA, Aseltine RH, Gore S. Adverse childhood experiences and mental health in young adults: a longitudinal survey. *BMC Public Health*. 2007;7:30. https://doi.org/10.1186/1471-2458-7-30.

5. Kerker BD, Zhang J, Nadeem E, et al. Adverse childhood experiences and mental health, chronic medical conditions, and development in young children. *Acad Pediatr*. 2015;15(5):510–517. https://doi.org/10.1016/j.acap.2015.05.005.

6. Blodgett C, Lanigan JD. The association between adverse childhood experience (ACE) and school success in elementary school children. *Sch Psychol Q*. 2018;33(1):137–146. https://doi.org/10.1037/spq0000256.

7. Kwong TY, Hayes DK. Adverse family experiences and flourishing amongst children ages 6–17 years: 2011/12 National Survey of Children's Health. *Child Abuse Negl*. 2017;70:240–246.

8. McGloin JM, Widom CS. Resilience among abused and neglected children grown up. *Dev Psychopathol*. 2001 Fall; 13(4):1021–1038.

Students of color are statistically more likely to live in a lower SES household. According to the Department of Education's National Center for Education Statistics,[11] in 2014, 37% of African American, 31% of Hispanic, and only 12% each of White and Asian students lived in poverty. Students of color also tend to go to high-poverty schools, which generally offer fewer resources and a lower quality of education than schools attended by White and middle-class students.[12,13]

Furthermore, research has indicated that while students of color generally are overrepresented among children with LD,[14,15] early childhood special education and early intervention programs remain underrepresented for students of color.[16,17] Recent debate has emerged regarding whether and to what extent students of color are disproportionately overdiagnosed with LD. Some researchers have argued, contrary to common assumption, that minority students have been neglected in the assessment process and are less likely to receive special education services than their White peers.[18] Accordingly, recent research has advocated for strident use of ethical codes and standards to identify LD; application of higher identification standards would ensure equal access to services for minority and socioeconomically disadvantaged students.[19]

## BEHAVIORAL INDICATORS OF LEARNING DISABILITIES

According to the US Department of Education's *39th Annual Report to Congress on the Implementations of the Individuals with Disabilities Education Act, 2017*, in 2015–16, 6.7 million students ages 3–21 received special education services, with 34% identified as having specific learning disabilities.[14] For more than 50 years, the extensive debate has persisted about the causes of and categorization criteria for LD as well as how to best assess for them.[20,21] Even assessment professionals' viewpoints on causes and indicators can vary. For example, in a 2017 survey, Cottrell and Barrett found a significant correlation between school psychologists' perspectives (i.e., biological vs. environmental causes of LD) and the best identification methods. These findings underscore a broader concern about how differences in viewpoints among those assessing for learning challenges can impact identification methods, influence assessment practice, and contribute to inconsistency in students' access to services.[20]

As Miciak, Taylor, Stuebing, and Fletcher[22] pointed out, "There is no blood test or brain scan available that would differentiate which students truly demonstrate LDs from those who do not" (p. 22). Per the Individuals with Disabilities in Education Act of 2004,[23] the main methods for identifying LD are IQ–achievement discrepancy, *Response-to-Intervention* (RtI) method, and other procedures such as examining the student's *Pattern of Strengths and Weaknesses*.[20,23]

Quality of student work and academic performance that falls below grade level or developmental standards are certainly two important indicators of learning challenges.[24,25] Other indicators include difficulty with instructions; memory impairments; lack of mastery by expected age/grade in certain skills; poor coordination; difficulty with comprehension of words or concepts; problems with attention; poor organizational skills; inappropriate or disruptive behavior; variability in school performance; nonparticipation; difficulty listening; speaking in an age-inappropriate way; delayed or immature speech, etc. These indicators should prompt a comprehensive assessment to determine if the student meets the diagnostic criteria for LD.[26,27]

## NEUROBIOLOGICAL RISK FACTORS

### Neurodevelopmental Disorders

The number of LD-diagnosed children has increased significantly as the definitional expansion of learning disorder types has been classified.[28] The American Psychiatric Association identifies neurodevelopmental disorders in the DSM-5 as a group of conditions with onset in the developmental period. The disorders typically manifest early in development, often before the child enters grade school, and are characterized by developmental deficits that produce impairments of personal, social, academic, or occupational functioning. The range of developmental deficits varies from very specific limitations of learning or control of executive functions to global impairments of social skills or intelligence[29(p31)].

Within neurodevelopmental disorders, the DSM-5 classifications include intellectual disabilities, communication disorders (e.g., language disorder, speech sound disorder, childhood-onset fluency disorder/stuttering, and social/pragmatic communication disorder), autism spectrum disorder, attention deficit/hyperactivity disorder, specific learning disorder (e.g., reading, written expression, mathematics), motor disorders (e.g., developmental coordination disorder, stereotypic movement disorder, Tic disorders (e.g., Tourette's disorder, persistent/chronic motor or vocal tic disorder, provisional tic disorder), and other neurodevelopmental disorders (2013).

Neurodevelopmental disorders frequently cooccur.[29] Older children and adolescents with neurodevelopmental disorders are at higher than average risk for mood disorders, disruptive behavioral disorders, and attentional problems.[28] All neurodevelopmental disorders are more likely to be diagnosed in males than in females.[28–30] This gender difference may be attributed to behavioral problems more often recognized in young males,[28] while females with neurodevelopmental disorders tend to have higher rates of comorbid anxiety and depression.[29,31] This gender difference also may be attributed to genetic and structural vulnerabilities present in the male brain.[29,30]

## Etiology

Although all neurodevelopmental disorders have shown a genetic origin,[29] the focus here is narrowed to risks or predispositions related to learning challenges. A family history of learning difficulties is considered a risk factor for learning challenges in children and adolescents.[32] Educating parents about this genetic predisposition heightens awareness and increases motivation to seek support.[33] Some research has indicated that family history is not the most important predictor of learning difficulties. For example, a longitudinal study[33a] found that brain structure, specifically the development of left-brain white matter, was a more significant predictor than a family risk for atypical reading.[34] Relatedly, researchers[35] found that reading and math are processed in opposite hemispheres: Reading relies heavily on the left hemisphere, and math relies heavily on the right hemisphere. Differences in brain development, specifically in left-hemispheric connectivity, have been identified in children as young as 18 months.[36]

## Traumatic Brain Injury

Although considerable evidence has indicated that genetic vulnerability is associated with LD in adolescents,[34–36] head trauma due to physical injury also influences the developing brain.[37] *Traumatic Brain Injury* (TBI) is when typical utility of the brain is altered due to a jolt to the head.[38] A mild TBI, often classified as such if the loss of consciousness and/or disorientation is no longer than 30 min, also may be referred to as a concussion, minor head trauma, minor TBI, minor head injury, or minor brain injury. Generally, a loss of consciousness for 1–24 h indicates a moderate TBI and a loss of consciousness or coma for more than 24 h indicates a severe TBI.[38] TBI severity is also determined by the level of brain abnormality.[38]

TBI is the leading cause of death and disability for children in the United States,[38] with over half a million children under the age of 15 sustaining a TBI each year.[39] Boys ages 0–9 are 1.4 times more likely to sustain a TBI than girls, and boys ages 10–20 are 2.2 times more likely to sustain a TBI than girls the same age.[40] The effects of TBI and related recovery vary depending on severity and location of the injury.

Impacts of TBI in children include academic underachievement,[41,42] behavioral impairments[43,43a], deficits in social competence,[44–46] fatigue,[47,48] and sleep disturbances.[49,50] Fulton and colleagues[42] found that preschool-age children with a TBI had lower arithmetic faculty and school readiness skills when compared to children with an orthopedic injury and no TBI. They also found that later academic achievement was related significantly to intellectual functioning post-TBI.[42]

The age of the child when the head trauma occurred is significant to the overall impact of the TBI on the individual.[37,51] Young age at injury has been linked to higher severity of outcome impairment.[45] Landry-Roy, Bernier, Gravel, and Beauchamp[50] explained, "If the integrity of the brain is altered during early childhood, a critical time for the establishment and emergence of executive skills, there is likely to be increased risk for EF [executive function] impairments and cumulative deficits" (p. 1). Furthermore, individuals that sustained a TBI in early childhood still required or were utilizing academic services 7 years postinjury.[52] Therefore, when assessing adolescents for learning challenges, providers should screen for a history of head trauma to identify possible TBI symptoms.

## Risks Related to Biological Stressors

In addition to genetic predispositions for neurological and biological concerns, environmental stressors can influence neurology and biology. Life experience, in other words, can trigger lasting changes to brain structure and neurochemistry. Childhood chronic stress resulting from maltreatment, for example, impacts the developing adolescent brain (Cicchetti, Tykra, Ridout, & Parade, 2016).[53] Although it may not be entirely clear how early hardship affects physical health, research increasingly has found neurobiological differences between those who have experienced childhood adversity and those who have not.[53,54,54a] When assessing for learning challenges, the impact of maltreatment on the hippocampus—the area of the brain responsible for learning and various aspects of memory—should be considered.[53,54]

Biological stressors and medical conditions are risk factors that can interfere with adolescent learning and development as well. A child's capacity for processing and retaining information is impaired when struggling with health concerns.[55] Potential physical health barriers to learning include vision, hearing, asthma, and dental pain.[55] Another significant stressor that can impair health and learning is limited access to food. In 2015, an estimated 17.7% of households in the United States experienced *food insecurity* throughout the year,[55,56] meaning that one or more household members had to reduce food intake because money or other resources were lacking. Children identified as coming from food-insecure households are more likely to have repeated a grade and have significantly lower scores in math, while adolescents were more likely to have been suspended from school.[55,57] Both children and adolescents were more likely to have seen a psychologist and to have experienced interpersonal conflicts with peers.[55,57] Furthermore, children with food insecurity had higher rates of homelessness, chronic illness, as well as behavioral, academic, and emotional difficulties from infancy to adolescence.[58,59]

Although neurodevelopmental disorders typically are diagnosed during childhood, providers nevertheless should consider neurodevelopmental factors (e.g., chronic illness or food insecurity) that might undermine adolescent achievement to determine specific needs and maximize learning potential.

## PSYCHOSOCIAL RISK FACTORS

Research has identified a number of psychosocial factors that directly and indirectly threaten academic achievement. These factors are dynamically interrelated within individual adolescents and are not discrete processes. For the purposes of adolescent screening, identifying any of the following risk factors will provide professionals with data relevant toward determining the need for further exploration, psychoeducational evaluation, and intervention to promote future academic success and healthy adult functioning.

### Individual Risk Factors

Considerable research has focused on understanding the connection between individual factors and educational outcomes. How and to what extent these constructs interact and mutually reinforce one another to impact academic achievement is a complex question and a topic of empirical debate. For the purposes of assessment, only an overview of relevant results is presented here with the aim of recognizing those individual factors that may place adolescents at risk for poor educational outcomes.

**Poor academic self-concept**. According to Prince and Nurius (2014)[59a], students who develop a negative academic self-concept—particularly following persistent academic difficulties—tend to filter input from peers, teachers, and the wider sociocultural environment for content that reinforces their negative perceptions and reject any positive data that challenge their perspective. As this pattern becomes "progressively elaborated, organized, and interwoven with other related self-conceptions"[59a], students often make decisions that undermine school success and forego the increases in motivation, drive, and accomplishments that are aligned with a positive academic self-concept.[60,61,61a–c]

In a meta-analysis of 39 longitudinal studies, Huang[62] substantiated that students' prior overall academic self-perceptions were correlated significantly with subsequent academic achievement. Independent investigations also have demonstrated the direct and indirect significance and developmental effects of academic self-concept (broadly defined) on achievement and a range of educational outcomes (e.g., academic aspirations, access to guidance, and better grades), even after controlling for factors such as previous achievement histories.[63–71]

**Low motivation and negative school attitude**. Extensive empirical research has established that students with high educational motivation and a positive orientation toward school are more likely to exhibit self-regulatory and achievement-oriented behaviors and succeed academically.[60,72–80] Other studies have emphasized further the likely contribution of behavioral engagement as mediating the effects of school attitude on achievement: Students who are positively oriented toward school and learning are more actively engaged in class, receive better grades, and are absent less frequently.[81] By contrast and pertinent to adolescent screening, negative views of teachers, education, and high school predicted absenteeism[82] and dropout behavior,[83] both of which are associated with academic failure.

**Lack of school engagement**. Screening adolescents for a low sense of control with respect to academic performance is useful for assessing their risk for future educational challenges. School engagement is a multidimensional concept that reflects a commitment to learning and successful academic performance.[84] Specifically, school engagement involves behavioral engagement (e.g., attendance, completion of schoolwork, participation in academic and extracurricular activities, and other positive conduct that promotes learning), emotional engagement (e.g., attitudes about and feelings toward school, a sense of school belonging or identification with school), and cognitive engagement (e.g., self-regulatory and metacognitive approaches to learning such as moderating attention and effort, connecting new information to existing knowledge, and monitoring progress) as described in extensive research.[85–94]

School engagement and its connection with educational outcomes and other developmental trajectories have been an important area of empirical investigation.[84,93,95–100] Past research has identified significant positive correlations between school engagement and school success.[101] However, Wang and Eccles[93] emphasized that whether or not students feel emotionally connected to the school, they are likely to underachieve if their behavior reflects the lack of motivation, active participation, and self-regulated learning strategies necessary to attend classes and study effectively to improve academic performance.[95,102]

Disengaged students are more likely to underachieve and drop out of school.[103] Behavioral, emotional, and cognitive markers of school engagement are particularly significant for screening during early adolescence because they correspond with the need for "competency, autonomy, and relatedness in school" that is consistent with this stage of psychosocial development[86(p80)]. School plays a central role in adolescents' everyday lives; accordingly, negative identification with school may facilitate behavior that leads to poorer academic outcomes and likely signals a misalignment between students' developmental needs and the school environment.[92,104–106] In fact, school disengagement increases markedly during the middle and high school years.[107] Therefore, early identification of school disengagement and intervention may prevent dropout, delinquency, and other maladaptive behaviors.[100,108,109]

Both correlational and longitudinal studies examining the connection between perceived control and academic achievement have demonstrated a positive correlation between the two.[107,110–112] Students with a higher level of perceived control (i.e., an internal vs. external locus of control) have better academic outcomes, even across different age groups and SES.[103,111–114] Conversely, Sisney et al.[115] found a significant association between external locus of control and academic underachievement as well as higher dropout rates for high school students.

**Behavioral challenges.** Empirical investigations into the longitudinal trajectories between mental health and academic performance in children and adolescents have been an area of interest for several years,[116–119] particularly in research looking at how functioning in one domain of behavior unfolds in other domains, both directly and indirectly from childhood into adulthood. Moilanen et al.[119] have suggested that externalizing problems (e.g., impulsivity, hostility) and/or internalizing symptoms (e.g., anxiety and depression) undermine learning through a process of maladjustment.

For example, longitudinal research spanning 20 years—from childhood and adolescence through early adulthood—has described a link between externalizing problems and difficulties that extend across multiple domains of functioning, which impede academic achievement and social competence.[120] Similarly, Moilanen, Shaw, and Maxwell[119] found that externalizing behaviors forecasted low academic achievement over a 6-year period from middle childhood to early adolescence. Externalizing behaviors, in particular, appeared to directly hamper students' ability to effectively engage in class[121,122]; disruptive behavior often leads to disciplinary action (e.g., removal from class, suspension) that diminishes learning opportunities and hinders motivation. Consequently, externalizing students may develop persistent negative reactions to the school setting that compromise their academic performance.[123]

Internalizing symptoms similarly predicted a decline in academic competence in adolescents,[124] primarily during the transition from middle childhood to adolescence and following a period of escalating externalizing problems.[119] These results are consistent with research covering similar developmental periods[125] and over longer trajectories,[126,127] which have observed that externalizing problems weaken performance in the academic domain by adolescence that then contributes to internalizing problems in the domain of adaptation by early adulthood. This pattern was consistent across gender while controlling for IQ, parenting, and SES. Deighton et al.'s recent study[128] also supported these earlier investigations and found that higher levels of both internalizing and externalizing difficulties led to successive reductions in educational attainment.

In general, limited academic progress interacts with intensifying negative feelings about school to create overwhelming hurdles for students to reach meaningful achievements academically. Relevant to screening, as educational difficulties accumulate for adolescents with externalizing and/or internalizing symptoms, students become increasingly vulnerable to academic failure and associated outcomes (e.g., delinquency, drug use, teenage pregnancy).

**Low socioemotional competence**. In early adolescence, students begin to turn their attention away from family and toward their peer group.[129] Socioemotional skills are essential during this developmental phase as they support positive classroom functioning, interpersonal effectiveness, and facilitate healthy momentum along the later adolescent developmental trajectory.[130–132]

Past theoretical and empirical investigations have indicated that socioemotional aspects of development such as socioemotional competence (SEC) are inextricably connected to and predict academic success.[133–149] For example, in recent research,[150] teacher-reported SEC in early adolescence predicted higher scores in math and reading on standardized tests a year later.

Relevant to adolescent screening, poor SEC has been found to be negatively linked to a number of indicators of academic success, including less academic connectedness, engagement, achievement, and an increased risk for dropout.[135,148,151–154]

**Substance use**. Considerable evidence has found that substance use is associated with academic problems.[100] Although the impact of drug use on school performance varies by drug type, generally adolescents who use substances are vulnerable to educational underachievement via the following mechanisms: (1) the harmful effects of substances on neuropsychological and cognitive functioning,[155–157] (2) the tendency to affiliate with deviant, drug-using peers and high-risk groups,[158–161] (3) adopting behaviors and attitudes that devalue education and undermine academic success,[162] (4) poorer attendance and classroom performance,[163,164] and (5) school disengagement.[165,166]

Research to date has centered primarily on cannabis and alcohol use which—in addition to tobacco—represent the drugs most frequently used by adolescents.[167] Studies consistently have demonstrated that adolescent cannabis use is associated with school noncompletion,[168–173] and these effects were amplified for socioeconomically disadvantaged youth.[172,174] Similarly, tobacco use has been linked with failure to complete school,[162,172,175,176] with smaller effect sizes than for cannabis. Alcohol use similarly has predicted later school disconnection and academic underperformance.[175,177] Notably, these associations were strengthened by peer alcohol use.[178] Register, Williams, and Grimes[179] found that other illicit drug use reduced grade level attainment by 1 year. In a longitudinal study of Australian mid-adolescents, Kelly, Chan, Mason, and Williams[180] found that relative to nonusers and mainly alcohol users, polydrug (i.e., alcohol, tobacco, and cannabis) users were at substantially greater risk for school noncompletion even after accounting for confounds such as school commitment, academic failure, and peer drug use. For further discussion, see the chapter on substance abuse.

**Gender identity and sexuality concerns**. Sexual minority students (i.e., LGBTQ and gender-nonconforming youth) are at increased risk of poor school outcomes (e.g., truancy, negative school attitudes, lower grade point averages, reports of victimization) in comparison with students identifying as heterosexual.[181–184,184a]

**Involvement in the juvenile justice system**. Both engaging in unlawful activities and spending time in juvenile detention facilities are linked with academic underachievement.[185,186] In general, the academic performance of adolescents incarcerated in juvenile correctional detention facilities corresponds developmentally with students who are 5 years younger.[187] According to Stone and Zibulsky,[188] system involved youth are at greater risk for failing courses, being involved in special education, and dropping out. The educational experiences of remanded youth are often interrupted, sometimes indefinitely, and poor educational outcomes are likely due to variable school attendance, multiple transitions and academic discontinuity, inconsistencies in the quality of instruction, and unreliable efforts to assess academic needs due to challenges with recordkeeping and data sharing.

Important to consider is that the academic challenges of these adolescents often precede involvement in the juvenile justice system.[187] This population of students overlaps significantly with those involved in the child welfare system given the fact that childhood maltreatment appreciably increases the probability of later delinquency.[189–191] The sociodemographic risk factors associated with involvement in both systems also intersect. For instance, poor males of color are overrepresented in the juvenile justice system[192] and are more likely to be arrested than their White peers.[193]

**Low participation in extracurricular activities**. Research has presented conflicting data regarding beneficial amounts of time that students should spend engaged in extracurricular activity.[194] Although extracurricular involvement certainly has positive influences on academic achievement, overscheduled students have demonstrated adverse effects.[194–196] Overall, relevant research has indicated that a reasonable (i.e., not excessive and not sparse) amount of time spent in extracurricular activity yields the most beneficial outcomes.[194]

**Earlier school challenges**. The longitudinal consequences of learning challenges can be mitigated by early identification and treatment; however, without intervention, children are at risk for developing emotional and behavioral difficulties as they encounter persistent academic failure. Research has established that at-risk children generally perform poorly across the developmental trajectory.[197–199] Montague et al.[198] found that reading and math achievement, in particular, heralded later academic outcomes in middle and high school. Similarly, their findings established that teacher evaluations identifying early childhood behavioral challenges were reliable predictors of behavioral problems in adolescence.

## Family and Household Factors

**Childhood maltreatment and exposure to trauma.** Childhood trauma is central to understanding adolescent outcomes as well as their influence on school experiences. A preponderance of empirical evidence—including neurobiological, epigenetic, and biosocial studies—substantiates that exposure to maltreatment in childhood (e.g., emotional, physical, sexual abuse and/or neglect, parent separation, witnessing domestic violence, household substance abuse, household mental illness, household member incarceration, etc.) is a risk marker for academic underachievement and maladjustment.[188,200–212] Notably, Leiter and Johnsen[206] found that among children who had experienced childhood maltreatment, those who had been exposed to intimate partner violence had the poorest academic outcomes.

The toxic stress and the associated release of cortisol and adrenaline connected to cumulative trauma cause structural and functional damage to the brain[213,213a], which is often expressed in ways that challenge students' capacity to learn and, by extension, achieve academically. According to a recent analysis by Johnson,[214] traumatic experiences trigger both social and neurophysiological adaptations that undercut the cognitive functioning, emotional and behavioral adjustment, coping strategies, and interpersonal effectiveness that are essential for school success. Johnson[214] also has asserted that trauma is linked to unhealthy coping mechanisms and the onset of substance abuse disorders. Effectively, the traumatized brain focuses its energy on survival and wrenches its resources away from the cognitive activities that are essential to learning[215]: Traumatic experiences in childhood can diminish comprehension, memory, trust, language abilities, and self-regulation.[216,217]

Specifically, neurophysiological responses to trauma—including hyperarousal (known colloquially as *fight, flight*, or *freeze*) and dissociation—often evolve into emotional and behavioral challenges that undermine academic achievement.[215,218,219] Children are likely to model the problematic behavior associated with their traumatic experiences or pursue a connection with deviant peers, adversely affecting academic performance.[216] Children exposed to maltreatment also can develop negative attitudes toward adults, negatively impacting interpersonal interactions with teachers and other authority figures.[216,220] Most observably, fight or flight reactions and externalizing behaviors such as aggression or defiance undermine critical relationships with school personnel and result in disciplinary actions that compromise learning.[221,222] Similarly, teachers may perceive students' internalizing behaviors, including cognitive and physical unresponsiveness (freeze reactions), as defiance or disrespect, leading to conflicts and disciplinary consequences; freeze responses also are associated with falling behind academically and performing poorly on standardized assessments.[218] Even the more nuanced dissociative responses to trauma, including memory suppression, distraction, and/or confusion, often lead to seemingly defiant or apathetic behavior, academic underperformance, and disengagement.[219]

**Permissive or authoritarian parenting style**. A meta-analysis[223] of 308 empirical studies on parenting styles indicated that while certain styles (i.e., responsiveness or autonomy-granting) were associated with higher academic achievement; others (i.e., psychological control or permissiveness) had lesser associations to academic achievement than did school-specific parental involvement.

**Parental divorce, separation, or conflict**. Research has determined that younger children's (e.g., between 6 and 14 years) academic achievement is more affected by parental marital dissolution than older children.[224,225] Other studies have established that parental conflict adversely affects school behavior, grades, and self-concept because of disruptions to the relational support and communication necessary to meet their emotional, socialization, and educational needs.[147,148,226–235] Relatedly, students who reside with single mothers reportedly have a 14%

less chance for academic success and advancing to higher educational levels than children from intact families[236,237]; and this result is amplified in circumstances under which the custodial mother is less educated.[238]

**Foster or adoptive status**. Students involved in the foster care system often struggle academically, and the implications of risk for academic failure are compelling given that school engagement, performance, and attainment are intimately tied to their well-being across the developmental trajectory.[188] Important to consider is that childhood maltreatment is connected to both academic difficulty and formal system involvement.

Narrative reviews have indicated that preschool children enter foster care with low average intellectual functioning and fundamental prereading deficits—academic challenges that likely existed before their introduction to the foster care system and formal schooling.[239,240] Once matriculated, foster students generally perform below grade expectations, show significant differences between measured IQ and achievement, and fall behind demographically similar peers in reading and mathematics achievement. Students in foster care also tend to take fewer honors (vs. general), track coursework, enroll in less college preparatory classes, spend less time on homework, exhibit more disciplinary problems, and express lower academic expectations.[241] Foster care data sources have revealed a disproportionate representation of foster youth under the emotionally disturbed, learning disabled, and mental retardation designations of special education.[242,243]

In a 2007 meta-analysis of 31 studies, Scherr reported that foster children also are at a uniquely elevated risk for grade retention and disciplinary actions. Studies[239,240] also have found that placement restrictiveness and stability, as well as transitions surrounding care, are linked to foster students' academic performance: Specifically, students in the most restrictive placements experienced greater academic challenges. Placement transfers also increased the probability of school transfers and adversely impacted attendance within a year after placement.[244] Other research has concluded that both lengths of and transitions surrounding care are associated with foster students' academic performance, including an increased likelihood of nonschool transfers,[245] lower test scores,[244] and lower subsequent attendance. In a study by Smithgall, Gladden, Howard, George, and Courtney,[246] the author determined that children and adolescents in foster care are at a higher risk of being retained in the year following placement.

With respect to adoption status, in a meta-analysis, Van IJzendoorn and Juffer[247] determined that adopted children academically outperformed siblings who remained in institutional settings as well as their nonadopted peers. A conflicting analysis indicated that adopted children underperformed compared to their nonadopted peers, particularly if they were adopted after 12 months old.[248] Adopted children, whose academic achievement lagged behind that of their nonadopted peers also exhibited higher levels of hyperactivity,[249] were more likely to have a learning disorder,[247] and both of these factors might explain their educational challenges. Overall, research has indicated that most adopted children placed before 4 years old enjoy academic success similar to that of their nonadopted peers, regardless of country of origin.

**Caregiver educational attainment and involvement**. Research has indicated that students' perceptions of teacher and parental involvement impact their view of academic potential. In a study by You, Hong, and Ho,[250] results indicated that when students feel supported and when their academic efforts are positively reinforced, their confidence and sense of control regarding future educational success and academic achievement is positively influenced.

Parents' educational background also impacts students' view of their educational futures. In a study that examined long-term effects of parents' educational and occupational success, researchers found that higher levels of parental education were associated with higher levels of educational aspirations or educational pursuits.[251]

**Parental education and low family income**. Extensive empirical research has concluded that parental education and family income are reliable predictors of academic outcomes for youth across race, ethnic, and immigrant groups: Academic underachievement and limited academic attainment exemplify two principal by-products of growing up in a disadvantaged household.[252–255] These results are consistent with other literature.[190,202,209,256–261] The educational consequences associated with poverty are ascribed, in part, to limited access to educational enrichment activities and exposure to stressors, for example, a lack of structure and poor housing conditions.[262,263]

Research also has long established that educational differences related to family background increase as students advance academically.[264–270] Namely, among students of variable socioeconomic backgrounds, disparities in achievement remained stable during elementary school, expanded dramatically as they approached the transition to middle school, and accelerated leading up to high school. These shifts reflect minimal developmental progress toward academic parity across racial and ethnic populations, increasing inequalities between low and high-income students, and ineffective policy efforts to remedy these disparities once children begin school.[271,272]

According to Caro, McDonald, and Willms,[273] the literature has demonstrated that the socioeconomic challenges surrounding students' early educational experiences have enduring consequences. Generally, as low SES children mature, their academic picture becomes bleaker over the course of their development. For example, they tend to drop out early,[274–279] are less likely to follow a college preparatory path,[280–283,283a] are less inclined to pursue postsecondary education or successfully enter the labor force,[284–286] and struggle with socioemotional difficulties.[262,263]

## Sociocultural Factors

**Ethnic minority or immigrant status**. Racial and ethnic discrepancies in academic performance and attainment have declined over the past 30 years by conventional measures, while the poverty gap has expanded.[270,287,288] In general, academic ambitions have remained elevated for all racial and ethnic groups indicating that the majority of adolescents intend to go to college.[289–291] However, remarkable differences have persisted, particularly between the least advantaged populations (e.g., African Americans, Hispanics, and Native Americans) and more privileged groups (e.g., Whites and Asian Americans). This hierarchy in academic achievement has been evident across several measures of academic experience, including grades,[292] test scores,[4,4a] course taking,[293–295] and college preparatory paths,[296–300] particularly through secondary education.[287] In recent studies, when children from low-income families as well as African-American and Hispanic/Latino families enter kindergarten, most are already behind their White classmates.[301] These gaps in reading and math skills have been found to persist past fourth grade and increase by eighth grade.[9]

Similarly, past research has found that school incompletion is unevenly distributed racially, economically, and geographically.[302] Researchers historically have found that Blacks, Hispanics, and Native Americans are significantly more likely than White or other minority students to drop out of school.[303–306] Researchers also have investigated factors that forecast school dropout for various racial and ethnic populations and reported that immigrants drop out at a higher rate than native-born individuals of native parentage; this is particularly the case for recent immigrants.[306] Certainly, immigrants enhance the complexity of the US minority population, including youth along the SES continuum. Overwhelmingly, research has indicated that immigrant children perform better than their same-ethnic counterparts with comparable parental backgrounds.[291,307–311]

## Peer Factors

**Peer victimization**. Peer-relatedness has been shown to have beneficial effects on students' learning through comfort with engagement[311a] and comfort with taking learning risks.[312] Conversely, youth who have had multiple victimization experiences have demonstrated more significant academic problems than those with fewer experiences.[205,210,313–317]

**Negative peer influences**. Research has highlighted that students experience remarkable social pressure to share the same attitudes as their peers. Thus, students' academic interest, engagement, and achievement may be compromised significantly by their peers' negative attitude toward school.[210]

## School Factors

**Poor teacher-student relationship and ineffective teachers**. Teachers can profoundly influence student learning and achievement, and the nature of the teacher-student relationship has been found to significantly impact students' academic success.[318,319] Teacher quality, relatedly, significantly influences academic success[318,320,320a]; therefore, the implications of teacher-student misalignment are likely to have a meaningfully deleterious effect on students' educational outcomes.

## Work Factors

**Work intensity and early engagement in work**. Research has indicated contradictory data regarding the relationship between student employment and school performance, with some data having revealed variance depending on multiple factors, such as gender or type of employment.[321,322] Although research has indicated that intensity of engagement in employment is negatively correlated with academic performance, less intensive engagement was positively correlated with academic performance.[322,323]

## Community Factors

**Neighborhood poverty**. Research has shown that neighborhood poverty, such as family poverty, consistently and significantly has predicted academic achievement, showing clear negative effects.[208,257]

**Neighborhood violence**. Research has substantiated that exposure to violence has a negative impact on academic functioning,[324,325] and one notable predictive factor is friendship with peers who are not actively engaged in academics.[326]

### Technology Factors

**Videogaming and mobile device use**. Appropriate and thoughtful use of technology can support students' learning, positively impact academic performance, and help to prepare them for future success.[327] However, utilizing technology also can undermine students' educational outcomes when appropriate use evolves into preoccupation or addiction and is accompanied by symptoms predictive of mental health concerns.[328] For a more detailed discussion, see the chapter on Screening for Screen Time.

**Social media and cyber-victimization**. Interactive social media use among youth continues to accelerate.[329,330] Adolescents are increasingly at risk for victimization experiences given their growing access to the Internet and the myriad ways perpetrators can bully in a sometimes dangerously unregulated online environment.[331,332]

## DISCUSSION

Sometimes questions about how adolescents can achieve their fullest academic potential cannot be answered without greater clarification and comprehensive planning. As Cantor, Osher, Berg, Steyer, and Rose[333] described, students learn contextually, and neural malleability allows for ongoing influence from those with whom they have relationships. Given the enduring influence of dynamic systems and relationship security on development, an individualized and collaborative assessment process led by encouraging, empathic, and respectful providers can support students in developing more accurate, compassionate, and useful stories about the obstacles they have encountered and strengthening their resilience vis à vis risk factors.[334,335]

Despite civil rights victories that helped to establish educational rights for all, there is still a substantial achievement gap between students with learning challenges and those without.[336] There are many theories about the best way to close educational gaps and help students achieve their academic potential. *Growth mindset* theory, for example, promotes increasing academic performance by shifting students' view of intellectual ability from something that is fixed to something that can be improved.[337,338,338a] As Blackwell et al.[337] stated, "Children's beliefs become the mental 'baggage' that they bring to the achievement situation" (p. 259). The results from a study utilizing a growth mindset intervention with 10th-grade females (38% White, 25% Black, 29% Hispanic) in rural, low-income areas indicated stronger growth mindsets at both posttest and 4-month follow-up and correlated with improved final grades (Burnette et al., 2018). In another study, a growth mindset intervention program was shown to improve standardized test scores in stereotyped students, including female students completing standardized tests in mathematics.[339]

A glaring weakness of conventional methods of educational assessments is that the process itself is often stigmatizing and marginalizing.[340] Assessment measures should be nonpathologizing and even empowering to the individual student in terms of seeking beneficial information about what the student needs to succeed. Just as schools fail students by not developing curricula that consider student differences,[340] assessment practices can fail students by dismissing the nuanced differences in each student's learning obstacles and strengths. Ideally, assessment questions, activities, and prompts should encourage the possibility of increased academic achievement and learning confidence. Accordingly, the assessment experience would reflect growth mindset theory by reinforcing the understanding that intelligence is malleable rather than fixed. Beyond attending to risk factors for and current concerns about learning challenges, professionals should emphasize resiliency factors and learning strengths.

An effective assessment model for identifying learning challenges must prioritize collaborative input from everyone involved in the student's learning (e.g., student, teacher, classroom aides, school psychologist, etc.) with special attention to empowering the caregivers and the family system itself. Galvanizing advocacy by caregivers for improving their children's education has been shown to ignite students' sense of efficacy toward securing academic success.[341] A recent study exploring a *parent empowerment framework* using a national sample of 9,982 parents indicated that parent empowerment interventions should consider sociocultural factors (e.g., race, ethnicity, SES, parent educational background, and language) and should be implemented with attention to any structural barriers within the school.[341] This study also highlighted the importance of parents' relationships with teachers, counselors, and peer-parents. In this context, parents are emboldened via "relational power through a diversity of relationships" (p. 177).

This need for parental empowerment and increased communication between school and caregivers is further supported by a recent survey and mixed-method design study.[342] Parents reported a lack of understanding about RtI, a commonly used assessment and intervention approach for students who may have LD and who may require special education services. The parents in this study also reported that they had not been given sufficient information about this approach to addressing their children's needs.

Historically, deficit-based and decontextualized approaches to defining and assessing learning challenges have had an adverse effect on many students; moving toward a strengths-based, individualized, and culturally responsive approach to evaluation can provide students and professionals with more effective means for developing and implementing interventions that facilitate academic progress.[343] In contrast to a deficiency-based assessment process that reinforces students' negative self-perceptions of incompetence, collaborative assessment can serve as a meaningful and therapeutic intervention in and of itself.

## REFERENCES


1. Kotok S. Unfulfilled potential: high-achieving minority students and the high school achievement gap in math. *High Sch J.* 2017;100(3):183–202. https://doi.org/10.1353/hsj.2017.0007.
2. *Achievement Gaps*; 2015. Retrieved from https://nces.ed.gov/nationsreportcard/studies/gaps/.
3. Minor EC. Racial differences in mathematics test scores for advanced mathematics students. *High Sch J.* 2016; 99(3):193–210.
4. Jencks C, Phillips M. *The Black-White Test Score Gap.* Washington, D.C.: Brookings Institution Press; 1998.

4a. Miller LS. *An American imperative: Accelerating minority educational advancement.* New Haven, CT: Yale University Press; 1995.

5. National Education Association (n.d.). Students Affected by Achievement Gaps. Retrieved from www.nea.org/home/20380.htm.
6. Kim R. *A Report on the Status of Gay, Lesbian, Bisexual and Transgender People in Education: Stepping Out of the Closet, into the Light;* 2009. Retrieved from www.nea.org/assets/docs/HE/glbtstatus09.pdf.
7. Rosado S, Toya GJ. Applied critical leadership and sense of belonging: lessons learned from cultural center staff and lesbian, gay, and bisexual Latino/a students. In: Santamaría LJ, Santamaría AP, Santamaría LJ, Santamaría AP, eds. *Culturally Responsive Leadership in Higher Education: Promoting Access, Equity, and Improvement.* New York, NY, US: Routledge/Taylor & Francis Group; 2016:31–43. https://doi.org/10.2307/2673234.
8. *Closing Early Learning Opportunity Gaps under ESSA;* 2018. Retrieved from http://www.ncsl.org/research/education/equity-and-the-opportunity-gap.aspx.
9. Solano IS, Weyer M. Closing the opportunity gap in early childhood education. *NCSL Legisbrief.* 2017;25(25):1–2.
10. *Closing the Opportunity Gap;* 2016. Retrieved from http://www.theopportunitygap.com/wp-content/uploads/2015/08/2016-Working-Group-Report.pdf#page=74.
11. National Center for Education Statistics. *Status and Trends in the Education of Racial and Ethnic Groups;* 2017. Retrieved from https://nces.ed.gov/programs/raceindicators/indicator_rad.asp.
12. Blanchett WJ, Klingner JK, Harry B. The intersection of race, culture, language, and disability: implications for urban education. *Urban Educ.* 2009;44(4):389–409. https://doi.org/10.1177/0042085909338686.
13. Kozol J. *The Shame of the Nation: The Restoration of Apartheid Schooling in America.* New York, NY, US: Crown Trade Paperbacks/Crown Publishers; 2005.
14. *39th Annual Report to Congress on the Implementations of the Individuals with Disabilities Education Act, 2017;* 2018. Retrieved from https://www2.ed.gov/about/reports/annual/osep/2017/parts-b-c/39th-arc-for-idea.pdf.
15. Zhang D, Katsiyannis A, Ju S, Roberts E. Minority representation in special education: 5-year trends. *J Child Fam Stud.* 2014;23(1):118–127. https://doi.org/10.1007/s10826-012-9698-6.
16. Morgan PL, Farkas G, Hillemeier MM, Maczuga S. Are minority children disproportionately represented in early intervention and early childhood special education? *Educ Res.* 2012;41(9):339–351. https://doi.org/10.3102/0013189X12459678.
17. Morgan PL, Farkas G, Hillemeier MM, et al. Minorities are disproportionately underrepresented in special education: longitudinal evidence across five disability conditions. *Educ Res.* 2015;44(5):278–292. https://doi.org/10.3102/0013189X15591157.
18. Morgan PL, Farkas G, Hillemeier MM, Maczuga S. Replicated evidence of racial and ethnic disparities in disability identification in U.S. schools. *Educ Res.* 2017;46(6): 305–322. https://doi.org/10.3102/0013189X17726282.
19. Dombrowski SC, Gischlar KL. Ethical and empirical considerations in the identification of learning disabilities. *J App Sch Psychol.* 2014;30(1):68–82. https://doi.org/10.1080/15377903.2013.869786.
20. Cottrell JM, Barrett CA. Examining school psychologists' perspective about specific learning disabilities: implications for practice. *Psychol Sch.* 2017;54(3):294–308. https://doi.org/10.1002/pits.21997.
21. Hammill DD. On defining learning disabilities: an emerging consensus. *J Learn Disabil.* 1990;23(2):74–84. Retrieved from http://ldx.sagepub.com.paloaltou.idm.oclc.org/.
22. Miciak J, Taylor WP, Stuebing KK, Fletcher JM. Simulation of LD identification accuracy using a pattern of processing strengths and weaknesses method with multiple measures. *J Psychoeducational Assess.* 2018;36(1):21–33. https://doi.org/10.1177/0734282916683287.

23. 20 U.S.C. § 1400. *Individuals with Disabilities in Education Act (IDEA) of 2004*; 2004. Retrieved from http://idea.ed.gov/download/statute.html.
24. Hale J, Alfonso V, Berninger V, et al. Critical issues in response-to- intervention, comprehensive evaluation, and specific learning disabilities identification and intervention: an expert white paper consensus. *Learn Disabil Q*. 2010;33(3):223–236. https://doi.org/10.1177/073194871003300310.
25. Maddocks DS. The identification of students who are gifted and have a learning disability: a comparison of different diagnostic criteria. *Gifted Child Q*. 2018;62(2):175–192. https://doi.org/10.1177/0016986217752096.
26. American Academy of Child and Adolescent Psychiatry. *Learning Disorders*; 2013. Retrieved from http://www.aacap.org/AACAP/Families_and_Youth/Facts_for_Families/FFF-Guide/Children-With-Learning-Disorders-016.aspx External Web Site Policy.
27. US Department of Health and Human Services (n.d.). What are the Indicators of Learning Disabilities? Retrieved from https://www.nichd.nih.gov/health/topics/learning/conditioninfo/symptoms.
28. Sadock B, Kaplan H, Sadock V. *Kaplan & Sadock's Synopsis of Psychiatry: Behavioral Sciences/clinical Psychiatry*. Philadelphia: Wolter Kluwer/Lippincott Williams & Wilkins; 2007.
29. American Psychiatric Association. *Diagnostic and Statistical Manual of Mental Disorders*. 5th ed. Arlington, VA: American Psychiatric Publishing; 2013.
30. Creswell CS, Skuse DH. Autism in association with turner syndrome: genetic implications for male vulnerability to pervasive developmental disorders. *Neurocase*. 1999;5(6):511–518. https://doi.org/10.1080/13554799908402746.
31. Pinares-Garcia P, Stratikopoulos M, Zagato A, Loke H, Lee J. Sex: a significant risk factor for neurodevelopmental and neurodegenerative disorders. *Brain Sci*. 2018;8(8):E154. https://doi.org/10.3390/brainsci8080154.
32. Powers SJ, Wang Y, Beach SD, Sideridis GD, Gaab N. Examining the relationship between home literacy environment and neural correlates of phonological processing in beginning readers with and without a familial risk for dyslexia: an fMRI study. *Ann Dyslexia*. 2016;66(3):337–360. https://doi.org/10.1007/s11881-016-0134-2.
33. Muter V, Snowling MJ. Children at familial risk of dyslexia: practical implications from an at-risk study. *Child Adolesc Mental Health*. 2009;14(1):37–41. https://doi.org/10.1111/j.1475-3588.2007.00480.x.
33a. Muter V, Snowling MJ. Children at Familial Risk of Dyslexia: Practical Implications from an At-Risk Study. *Child & Adolescent Mental Health*. 2009;14(1):37–41. https://doi.org/10.1111/j.1475-3588.2007.00480.x.
34. Wang Y, Mauer MV, Raney T, et al. Development of tract-specific white matter pathways during early reading development in at-risk children and typical controls. *Cereb Cortex*. 2017;27(4):2469–2485.
35. Ashkenazi S, Black JM, Abrams DA, Hoeft F, Menon V. Neurobiological underpinnings of math and reading learning disabilities. *J Learn Disabil*. 2013;46(6):549–569. https://doi.org/10.1177/0022219413483174.
36. Langer N, Peysakhovich B, Zuk J, et al. White matter alterations in infants at risk for developmental dyslexia. *Cereb Cortex*. 2017;27(2):1027–1036.
37. Dunning DL, Westgate B, Adlam AR. A meta-analysis of working memory impairments in survivors of moderate-to-severe traumatic brain injury. *Neuropsychology*. 2016;30(7):811–819. https://doi.org/10.1037/neu0000285.
38. Centers for Disease Control and Prevention. *Report to Congress on Traumatic Brain Injury in the United States: Epidemiology and Rehabilitation*. Atlanta, GA: Author; 2015.
39. Faul M, Xu L, Wald MM, Coronado VG. *Traumatic Brain Injury in the United States: Emergency Department Visits, Hospitalizations and Deaths 2002–2006*. Atlanta, GA: Centers for Disease Control and Prevention, National Center for Injury Prevention and Control; 2010. https://doi.org/10.15620/cdc.5571.
40. Thurman DJ. The epidemiology of traumatic brain injury in children and youths: a review of research since 1990. *J Child Neurol*. 2016;31(1):20–27. https://doi.org/10.1177/0883073814544363.
41. Catroppa C, Anderson VA, Muscara F, et al. Educational skills: long-term outcome and predictors following paediatric traumatic brain injury. *Neuropsychol Rehabil*. 2009;19(5):716–732. https://doi.org/10.1080/09602010902732868.
42. Fulton JB, Yeates KO, Taylor HG, Walz NC, Wade SL. Cognitive predictors of academic achievement in young children 1 year after traumatic brain injury. *Neuropsychology*. 2012;26(3):314–322. https://doi.org/10.1037/a0027973.
43. Li L, Liu J. The effect of pediatric traumatic brain injury on behavioral outcomes: a systematic review. *Dev Med Child Neurol*. 2013;55(1):37–45. https://doi.org/10.1111/j.1469-8749.2012.04414.x.
43a. Gagner C, Landry-Roy C, Bernier A, Gravel J, Beauchamp M. Behavioral consequences of mild traumatic brain injury in preschoolers. *Psychol Med*. 2018;48(9):1551–1559. https://doi.org/10.1017/S0033291717003221.
44. Yeates KO, Swift E, Taylor HG, et al. Short- and long-term social outcomes following pediatric traumatic brain injury. *J Int Neuropsychol Soc*. 2004;10(3):412–426. https://doi.org/10.1017/S1355617704103093.
45. Anderson V, Beauchamp MH, Yeates KO, et al. Social competence at two years after childhood traumatic brain injury. *J Neurotrauma*. 2017;34(14):2261–2271. https://doi.org/10.1089/neu.2016.4692. Retrieved from.
46. Ganesalingam K, Yeates KO, Taylor HG, Walz NC, Stancin T, Wade S. Executive functions and social competence in young children 6 months following traumatic brain injury. *Neuropsychology*. 2011;25(4):466–476. https://doi.org/10.1037/a0022768.
47. Crichton A, Oakley E, Babl FE, et al. Predicting fatigue 12 months after child traumatic brain injury: child factors and postinjury symptoms. *J Int Neuropsychol Soc*. 2018;24(3):224–236. https://doi.org/10.1017/S1355617717000893.

48. Wilkinson J, Marmol NL, Godfrey C, et al. Fatigue following paediatric acquired brain injury and its impact on functional outcomes: a systematic review. *Neuropsychol Rev.* 2018;28(1):73–87. https://doi.org/10.1007/s11065-018-9370-z.
49. Gagner C, Landry-Roy C, Lainé F, Beauchamp MH. Sleep-wake disturbances and fatigue after pediatric traumatic brain injury: a systematic review of the literature. *J Neurotrauma.* 2015;32(20):1539–1552. https://doi.org/10.1089/neu.2014.3753.
50. Landry-Roy C, Bernier A, Gravel J, Beauchamp MH. Executive functions and their relation to sleep following mild traumatic brain injury in preschoolers. *J Int Neuropsychol Soc.* 2018. https://doi.org/10.1017/S1355617718000401.
51. Krasny-Pacini A, Chevignard M, Lancien S, et al. Executive function after severe childhood traumatic brain injury - age-at-injury vulnerability periods: the TGE prospective longitudinal study. *Ann Phys Rehabil Med.* 2017;60(2):74–82. https://doi.org/10.1016/j.rehab.2016.06.001.
52. Kingery KM, Narad ME, Taylor HG, Yeates KO, Stancin T, Wade SL. Do children who sustain traumatic brain injury in early childhood need and receive academic services 7 years after injury? *J Dev Behav Pediatrics.* 2017;38(9):728–735. https://doi.org/10.1097/DBP.0000000000000489.
53. McCrory E, De Brito SA, Viding E. Research review: the neurobiology and genetics of maltreatment and adversity. *J Child Psychol Psychiatry Allied Discipl.* 2010;51(10):1079–1095. https://doi.org/10.1111/j.1469-7610.2010.02271.x.
54. Mizomuri SJY, Smith DM, Puryear CB. Mnemonic contributions of hippocampal place cells. In: Martinez J, Kesner R, eds. *Neurobiology of Learning and Memory.* Burlington, MA: Elsevier; 2007:155–189. https://doi.org/10.1016/B978-012372540-0/50006-6.
54a. Cicchetti D, Tyrka AR, Ridout KK, Parade SH. Childhood adversity and epigenetic regulation of glucocorticoid signaling genes: Associations in children and adults. *Development & Psychopathology.* 2016;28(4pt2):1319–1331. https://doi.org/10.1017/S0954579416000870.
55. Gracy D, Fabian A, Basch CH, et al. Missed opportunities: do states require screening of children for health conditions that interfere with learning? *PLoS One.* 2018;13(1):e0190254. https://doi.org/10.1371/journal.pone.0190254.
56. Coleman-Jensen A, Rabbitt M, Gregory C, Singh A. *Household Food Security in the United States in 2015, ERR-215;* 2016. Retrieved from www.ers.usda.gov/webdocs/publications/79761/err-215.pdf37.
57. Alaimo K, Olson CM, Frongillo Jr EA. Food insufficiency and American school-aged children's cognitive, academic, and psychosocial development. *Pediatrics.* 2001;108(1):44–53.
58. Shankar P, Chung R, Frank DA. Association of food insecurity with children's behavioral, emotional, and academic outcomes: a systematic review. *J Dev Behav Pediatrics.* 2017;38(2):135–150.
59. Weinreb L, Wehler C, Perloff J, et al. Hunger: its impact on children's health and mental health. *Pediatrics.* 2002;110(4):e41. https://doi.org/10.1542/peds.110.4.e41.
59a. Prince D, Nurius PS. The role of positive academic self-concept in promoting school success. *Child Youth Serv Rev.* 2014;43:145–152. https://doi.org/10.1016/j.childyouth.2014.05.003.
60. Green J, Liem GA, Martin AJ, Colmar S, Marsh HW, McInerney D. Academic motivation, self-concept, engagement, and performance in high school: key processes from a longitudinal perspective. *J Adolesc.* 2012;35(5):1111–1122. https://doi.org/10.1016/j.adolescence.2012.02.016.
61. Yeung AS, Craven RG, Kaur G. Mastery goal, value and self-concept: what do they predict? *Educ Res.* 2012;54(4):469–482. https://doi.org/10.1080/00131881.2012.734728.
61a. Fiske ST, Taylor SE. *Social cognition: From brains to culture.* 2nd ed. Los Angeles, CA: Sage; 2013. https://doi.org/10.4135/9781446286395.
61b. Marsh HW, Craven RG. Reciprocal effects of self-concept and performance from a multidimensional perspective: Beyond seductive pleasure and unidimensional perspectives. *Perspectives on Psychological Science.* 2006;1:95–180.
61c. Nurius PS, Macy RJ. Cognitive behavioral theory. Human behavior in the social environment. In: Sowers KM, Dulmus CN, eds. *Comprehensive handbook of social work and social welfare.* 2nd ed. New York: Wiley; 2012:101–133; Vol. 2.
62. Huang C. Self-concept and academic achievement: a meta-analysis of longitudinal relations. *J Sch Psychol.* 2011;49(5):505–528. https://doi.org/10.1016/j.jsp.2011.07.001.
63. Hansford B, Hattie J. The relationship between self and achievement/performance measures. *Rev Educ Res.* 1982;52(1):123–142. https://doi.org/10.3102/00346543052001123.
64. Hattie JA. *Self-Concept.* Hillsdale, NJ: Lawrence Erlbaum; 1992.
65. Liu KS, Cheng YY, Chen YL, Wu YY. Longitudinal effects of educational expectations and achievement attributions on adolescents' academic achievements. *Adolescence.* 2009;44(176):911–924.
66. Marsh HW, O'Mara A. Reciprocal effects between academic self-concept, self-esteem, achievement, and attainment over seven adolescent years: unidimensional and multidimensional perspectives of self-concept. *Personal Social Psychol Bull.* 2008;34(4):542–552. https://doi.org/10.1177/0146167207312313.
67. Valentine JC, DuBois DL, Cooper H. The relation between self-beliefs and academic achievement: a meta-analytic review. *Educ Psychol.* 2004;39(2):111–133. https://doi.org/10.1207/s15326985ep3902_3.
68. West CK, Fish JA, Stevens RJ. General self-concept, self-concept of academic ability and school achievement:

implications for "causes" of self-concept. *Austr J Educ.* 1980;24(2):194–213. https://doi.org/10.1177/000494418002400207.

69. Wouters S, Germeijs V, Colpin H, Verschueren K. Academic self-concept in high school: predictors and effects on adjustment in higher education. *Scand J Psychol.* 2011;52(6):586–594. https://doi.org/10.1111/j.1467-9450.2011.00905.x.
70. Wylie RC. *Measures of Self-Concept.* U of Nebraska Press; 1989.
71. Zimmerman BJ. Self-efficacy and educational development. In: *Self-efficacy in Changing Societies.* 1995:202–231.
72. Bandura A, Barbaranelli C, Caprara GV, Pastorelli C. Self-efficacy beliefs as shapers of children's aspirations and career trajectories. *Child Dev.* 2001;72(1):187–206. https://doi.org/10.1111/1467-8624.00273.
73. Linnenbrink EA, Pintrich PR. Motivation as an enabler for academic success. *School Psychol Rev.* 2002;31(3):313–327.
74. Ma X, Kishor N. Attitude toward self, social factors, and achievement in mathematics: a meta-analytic review. *Educ Psychol Rev.* 1997;9(2):89–120. https://doi.org/10.1023/A:1024785812050.
75. Martin AJ. Examining a multidimensional model of student motivation and engagement using a construct validation approach. *Br J Educ Psychol.* 2007;77(Pt 2):413–440. https://doi.org/10.1348/000709906X118036.
76. Martin AJ. Motivation and engagement across the academic life span: a developmental construct validity study of elementary school, high school, and university/college students. *Educ Psychol Measurement.* 2009;69(5):794–824. https://doi.org/10.1177/0013164409332214.
77. Meece JL, Wigfield A, Eccles JS. Predictors of math anxiety and its influence on young adolescents' course enrollment intentions and performance in mathematics. *J Educ Psychol.* 1990;82(1):60–70. https://doi.org/10.1037/0022-0663.82.1.60.
78. Pekrun R, Goetz T, Titz W, Perry RP. *Positive Emotions in Education.* 2002.
79. Pintrich PR. A motivational science perspective on the role of student motivation in learning and teaching contexts. *J Educ Psychol.* 2003;95(4):667–686. https://doi.org/10.1037/0022-0663.95.4.667.
80. Schunk DH, Pintrich PR, Meece JL. *Motivation in Education: Theory, Research, and Applications.* 2008.
81. Valiente C, Lemery-Chalfant K, Swanson J, Reiser M. Prediction of children's academic competence from their effortful control, relationships, and classroom participation. *J Educ Psychol.* 2008;100(1):67–77. https://doi.org/10.1037/0022-0663.100.1.67.
82. Attwood G, Croll P. Truancy in secondary school pupils: prevalence, trajectories and pupil perspectives. *Res Pap Educ.* 2006;21(4):467–484. https://doi.org/10.1080/02671520600942446.
83. Vallerand RJ, Fortier MS, Guay F. Self-determination and persistence in a real-life setting: toward a motivational model of high school dropout. *J Pers Soc Psychol.* 1997;72(5):1161–1176. https://doi.org/10.1037/0022-3514.72.5.1161.
84. Caraway K, Tucker CM, Reinke WM, Hall C. Self-efficacy, goal orientation, and fear of failure as predictors of school engagement in high school students. *Psychol Sch.* 2003;40(4):417–427. https://doi.org/10.1002/pits.10092.
85. Connell JP. Context, self, and action: a motivational analysis of self-system processes across the life span. *Self Transition.* 1990;8:61–97.
86. Fredricks JA, Blumenfeld PC, Paris AH. School engagement: potential of the concept, state of the evidence. *Rev Educ Res.* 2004;74(1):59–109. https://doi.org/10.3102/00346543074001059.
87. Finn JD. *School Engagement and Students at Risk.* Washington, DC: National Center for Education Statistics; 1993.
88. Finn JD, Pannozzo GM, Voelkl KE. Disruptive and inattentive-withdrawn behavior and achievement among fourth graders. *Elem Sch J.* 1995;95(5):421–434. https://doi.org/10.1086/461853.
89. Furrer C, Skinner E. Sense of relatedness as a factor in children's academic engagement and performance. *J Educ Psychol.* 2003;95(1):148–162. https://doi.org/10.1037/0022-0663.95.1.148.
90. Jimerson SR, Campos E, Greif JL. Toward an understanding of definitions and measures of school engagement and related terms. *California Sch Psychol.* 2003;8(1):7–27. https://doi.org/10.1007/BF03340893.
91. Skinner EA, Belmont MJ. Motivation in the classroom: reciprocal effects of teacher behavior and student engagement across the school year. *J Educ Psychol.* 1993;85(4):571–581. https://doi.org/10.1037/0022-0663.85.4.571.
92. Voelkl KE. Identification with school. *Am J Educ.* 1997;105(3):294–318. https://doi.org/10.1086/444158.
93. Wang MT, Eccles JS. Adolescent behavioral, emotional, and cognitive engagement trajectories in school and their differential relations to educational success. *J Res Adolesc.* 2012;22(1):31–39. https://doi.org/10.1111/j.1532-7795.2011.00753.x.
94. Zimmerman BJ. Attaining self-regulation: a social cognitive perspective. In: *Handbook of Self-Regulation.* 2000:13–39.
95. Archambault I, Janosz M, Fallu J, Pagani LS. Student engagement and its relationship with early high school dropout. *J Adolesc.* 2009;32(3):651–670. https://doi.org/10.1016/j.adolescence.2008.06.007.
96. Marks HM. Student engagement in instructional activity: patterns in the elementary, middle, and high school years. *Am Educ Res J.* 2000;37(1):153–184. https://doi.org/10.3102/00028312037001153.
97. McDermott PA, Mordell M, Stoltzfus JC. The organization of student performance in American schools: discipline, motivation, verbal learning, nonverbal learning. *J Educ Psychol.* 2001;93(1):65–76. https://doi.org/10.1037/0022-0663.93.1.65.
98. Skinner EA, Kindermann TA, Connell JP, Wellborn JG. Engagement and disaffection as organizational constructs in the dynamics of motivational development. In: *Handbook of Motivation at School.* 2009:223–245.

99. Wang MT, Holcombe R. Adolescents' perceptions of school environment, engagement, and academic achievement in middle school. *Am Educ Res J*. 2010;47(3): 633–662. https://doi.org/10.3102/0002831209361209.
100. Henry KL, Knight KE, Thornberry TP. School disengagement as a predictor of dropout, delinquency, and problem substance use during adolescence and early adulthood. *J Youth Adolesc*. 2012;41(2):156–166. https://doi.org/10.1007/s10964-011-9665-3.
101. Appleton JJ, Christenson SL, Kim D, Reschly AL. Measuring cognitive and psychological engagement: validation of the student engagement instrument. *J Sch Psychol*. 2006;44(5):427–445. https://doi.org/10.1016/j.jsp.2006.04.002.
102. Finn JD. Withdrawing from school. *Rev Educ Res*. 1989; 59(2):117–142. https://doi.org/10.3102/00346543059002117.
103. Finn JD, Rock DA. Academic success among students at risk for school failure. *J Appl Psychol*. 1997;82(2):221. https://doi.org/10.1037/0021-9010.82.2.221.
104. Eccles JS, Midgley C. Stage/environment fit: developmentally appropriate classrooms for early adolescents. In: Ames R, Ames C, eds. *Research on Motivation in Education*. New York: Academic Press; 1989:139–181. Vol. 3.
105. Roeser RW, Eccles JS, Sameroff AJ. Academic and emotional functioning in early adolescence: longitudinal relations, patterns, and prediction by experience in middle school. *Dev Psychopathol*. 1998;10(2):321–352. https://doi.org/10.1017/S0954579498001631.
106. Schiefele J, Krapp A, Winteler A. Interest as a predictor of academic achievement: a meta-analysis of research. In: Renninger KA, Hidi S, Krapp A, eds. *The Role of Interest in Learning and Development*. Hillsdale, NJ: Lawrence Erlbaum; 1992.
107. Wigfield A, Eccles JS, Schiefele U, Roeser RW, Davis-Kean P. Development of achievement motivation. In: Eisenberg N, Damon W, Lerner RM, eds. *Social, Emotional, and Personality Development*. Hoboken, NJ, US: John Wiley & Sons Inc; 2006:933–1002. Handbook of Child Psychology.
108. Heppen JB, Therriault SB. *Developing Early Warning Systems to Identify Potential High School Dropouts*. National High School Center; 2008. Issue Brief.
109. Neild RC, Balfanz R, Herzog L. An early warning system. *Educ Leadersh*. 2007;65(2):28–33.
110. Crosnoe R, Huston AC. Socioeconomic status, schooling, and the developmental trajectories of adolescents. *Dev Psychol*. 2007;43(5):1097–1110. https://doi.org/10.1037/0012-1649.43.5.1097.
111. Findley MJ, Cooper HM. Locus of control and academic achievement: a literature review. *J Personal Soc Psychol*. 1983;44(2):419–427. https://doi.org/10.1037/0022-3514.44.2.419.
112. Ross CE, Broh BA. The role of self-esteem and the sense of personal control in the academic achievement process. *Sociol Educ*. 2000;73(4):270–284.
113. Sterbin A, Rakow E. Self-esteem, locus of control, and student achievement. In: *Paper Presented at the Annual Meeting of the Mid-south Educational Research Association, Tuscaloosa, Alabama*. 1996. ERIC Document Reproduction Service No. ED406 429.
114. Stipek DJ, Weisz JR. Perceived personal control and academic achievement. *Rev Educ Res*. 1981;51(1):101–137. https://doi.org/10.3102/00346543051001101.
115. Sisney S, Strickler B, Tyler MA, Wilhoit C, Duke M, Nowicki Jr S. *Reducing the Drop Out Rates of At-Risk High School Students: The Effective Learning Program*. Emory University; 2000.
116. Ansary NS, Luthar SS. Distress and academic achievement among adolescents of affluence: a study of externalizing and internalizing problem behaviors and school performance. *Develop Psychopathol*. 2009;21(1):319–341.
117. Bennett KJ, Brown KS, Boyle M, Racine Y, Offord D. Does low reading achievement at school entry cause conduct problems? *Social Sci Med*. 2003;56(12):2443–2448. https://doi.org/10.1016/S0277-9536(02)00247-2.
118. McCarty CA, Mason WA, Kosterman R, Hawkins JD, Lengua LJ, McCauley E. Adolescent school failure predicts later depression among girls. *J Adolesc Health*. 2008; 43(2):180–187. https://doi.org/10.1016/j.jadohealth.2008.01.023.
119. Moilanen KL, Shaw DS, Maxwell KL. Developmental cascades: externalizing, internalizing, and academic competence from middle childhood to early adolescence. *Dev Psychopathol*. 2010;22(3):635–653. https://doi.org/10.1017/S0954579410000337.
120. Breslau J, Miller E, Breslau N, Bohnert K, Lucia V, Schweitzer J. The impact of early behavior disturbances on academic achievement in high school. *Pediatrics*. 2009;123(6):1472–1476. https://doi.org/10.1542/peds.2008-1406.
121. Chen X, Rubin KH, Li D. Relation between academic achievement and social adjustment: evidence from Chinese children. *Dev Psychol*. 1997;33(3):518–525.
122. Dishion TJ, Patterson GR, Stoolmiller M, Skinner ML. Family, school, and behavioral antecedents to early adolescent involvement with antisocial peers. *Dev Psychol*. 1991;27(1):172–180. https://doi.org/10.1037/0012-1649.27.1.172.
123. Roeser RW, van der Wolf K, Strobel KR. On the relation between social–emotional and school functioning during early adolescence: preliminary findings from Dutch and American samples. *J Sch Psychol*. 2001;39(2):111–139. https://doi.org/10.1016/S0022-4405(01)00060-7.
124. Obradović J, Burt KB, Masten AS. Testing a dual cascade model linking competence and symptoms over 20 years from childhood to adulthood. *J Clin Child Adolesc Psychol*. 2010;39(1):90–102.
125. Chen X, Huang X, Chang L, Wang L, Li D. Aggression, social competence, and academic achievement in Chinese children: a 5-year longitudinal study. *Dev Psychopathol*. 2010;22(3):583–592. https://doi.org/10.1017/S0954579410000295.

126. Lewis GJ, Asbury K, Plomin R. Externalizing problems in childhood and adolescence predict subsequent educational achievement but for different genetic and environmental reasons. *J Child Psychol Psychiatry Allied Discipl.* 2017;58(3):292–304. https://doi.org/10.1111/jcpp.12655.
127. Masten AS, Roisman GI, Long JD, et al. Developmental cascades: linking academic achievement and externalizing and internalizing symptoms over 20 years. *Dev Psychol.* 2005;41(5):733–746. https://doi.org/10.1037/0012-1649.41.5.733.
128. Deighton J, Humphrey N, Belsky J, Boehnke J, Vostanis P, Patalay P. Longitudinal pathways between mental health difficulties and academic performance during middle childhood and early adolescence. *Br J Dev Psychol.* 2018;36(1):110–126. https://doi.org/10.1111/bjdp.12218.
129. Eccles JS, Roeser RW. Schools, academic motivation, and stage-environment fit. In: *Handbook of Adolescent Psychology*. Vol. 1. 2009:404–434.
130. Graber JA, Brooks-Gunn J. Transitions and turning points: navigating the passage from childhood through adolescence. *Dev Psychol.* 1996;32(4):768–776. https://doi.org/10.1037/0012-1649.32.4.768.
131. McLaughlin C, Clarke B. Relational matters: a review of the impact of school experience on mental health in early adolescence. *Educ Child Psychol.* 2010;27(1):91–103.
132. Wentzel KR. Peers and academic functioning at school. In: Rubin KH, Bukowski WM, Laursen B, eds. *Social, Emotional, and Personality Development in Context. Handbook of Peer Interactions, Relationships, and Groups*. New York, NY, US: Guilford Press; 2009:531–547.
133. Caprara GV, Barbaranelli C, Pastorelli C, Bandura A, Zimbardo PG. Prosocial foundations of children's academic achievement. *Psychol Sci.* 2000;11(4):302–306. https://doi.org/10.1111/1467-9280.00260.
134. Durlak JA, Weissberg RP, Dymnicki AB, Taylor RD, Schellinger KB. The impact of enhancing students' social and emotional learning: a meta-analysis of school-based universal interventions. *Child Dev.* 2011;82(1):405–432. https://doi.org/10.1111/j.1467-8624.2010.01564.x.
135. Elias MJ, Haynes NM. Social competence, social support, and academic achievement in minority, low-income, urban elementary school children. *Sch Psychol Q.* 2008;23(4):474–495. https://doi.org/10.1037/1045-3830.23.4.474.
136. Elliott SN, Malecki CK, Demaray MK. New directions in social skills assessment and intervention for elementary and middle school students. *Exceptionality*. 2001;9(1–2):19–32. https://doi.org/10.1080/09362835.-2001.9666989.
137. Márquez PGO, Martín RP, Brackett MA. Relating emotional intelligence to social competence and academic achievement in high school students. *Psicothema*. 2006;18(suppl):118–123.
138. Greenberg MT, Weissberg RP, O'Brien MU, et al. Enhancing school-based prevention and youth development through coordinated social, emotional, and academic learning. *Am Psychol.* 2003;58(6–7):466–474. https://doi.org/10.1037/0003-066X.58.6-7.466.
139. Hawkins JD, Kosterman R, Catalano RF, Hill KG, Abbott RD. Effects of social development intervention in childhood 15 years later. *Arch Pediatrics Adolesc Med.* 2008;162(12):1133–1141. https://doi.org/10.1001/archpedi.162.12.1133.
140. Izard C, Fine S, Schultz D, Mostow A, Ackerman B, Youngstrom E. Emotion knowledge as a predictor of social behavior and academic competence in children at risk. *Psychol Sci.* 2001;12(1):18–23. https://doi.org/10.1111/1467-9280.00304.
141. Jones SM, Bouffard SM. Social and emotional learning in schools: from programs to strategies [Society for Research in Child Development.] *Soc Policy Rep.* 2012;26(4):1–33. https://doi.org/10.1002/j.2379-3988.2012.tb00073.x.
142. Jones SM, Brown JL, Lawrence Aber J. Two-year impacts of a universal school-based social-emotional and literacy intervention: an experiment in translational developmental research. *Child Dev.* 2011;82(2):533–554. https://doi.org/10.1111/j.1467-8624.2010.01560.x.
143. Malecki CK, Elliot SN. Children's social behaviors as predictors of academic achievement: a longitudinal analysis. *Sch Psychol Q.* 2002;17(1):1–23. https://doi.org/10.1521/scpq.17.1.1.19902.
144. Seider S, Gilbert JK, Novick S, Gomez J. The role of moral and performance character strengths in predicting achievement and conduct among urban middle school students. *Teach Coll Rec.* 2013;115(8):1–19.
145. Taylor RD, Dymnicki AB. Empirical evidence of social and emotional learning's influence on school success: a commentary on "building academic success on social and emotional learning: what does the research say?" a book edited by Joseph E. Zins, Roger P. Weissberg, Margaret C. Wang, and Herbert J. Walberg. *J Educ Psychol Consult.* 2007;17(2–3):225–231.
146. Welsh M, Parke RD, Widaman K, O'Neil R. Linkages between children's social and academic competence: a longitudinal analysis. *J Sch Psychol.* 2001;39(6):463–482. https://doi.org/10.1016/S0022-4405(01)00084-X.
147. Wentzel KR. Relations between social competence and academic achievement in early adolescence. *Child Dev.* 1991a;62(5):1066–1078. https://doi.org/10.2307/1131152.
148. Wentzel KR. Social competence at school: relation between social responsibility and academic achievement. *Rev Educ Res.* 1991b;61(1):1–24. https://doi.org/10.3102/00346543061001001.
149. Zins JE, Bloodworth MR, Weissberg RP, Walberg HJ. The scientific base linking social and emotional learning to school success. In: *Building Academic Success on Social and Emotional Learning: What Does the Research Say*. 2004:3–22.
150. Oberle E, Schonert-Reichl KA, Hertzman C, Zumbo BD. Social–emotional competencies make the grade: predicting academic success in early adolescence. *J Appl Dev Psychol.* 2014;35(3):138–147. https://doi.org/10.1016/j.appdev.2014.02.004.

151. Appleton JJ, Christenson SL, Furlong MJ. Student engagement with school: critical conceptual and methodological issues of the construct. *Psychol Sch.* 2008;45(5): 369–386.
152. Libbey HP. Measuring student relationships to school: attachment, bonding, connectedness, and engagement. *J School Health.* 2004;74(7):274–283. https://doi.org/10.1111/j.1746-1561.2004.tb08284.x.
153. Whitted KS. Understanding how social and emotional skill deficits contribute to school failure. *Prev Sch Fail.* 2011;55(1):10–16. https://doi.org/10.1080/10459880903286755.
154. Zsolnai A. Relationship between children's social competence, learning motivation and school achievement. *Educ Psychol.* 2002;22(3):317–329. https://doi.org/10.1080/01443410220138548.
155. Eldreth DA, Matochik JA, Cadet JL, Bolla KI. Abnormal brain activity in prefrontal brain regions in abstinent marijuana users. *NeuroImage.* 2004;23(3):914–920. https://doi.org/10.1016/j.neuroimage.2004.07.032.
156. Lynskey M, Hall W. The effects of adolescent cannabis use on educational attainment: a review. *Addiction.* 2000; 95(11):1621–1630. https://doi.org/10.1046/j.1360-0443.2000.951116213.x.
157. Quickfall J, Crockford D. Brain neuroimaging in cannabis use: a review. *J Neuropsychiatry Clin Neurosc.* 2006;18(3): 318–332. https://doi.org/10.1176/jnp.2006.18.3.318.
158. Hall W, Pacula RL. *Cannabis Use and Dependence: Public Health and Public Policy.* UK: Cambridge University Press; 2003. https://doi.org/10.1017/CBO9780511470219.
159. Kelly AB, O'Flaherty M, Connor JP, et al. The influence of parents, siblings and peers on pre- and early-teen smoking: a multilevel model. *Drug Alcohol Rev.* 2011;30(4): 381–387. https://doi.org/10.1111/j.1465-3362.2010.00231.x.
160. Kelly AB, Chan GC, Toumbourou JW, et al. Very young adolescents and alcohol: evidence of a unique susceptibility to peer alcohol use. *Addict Behav.* 2012;37(4):414–419. https://doi.org/10.1016/j.addbeh.2011.11.038.
161. Verkooijen KT, de Vries NK, Nielsen GA. Youth crowds and substance use: the impact of perceived group norm and multiple group identification. *Psychol Addict Behav.* 2007;21(1):55–61. https://doi.org/10.1037/0893-164X.21.1.55.
162. Kandel DB, Davies M, Karus D, Yamaguchi K. The consequences in young adulthood of adolescent drug involvement. An overview. *Arch Gen Psychiatry.* 1986;43(8): 746–754. https://doi.org/10.1001/archpsyc.1986.01800080032005.
163. Presley CA, Pimentel ER. The introduction of the heavy and frequent drinker: a proposed classification to increase accuracy of alcohol assessments in postsecondary educational settings. *J Studies Alcohol.* 2006;67(2): 324–331. https://doi.org/10.15288/jsa.2006.67.324.
164. Townsend L, Flisher AJ, King G. A systematic review of the relationship between high school dropout and substance use. *Clin Child Fam Psychol Rev.* 2007;10(4):295–317. https://doi.org/10.1007/s10567-007-0023-7.
165. Eisenberg ME, Forster JL. Adolescent smoking behavior: measures of social norms. *Am J Prevent Med.* 2003;25(2):122–128. https://doi.org/10.1016/S0749-3797(03)00116-8.
166. Azagba S, Asbridge M. School connectedness and susceptibility to smoking among adolescents in Canada. *Nicotine Tob Res.* 2013;15(8):1458–1463. https://doi.org/10.1093/ntr/nts340.
167. Australian Institute of Health and Welfare (AIHW). *2010 National Drug Strategy Household Survey Report.* Canberra: AIHW; 2010. Cat no. PHE 145, Report no.: Data statistics series no. 25.
168. Macleod J, Oakes R, Copello A, et al. Psychological and social sequelae of cannabis and other illicit drug use by young people: a systematic review of longitudinal, general population studies. *Lancet.* 2004;363(9421):1579–1588. https://doi.org/10.1016/S0140-6736(04)16200-4.
169. Horwood LJ, Fergusson DM, Hayatbakhsh MR, et al. Cannabis use and educational achievement: findings from three Australasian cohort studies. *Drug Alcohol Depend.* 2010;110(3):247–253. https://doi.org/10.1016/j.drugalcdep.2010.03.008.
170. Bray JW, Zarkin GA, Ringwalt C, Qi J. The relationship between marijuana initiation and dropping out of high school. *Health Econ.* 2000;9(1):9–18. https://doi.org/10.1002/(SICI)1099-1050(200001)9:1<9::AID-HEC471>3.0.CO;2-Z.
171. Fergusson DM, Horwood LJ, Beautrais AL. Cannabis and educational achievement. *Addiction.* 2003;98(12): 1681–1692. https://doi.org/10.1111/j.1360-0443.2003.00573.x.
172. Lynskey MT, Coffey C, Degenhardt L, Carlin JB, Patton G. A longitudinal study of the effects of adolescent cannabis use on high school completion. *Addiction.* 2003;98(5): 685–692. https://doi.org/10.1046/j.1360-0443.2003.00356.x.
173. Fergusson DM, Boden JM. Cannabis use and later life outcomes. *Addiction.* 2008;103(6):969–976. https://doi.org/10.1111/j.1360-0443.2008.02221.x.
174. Cobb-Clark DA, Kassenboehmer SC, Le T, McVicar D, Zhang R. 'High'-school: the relationship between early marijuana use and educational outcomes. *Econ Rec.* 2015;91(293):247–266. https://doi.org/10.1111/1475-4932.12166.
175. Ellickson P, Bui K, Bell R, McGuigan KA. Does early drug use increase the risk of dropping out of high school? *J Drug Issues.* 1998;28(2):357–380. https://doi.org/10.1177/002204269802800205.
176. Newcomb MD, Abbott RD, Catalano RF, Hawkins JD, Battin-Pearson S, Hill K. Mediational and deviance theories of late high school failure: process roles of structural strains, academic competence, and general versus specific problem behavior. *J Couns Psychol.* 2002;49(2):172–186. https://doi.org/10.1037/0022-0167.49.2.172.
177. Crosnoe R, Benner AD, Schneider B. Drinking, socioemotional functioning, and academic progress in secondary school. *J Health Social Behav.* 2012;53(2):150–164. https://doi.org/10.1177/0022146511433507.

178. Crosnoe R, Muller C, Frank K. Peer context and the consequences of adolescent drinking. *Soc Prob*. 2004;51(2):288–304. https://doi.org/10.1525/sp.2004.51.2.288.
179. Register CA, Williams DR, Grimes PW. Adolescent drug use and educational attainment. *Educ Econ*. 2001;9(1):1–18. https://doi.org/10.1080/09645290124529.
180. Kelly AB, Chan GC, Mason WA, Williams JW. The relationship between psychological distress and adolescent polydrug use. *Psychol Addict Behav*. 2015;29(3):787–793. https://doi.org/10.1037/adb0000068.
181. Poteat VP, Scheer JR, Mereish EH. Factors affecting academic achievement among sexual minority and gender-variant youth. *Adv Child Dev Behav*. 2014;47:261–300. https://doi.org/10.1016/bs.acdb.2014.04.005.
182. Robinson JP, Espelage DL. Inequities in educational and psychological outcomes between LGBTQ and straight students in middle and high school. *Educ Res*. 2011;40(7):315–330. https://doi.org/10.3102/0013189X11422112.
183. Russell ST, Everett BG, Rosario M, Birkett M. Indicators of victimization and sexual orientation among adolescents: analyses from youth risk behavior surveys. *Am J Pub Health*. 2014;104(2):255–261. https://doi.org/10.2105/AJPH.2013.301493.
184. Russell ST, Seif H, Truong NL. School outcomes of sexual minority youth in the United States: evidence from a national study. *J Adolesc*. 2001;24(1):111–127. https://doi.org/10.1006/jado.2000.0365.
184a. Kann L, Kinchen S, Shanklin SL, Flint KH, Kawkins J, Harris WA, Zaza S. Youth risk behavior surveillance—United States, 2013. *MMWR. Surveillance Summaries*. 2014;63(4):1–168. the Centers for Disease Control and Prevention (CDC) http://www.jstor.org/stable/24806229.
185. Fergusson DM, Horwood LJ. Early disruptive behavior, IQ, and later school achievement and delinquent behavior. *J Abnorm Child Psychol*. 1995;23(2):183–199. https://doi.org/10.1007/BF01447088.
186. Katsiyannis A, Archwamety T. Academic remediation/achievement and other factors related to recidivism rates among delinquent youths. *Behav Disord*. 1999;24(2):93–101. https://doi.org/10.1177/019874299902400206.
187. Sander JB, Patall EA, Amoscato LA, Fisher AL, Funk C. A meta-analysis of the effect of juvenile delinquency interventions on academic outcomes. *Child Youth Serv Rev*. 2012;34(9):1695–1708. https://doi.org/10.1016/j.childyouth.2012.04.005.
188. Stone S, Zibulsky J. Maltreatment, academic difficulty, and systems-involved youth: current evidence and opportunities. *Psychol Sch*. 2015;52(1):22–39. https://doi.org/10.1002/pits.21812.
189. Bender K. Why do some maltreated youth become juvenile offenders?: a call for further investigation and adaptation of youth services. *Child Youth Serv Rev*. 2010;32(3):466–473. https://doi.org/10.1016/j.childyouth.2009.10.022.
190. Maxfield MG, Widom CS. The cycle of violence. Revisited 6 years later. *Arch Pediatrics Adolesc Med*. 1996;150(4):390–395. https://doi.org/10.1001/archpedi.1996.02170290056009.
191. Widom CS. The cycle of violence. *Science*. 1989;244(4901):160–166.
192. Sander JB. School psychology, juvenile justice, and the school to prison pipeline. *Communique*. 2010;39(4):4–6.
193. Herz DC, Ryan JP. Building multisystem approaches in child welfare and juvenile justice. In: *Bridging Two Worlds: Youth Involved in the Child Welfare and Juvenile Justice Systems: A Policy Guide for Improving Outcomes*. 2008:27–113.
194. Fredricks JA. Extracurricular participation and academic outcomes: testing the over-scheduling hypothesis. *J Youth Adolesc*. 2012;41(3):295–306. https://doi.org/10.1007/s10964-011-9704-0.
195. Busseri MA, Rose-Krasnor L, Willoughby T, Chalmers H. A longitudinal examination of breadth and intensity of youth activity involvement and successful development. *Dev Psychol*. 2006;42(6):1313–1326. https://doi.org/10.1037/0012-1649.42.6.1313.
196. Marsh H, Kleitman S. Extracurricular school activities: the good, the bad, and the nonlinear. *Harvard Educ Rev*. 2002;72(4):464–515. https://doi.org/10.17763/haer.72.4.051388703v7v7736.
197. Fletcher JM, Lyon GR, Fuchs LS, Barnes MA. *Learning Disabilities: From Identification to Intervention*. New York: Guilford; 2007.
198. Montague M, Enders C, Cavendish W, Castro M. Academic and behavioral trajectories for at-risk adolescents in urban schools. *Behav Disord*. 2011;36(2):141–156.
199. Shaywitz SE, Shaywitz BA. Reading disability and the brain. *Educ Leadersh*. 2004;61(6):6–11.
200. Boden JM, Horwood LJ, Fergusson DM. Exposure to childhood sexual and physical abuse and subsequent educational achievement outcomes. *Child Abuse Neglect*. 2007;31(10):1101–1114. https://doi.org/10.1016/j.chiabu.2007.03.022.
201. Chandy JM, Blum RW, Resnick MD. Gender-specific outcomes for sexually abused adolescents. *Child Abuse Neglect*. 1996;20(12):1219–1231. https://doi.org/10.1016/S0145-2134(96)00117-2.
202. Eckenrode J, Laird M, Doris J. School performance and disciplinary problems among abused and neglected children. *Dev Psychol*. 1993;29(1):53–62. https://doi.org/10.1037/0012-1649.29.1.53.
203. Einbender AJ, Friedrich WN. Psychological functioning and behavior of sexually abused girls. *J Consul Clin Psychol*. 1989;57(1):155–157. https://doi.org/10.1037/0022-006X.57.1.155.
204. Frothingham TE, Hobbs CJ, Wynne JM, Yee L, Goyal A, Wadsworth DJ. Follow up study eight years after diagnosis of sexual abuse. *Arch Dis Child*. 2000;83(2):132–134. https://doi.org/10.1136/adc.83.2.132.
205. Holt MK, Finkelhor D, Kantor GK. Multiple victimization experiences of urban elementary school students: associations with psychosocial functioning and academic performance. *Child Abuse Neglect*. 2007;31(5):503–515 https://doi.org/10.1016/j.chiabu.2006.12.006.

206. Leiter J, Johnsen MC. Child maltreatment and school performance. *Am J Educ.* 1994;102(2):154–189. https://doi.org/10.1086/444063.
207. Lisak D, Luster L. Educational, occupational, and relationship histories of men who were sexually and/or physically abused as children. *J Traumatic Stress.* 1994; 7(4):507–523. https://doi.org/10.1002/jts.2490070402.
208. Nikulina V, Widom CS, Czaja S. The role of childhood neglect and childhood poverty in predicting mental health, academic achievement and crime in adulthood. *Am J Commun Psychol.* 2011;48(3–4):309–321. https://doi.org/10.1007/s10464-010-9385-y.
209. Perez CM, Widom CS. Childhood victimization and long-term intellectual and academic outcomes. *Child Abuse Neglect.* 1994;18(8):617–633. https://doi.org/10.1016/0145-2134(94)90012-4.
210. Schwartz D, Lansford JE, Dodge KA, Pettit GS, Bates JE. The link between harsh home environments and negative academic trajectories is exacerbated by victimization in the elementary school peer group. *Dev Psychol.* 2013;49(2): 305–316. https://doi.org/10.1037/a0028249.
211. Shonk SM, Cicchetti D. Maltreatment, competency deficits, and risk for academic and behavioral maladjustment. *Dev Psychol.* 2001;37(1):3–17. https://doi.org/10.1037/0012-1649.37.1.3.
212. Wodarski JS, Kurtz PD, Gaudin Jr JM, Howing PT. Maltreatment and the school-age child: major academic, socioemotional, and adaptive outcomes. *Social Work.* 1990;35(6): 506–513. https://doi.org/10.1093/sw/35.6.506.
213. Karr-Morse R, Wiley MS. *Scared Sick: The Role of Childhood Trauma in Adult Disease.* New York, NY, US: Basic Books; 2012.
213a. Nakazawa DJ. *Childhood disrupted: How your biography becomes your biology, and how you can heal.* New York, NY: Atria Books National Education Association; 2015 (n.d.). Students affected by achievement gaps www.nea.org/home/20380.htm.
214. Johnson ME. The effects of traumatic experiences on academic relationships and expectations in justice-involved children. *Psychol Sch.* 2018;55(3):240–249. https://doi.org/10.1002/pits.22102.
215. Perry BD. Traumatized children: how childhood trauma influences brain development. *J California Alliance Mentally Ill.* 2000;11(1):48–51.
216. Cole SF, O'Brien JG, Gadd MG, Ristuccia J, Wallace DL, Gregory M. *Helping Traumatized Children Learn: Supportive School Environments for Children Traumatized by Family Violence.* Boston, MA: Massachusetts Advocates for Children; 2005.
217. De Bellis MD, Zisk A. The biological effects of childhood trauma. *Child Adolesc Psychiatric Clin North America.* 2014;23(2):185–222. https://doi.org/10.1016/j.chc.2014.01.002. vii.
218. Perry BD, Pollard RA, Blakley TL, Baker WL, Vigilante D. Childhood trauma, the neurobiology of adaptation, and "use-dependent" development of the brain: how "states" become "traits. *Infant Mental Health J.* 1995;16(4): 271–291. https://doi.org/10.1002/1097-0355(199524)16:4<271::AID-IMHJ2280160404>3.0.CO;2-B.
219. Schwarz ED, Perry BD. The post-traumatic response in children and adolescents. *Psychiatric Clin North America.* 1994;17(2):311–326. https://doi.org/10.1016/S0193-953X(18)30117-5.
220. Holt S, Buckley H, Whelan S. The impact of exposure to domestic violence on children and young people: a review of the literature. *Child Abuse Neglect.* 2008;32(8): 797–810.
221. Noltemeyer AL, Ward RM, McLoughlin C. Relationship between school suspension and student outcomes: a meta-analysis. *Sch Psychol Rev.* 2015;44(2):224–240. https://doi.org/10.17105/spr-14-0008.1.
222. Perry BL, Morris EW. Suspending progress: collateral consequences of exclusionary punishment in public schools. *Am Sociol Rev.* 2014;79(6):1067–1087. https://doi.org/10.1177/0003122414556308.
223. Pinquart M. Associations of parenting styles and dimensions with academic achievement in children and adolescents: a meta-analysis. *Educ Psychol Rev.* 2016; 28(3):475–493. https://doi.org/10.1007/s10648-015-9338-y.
224. Martinot D, Monteil JM. Use of the self-concept in forming preferences by French students of different levels of academic achievement. *J Soc Psychol.* 2000;140(1): 119–131. https://doi.org/10.1080/00224540009600450.
225. Molepo LS, Maunganidze L, Mudhovozi P, Sodi T. Teacher ratings of academic achievement of children between 6 and 12 years old from intact and non-intact families. *Perspec Educ.* 2010;28(1):44–51.
226. Atwood JD, Schuster D, Tempestini M. *Dealing With 'Broken' Homes;* 1994. Retrieved on 31 August 2018 from http://findarticles.com/.
227. Carnegie Council on Adolescent Development. *Great Transitions: Preparing Adolescents for a New Century.* New York: Carnegie Corp; 1995.
228. Downey DB. The school performance of children from single-mother and single- father families: economic or interpersonal deprivation? *J Fam Issues.* 1994;15(1): 129–147. https://doi.org/10.1177/019251394015001006.
229. Dryfoos JG. *Safe Passage: Making it Through Adolescence in a Risky Society.* New York: Oxford University Press; 1998.
230. Ermisch JF, Francesconi M. Family structure and children's achievements. *J Popul Econ.* 2001;14(2):249–270. https://doi.org/10.1007/s001480000028.
231. Jimerson S, Egeland B, Teo A. A longitudinal study of achievement trajectories: factors associated with change. *J Educ Psychol.* 1999;91(1):116–126. https://doi.org/10.1037/0022-0663.91.1.116.
232. Lleras C. Employment, work conditions, and the home environment in single-mother families. *J Fam Issues.* 2008;29(10):1268–1297. https://doi.org/10.1177/0192513X08318842.
233. Masten AS, Coatsworth JD. The development of competence in favorable and unfavorable environments. Lessons from research on successful children. *Am Psychol.*

1998;53(2):205–220. https://doi.org/10.1037/0003-066X.53.2.205.

234. Smit ME. Divorce: a typical feature of a contemporary anti-child culture. *Child Abuse Res South Africa*. 2010; 11(1):11–15.

235. Størksen I, Røysamb E, Holmen TL, Tambs K. Adolescent adjustment and well-being: effects of parental divorce and distress. *Scand J Psychol*. 2006;47(1):75–84. https://doi.org/10.1111/j.1467-9450.2006.00494.x.

236. Björklund A, Sundström M. Parental separation and children's educational attainment: a siblings analysis on Swedish register data. *Economica*. 2006;73(292):605–624. https://doi.org/10.1111/j.1468-0335.2006.00529.x.

237. Ermisch J, Francesconi M, Pevalin DJ. Parental partnership and joblessness in childhood and their influence on young people's outcomes. *J Royal Stat Soc*. 2004;167(1):69–101. https://doi.org/10.1111/j.1467-985X.2004.00292.x.

238. Albertini M, Dronkers J. Effects of divorce on children's educational attainment in a Mediterranean and Catholic society: evidence from Italy. *Europ Soc*. 2009;11(1): 137–159.

239. Stone S. Child maltreatment, out-of-home placement and academic vulnerability: a fifteen-year review of evidence and future directions. *Child Youth Serv Rev*. 2007; 29(2):139–161. https://doi.org/10.1016/j.childyouth.2006.05.001.

240. Wulczyn F, Smithgall C, Chen L. Child well-being: the intersection of schools and child welfare. *Rev Res Educ*. 2009;33(1):35–62. https://doi.org/10.3102/0091732X08327208.

241. Blome WW. What happens to foster kids: educational experiences of a random sample of foster care youth and a matched group of non-foster care youth. *Child Adoles Social Work J*. 1997;14(1):41–53. https://doi.org/10.1023/A:1024592813809.

242. George RM, Voorhis JV, Grant S, Casey K, Robinson M. Special education experiences of foster children: an empirical study. *Child Welfare*. 1992;11:419–437.

243. Jonson-Reid M, Drake B, Kim J, Porterfield S, Han L. A prospective analysis of the relationship between reported child maltreatment and special education eligibility among poor children. *Child Maltreat*. 2004;9(4): 382–394. https://doi.org/10.1177/1077559504269192.

244. Burley M, Halpern M. *Educational Attainment of Foster Youth: Achievement and Graduation Outcomes for Children in State Care*; 2001. Retrieved from http://findarticles.com.

245. Conger D, Rebeck A. *How Children's Foster Care Experiences Affect Their Education*. New York: New York City Administration for Children's Services; 2001. Retrieved from http://findarticles.com/.

246. Smithgall C, Gladden RM, Howard E, George R, Courtney ME. *Educational Experiences of Children in Out-Of-Home Care*. Chicago, IL: Chapin Hall Center for Children at the University of Chicago; 2004.

247. van Ijzendoorn MH, Juffer F. The Emanuel Miller Memorial Lecture 2006: adoption as intervention. Meta-analytic evidence for massive catch-up and plasticity in physical, socio-emotional, and cognitive development. *J Child Psychol Psychiatry Allied Discipl*. 2006;47(12):1228–1245. https://doi.org/10.1111/j.1469-7610.2006.01675.x.

248. van Ijzendoorn MH, Juffer F, Poelhuis CWK. Adoption and cognitive development: a meta-analytic comparison of adopted and non adopted children's IQ and school performance. *Psychol Bull*. 2005;131(2):301–316. https://doi.org/10.1037/0033-2909.131.2.301.

249. Dalen M, Rygvold AL. Educational achievement in adopted children from China. *Adop Q*. 2006;9(4): 45–58. https://doi.org/10.1300/J145v09n04_03.

250. You S, Hong S, Ho H. Longitudinal effects of perceived control on academic achievement. *J Educ Res*. 2011; 104(4):253–266. https://doi.org/10.1080/00220671003733807.

251. Dubow EF, Boxer P, Huesmann LR. Long-term effects of parents' education on children's educational and occupational success: mediation by family interactions, child aggression, and teenage aspirations. *Merrill-Palmer Q*. 2009;55(3):224.

252. Entwisle DR, Alexander KL, Olson LS. First grade and educational attainment by age 22: a new story. *Am J Sociol*. 2005;110(5):1458–1502. https://doi.org/10.1086/428444.

253. Pagani L, Boulerice B, Vitaro F, Tremblay RE. Effects of poverty on academic failure and delinquency in boys: a change and process model approach. *J Child Psychol Psychiatry*. 1999;40(8):1209–1219. https://doi.org/10.1111/1469-7610.00537.

254. Sirin SR. Socioeconomic status and academic achievement: a meta-analytic review of research. *Rev Educ Res*. 2005;75(3):417–453. https://doi.org/10.3102/00346543075003417.

255. White KR. The relation between socioeconomic status and academic achievement. *Psychol Bull*. 1982;91(3): 461–481. https://doi.org/10.1037/0033-2909.91.3.461.

256. Brooks-Gunn J, Klebanov PK, Liaw FR. The learning, physical, and emotional environment of the home in the context of poverty: the Infant Health and Development Program. *Child Youth Serv Rev*. 1995; 17(1–2):251–276. https://doi.org/10.1016/0190-7409(95)00011-Z.

257. Farrington DP. Multiple risk factors for multiple problem violent boys. In: Corrado RR, Roesch R, Hart SD, Gierowski JK, eds. *Multi-problem Violent Youth: A Foundation for Comparative Research on Needs, Interventions and Outcomes*. Amsterdam: IOS Press; 2002:23–34.

258. Grogan-Kaylor A, Otis MD. The effect of childhood maltreatment on adult criminality: a tobit regression analysis. *Child Maltreat*. 2003;8(2):129–137. https://doi.org/10.1177/1077559502250810.

259. Hsieh CC, Pugh MD. Poverty, income inequality, and violent crime: a meta-analysis of recent aggregate data studies. *Crim Justice Rev*. 1993;18(2):182–202. https://doi.org/10.1177/073401689301800203.

260. Kessler RC, Neighbors HW. A new perspective on the relationships among race, social class, and psychological distress. *J Health Soc Behav*. 1986;27(2):107–115. https://doi.org/10.2307/2136310PMID:3734380.

261. Sullivan A, Ketende S, Joshi H. Social class and inequalities in early cognitive scores. *Sociology*. 2013;47(6):1187–1206. https://doi.org/10.1177/0038038512461861.
262. Bradley RH, Corwyn RF. Socioeconomic status and child development. *Ann Rev Psychol*. 2002;53(1):371–399. https://doi.org/10.1146/annurev.psych.53.100901.135233.
263. Hetzner NP, Johnson AD, Brooks-Gunn J. Poverty, effects of on social and emotional development. *Int Encyclopedia Educ*. 2010:643–652. https://doi.org/10.1016/B978-0-08-044894-7.00617-5.
264. Bast J, Reitsma P. Analyzing the development of individual differences in terms of Matthew effects in reading: results from a Dutch Longitudinal study. *Dev Psychol*. 1998; 34(6):1373–1399. https://doi.org/10.1037/0012-1649.34.6.1373.
265. DiPrete TA, Eirich GM. Cumulative advantage as a mechanism for inequality: a review of theoretical and empirical developments. *Ann Rev Sociol*. 2006;32:271–297. https://doi.org/10.1146/annurev.soc.32.061604.123127.
266. Jensen AR. Cumulative deficit in compensatory education. *J Sch Psychol*. 1966;4(3):37–47. https://doi.org/10.1016/0022-4405(66)90006-9.
267. Jensen AR. Cumulative deficit: a testable hypothesis? *Dev Psychol*. 1974;10(6):996–1019. https://doi.org/10.1037/h0037246.
268. Neal DA. Why has black-white skill convergence stopped? In: Hanushek EA, Welch F, eds. *Handbook of the Economics of Education*. New York: Elsevier; 2006: 511–576. Vol. 1.
269. Phillips M, Brooks-Gunn J, Duncan GJ, Klebanov P, Crane J. Family background, parenting practices, and the black–white test score gap. In: Jencks C, Phillips M, eds. *The Black–White Test Score Gap*. Washington, DC: Brookings; 1998:103–144.
270. Reardon SF. The widening academic achievement gap between the rich and the poor: new evidence and possible explanations. *Whither Oppor*. 2011:91–116.
271. Reardon SF, Galindo C. The Hispanic-White achievement gap in math and reading in the elementary grades. *Am Educ Res J*. 2009;46(3):853–891. https://doi.org/10.3102/0002831209333184.
272. Reardon SF, Portilla XA. Recent trends in income, racial, and ethnic school readiness gaps at kindergarten entry. *AERA Open*. 2016;2(3):1–18. https://doi.org/10.1177/2332858416657343.
273. Caro D, McDonald T, Willms JD. Socio-economic status and academic achievement trajectories from childhood to adolescence. *Can J Educ*. 2009;32(3):558–590.
274. Alexander KL, Entwisle DR, Kabbani NS. The dropout process in life course perspective: early risk factors at home and school. *Teach Coll Rec*. 2001;103(5): 760–822.
275. Battin-Pearson S, Newcomb MD, Abbott RD, Hill KG, Catalano RF, Hawkins JD. Predictors of early high school dropout: a test of five theories. *J Educ Psychol*. 2000;92(3):568–582. https://doi.org/10.1037/0022-0663.92.3.568.
276. Cairns RB, Cairns BD, Neckerman HJ. Early school dropout: configurations and determinants. *Child Dev*. 1989;60(6):1437–1452. https://doi.org/10.2307/1130933.
277. Janosz M, LeBlanc M, Boulerice B, Tremblay RE. Disentangling the weight of school dropout predictors: a test on two longitudinal samples. *J Youth Adolesc*. 1997;26(6): 733–762. https://doi.org/10.1023/A:1022300826371.
278. Rumberger RW. Why students drop out of school. In: Orfield G, ed. *Dropouts in America: Confronting the Graduation Rate Crisis*. Cambridge, MA: Harvard Education Press; 2004:131–156.
279. Schargel FP. School dropouts: a national issue. In: *Helping Students Graduate: A Strategic Approach to Dropout Prevention*. Larchmont, NY: Eye on Education; 2004.
280. Condron DJ. Stratification and educational sorting: explaining ascriptive inequalities in early childhood reading group placement. *Social Problems*. 2007;54(1): 139–160. https://doi.org/10.1525/sp.2007.54.1.139.
281. Krahn H, Taylor A. "Streaming" in the 10th grade in four Canadian provinces in 2000. *Educ Mat*. 2007;4(2).
282. Maaz K, Trautwein U, Lüdtke O, Baumert J. Educational transitions and differential learning environments: how explicit between-school tracking contributes to social inequality in educational outcomes. *Child Dev Perspect*. 2008;2(2):99–106. https://doi.org/10.1111/j.1750-8606.2008.00048.x.
283. Schnabel KU, Alfeld C, Eccles JS, Köller O, Baumert J. Parental influence on students' educational choices in the United States and Germany: different ramifications—same effect? *J Vocat Behav*. 2002;60(2):178–198. https://doi.org/10.1006/jvbe.2001.1863.
283a. Davies S, Guppy N. *The schooled society: An introduction to the sociology of education*. New York, NY: Oxford University Press; 2010.
284. Cabrera AF, La Nasa SM. On the path to college: three critical tasks facing America's disadvantaged. *Res Higher Educ*. 2001;42(2):119–149. https://doi.org/10.1023/A:1026520002362.
285. Kerckhoff AC, Raudenbush SW, Glennie E. Education, cognitive skill, and labor force outcomes. *Sociol Educ*. 2001;74(1):1–24. https://doi.org/10.2307/2673142.
286. Raudenbush S, Kasim R. Cognitive skill and economic inequality: findings from the national adult literacy survey. *Harvard Educ Rev*. 1998;68(1):33–80. https://doi.org/10.17763/haer.68.1.1j47150021346123.
287. Kao G, Thompson JS. Racial and ethnic stratification in educational achievement and attainment. *Ann Rev Sociol*. 2003;29(1):417–442. https://doi.org/10.1146/annurev.soc.29.010202.100019.
288. Reardon SF, Robinson JP. Patterns and trends in racial/ethnic and socioeconomic academic achievement gaps. In: *Handbook of Research in Education Finance and Policy*. 2008:497–516.
289. Hauser R, Anderson D. Post-high school plans and aspirations of black and white high school seniors: 1976–86. *Sociol Educ*. 1991;64(4):263–277. https://doi.org/10.2307/2112707.

290. Kao G, Tienda M. Educational aspirations of minority youth. *Am J Educ*. 1998;106(3):349–384. https://doi.org/10.1086/444188.
291. Goyette K, Xie Y. Educational expectations of asian american youths: determinants and ethnic differences. *Sociol Educ*. 1999;72(1):22–36. https://doi.org/10.2307/2673184.
292. Kao G, Tienda M, Schneider B. Racial and ethnic variation in academic performance. *Res Sociol Educ Soc*. 1996;11: 263–297.
293. Braddock JH. Tracking the middle grades: national patterns of grouping for instruction. *Phi Delta Kappan*. 1990;71(6):445–449.
294. Oakes J. Limiting opportunity: student race and curricular differences in secondary vocational education. *Am J Educ*. 1983;91(3):328–355. https://doi.org/10.1086/443693.
295. Oakes J. Opportunities, achievement, and choice: women and minority students in science and mathematics. *Rev Res Educ*. 1990;16:153–222.
296. Ekstrom RB, Goertz ME, Rock DA. *Education and American Youth: The Impact of the High School Experience*. Taylor & Francis; 1988.
297. Kubitschek WN, Hallinan MT. Race, gender, and inequity in track assignments. *Res Sociol Educ Soc*. 1996;11:121–146.
298. Oakes J. *Keeping Track: How Schools Structure Inequality*. New Haven, CT: Yale University Press; 1985.
299. Oakes J, Guiton G. Matchmaking: the dynamics of high school tracking decisions. *Am Educ Res J*. 1995;32(1): 3–33. https://doi.org/10.3102/00028312032001003.
300. Slavin RE, Braddock III JH. Ability grouping: on the wrong track. *Coll Board Rev*. 1993;168:11–17.
301. Garcia E. *Inequalities at the Starting Gate: Cognitive and Noncognitive Skills Gaps between 2010–2011 Kindergarten Classmates*. Washington, DC: Economic Policy Institute; 2015. Retrieved from http://s4.epi.org/files/pdf/85032c.pdf.
302. McLaren P. Broken dreams, false promises, and the decline of public schooling. *J Educ*. 1988;170(1): 41–65. https://doi.org/10.1177/002205748817000105.
303. Teachman J, Paasch K, Carver K. Social capital and dropping out of school early. *J Marriage Fam*. 1996;58(3): 773–783. https://doi.org/10.2307/353735.
304. Velez W. High school attrition among hispanic and nonhispanic white youths. *Sociol Educ*. 1989;62(2):119–133. https://doi.org/10.2307/2112844.
305. Warren J. Educational inequality among white and mexican-origin adolescents in the american southwest: 1990. *Sociol Educ*. 1996;69(2):142–158. https://doi.org/10.2307/2112803.
306. White M, Kaufman G. Language usage, social capital, and school completion among immigrants and native-born ethnic groups. *Soc Sci Q*. 1997;78(2):385–398. Retrieved from http://www.jstor.org/stable/42864344.
307. Gibson MA, Ogbu JU. *Minority Status and Schooling: A Comparative Study of Immigrant and Involuntary Minorities*. New York, NY: Garland Publishing, Inc; 1991.
308. Kao G, Tienda M. Optimism and achievement: the educational performance of immigrant youth. *Soc Sci Q*. 1995; 76(1):1–19.
309. Rumbaut RG. *Immigrant Students in California Public Schools Microform: A Summary of Current Knowledge*. Baltimore, MD: Center for Research on Effective Schooling for Disadvantaged Students; 1990.
310. Suarez-Orozco MM. *Central American Refugees and U.S. High Schools: A Psychosocial Study of Motivation and Achievement*. Stanford University Press; 1989.
311. Zhou M. Growing up American: the challenge confronting immigrant children and children of immigrants. *Ann Rev Sociol*. 1997;23(1):63–95. https://doi.org/10.1146/annurev.soc.23.1.63.
311a. Mikami AY, Ruzek EA, Hafen CA, Gregory A, Allen JP. Perceptions of relatedness with classroom peers promote adolescents' behavioral engagement and achievement in secondary school. *Journal of Youth and Adolescence*. 2017; 46(11):2341–2354. https://doi.org/10.1007/s10964-017-0724-2.
312. Hamm JV, Faircloth BS. The role of friendship in adolescents' sense of school belonging. *New Dir Child Adolesc Dev*. 2005;2005(107):61–78. https://doi.org/10.1002/cd.121.
313. Appleyard K, Egeland B, van Dulmen MH, Sroufe LA. When more is not better: the role of cumulative risk in child behavior outcomes. *J Child Psychol Psychiatry*. 2005;46(3):235–245. https://doi.org/10.1111/j.1469-7610.2004.00351.x.
314. Holt MK, Espelage DL. A cluster analytic investigation of victimization among high school students: are profiles differentially associated with psychological symptoms and school belonging? In: Elias MJ, Zins JE, eds. *Bullying, Peer Harassment, and Victimization in the Schools: The Next Generation of Prevention*. New York: The Haworth Press, Inc; 2003:81–98.
315. Hughes HM, Parkinson D, Vargo M. Witnessing spouse abuse and experiencing physical abuse: a "double whammy"? *J Fam Viol*. 1989;4(2):197–209.
316. Naar-King S, Silvern L, Ryan V, Sebring D. Type and severity of abuse as predictors of psychiatric symptoms in adolescence. *J Fam Viol*. 2002;17(2):133–149. https://doi.org/10.1023/A:1015057416979.
317. Sternberg KJ, Lamb ME, Guterman E, Abbott CB. Effects of early and later family violence on children's behavior problems and depression: a longitudinal, multi-informant perspective. *Child Abuse Neglect*. 2006;30(3): 283–306. https://doi.org/10.1016/j.chiabu.2005.10.008.
318. Jimerson SR, Haddock AD. Understanding the importance of teachers in facilitating student success: contemporary science, practice, and policy. *Sch Psychol Q*. 2015; 30(4):488–493. https://doi.org/10.1037/spq0000134.
319. O'Connor E, McCartney K. Examining teacher–child relationships and achievement as part of an ecological model of development. *Am Educ Res J*. 2007;44(2): 340–369. https://doi.org/10.3102/0002831207302172.
320. Hattie JA. *Visible Learning: A Synthesis of 800+ Meta-Analyses on Achievement*. Abingdon: Routledge; 2009.
320a. Leigh A. Estimating teacher effectiveness from two-year changes in students' test scores. *Economics of Education Review*. 2010;29(3):480–488.

321. McNeal R. Are students being pulled out of high school? The effect of adolescent employment on dropping out. *Sociol Educ.* 1997;70(3):206–220. https://doi.org/10.2307/2673209.
322. Warren JR, LePore PC, Mare RD. Employment during high school: consequences for students' grades in academic courses. *Am Educ Res J.* 2000;37(4):943–969. https://doi.org/10.3102/00028312037004943.
323. Warren JR. Reconsidering the relationship between student employment and academic outcomes: a new theory and better data. *Youth Soc.* 2002;33(3):366–393. https://doi.org/10.1177/0044118X02033003002.
324. Borofsky LA, Kellerman I, Baucom B, Oliver PH, Margolin G. Community violence exposure and adolescents' school engagement and academic achievement over time. *Psychol Viol.* 2013;3(4):381–395. https://doi.org/10.1037/a0034121.
325. Lepore SJ, Kliewer W. Violence exposure, sleep disturbance, and poor academic performance in middle school. *J Abnorm Child Psychol.* 2013;41(8):1179–1189. https://doi.org/10.1007/s10802-013-9709-0.
326. Schwartz D, Kelly BM, Mali LV, Duong MT. Exposure to violence in the community predicts friendships with academically disengaged peers during middle adolescence. *J Youth Adolesc.* 2016;45(9):1786–1799. https://doi.org/10.1007/s10964-016-0485-3.
327. Tingir S, Cavlazoglu B, Caliskan O, Koklu O, Intepe-Tingir S. Effects of mobile devices on K–12 students' achievement: a meta-analysis. *J Comp Assist Learn.* 2017; 33(4):355–369. https://doi.org/10.1111/jcal.12184.
328. Lemola S, Perkinson-Gloor N, Brand S, Dewald-Kaufmann JF, Grob A. Adolescents' electronic media use at night, sleep disturbance, and depressive symptoms in the smartphone age. *J Youth Adolesc.* 2015;44(2): 405–418. https://doi.org/10.1007/s10964-014-0176-x.
329. Tang S, Patrick ME. Technology and interactive social media use among 8th and 10th graders in the US and associations with homework and school grades. *Comput Hum Behav.* 2018;86:34–44. https://doi.org/10.1016/j.chb.2018.04.025.
330. Valkenburg PM, Peter J. The differential susceptibility to media effects model. *J Commun.* 2013;63(2):221–243. https://doi.org/10.1111/jcom.12024.
331. Gardella JH, Fisher BW, Teurbe-Tolon AR. A systematic review and meta-analysis of cyber-victimization and educational outcomes for adolescents. *Rev Educ Res.* 2017;87(2):283–308. https://doi.org/10.3102/0034654316689136.
332. Louw AE, Winter M. The use and trends of information and communication technology (ICT) during middle childhood. *J Child Adolesc Mental Health.* 2011;23(1): 29–42. https://doi.org/10.2989/17280583.2011.594247.
333. Cantor P, Osher D, Berg J, Steyer L, Rose T. Malleability, plasticity, and individuality: how children learn and develop in context. *Appl Dev Sci.* 2018. https://doi.org/10.1080/10888691.2017.1398649.
334. Fischer KW, Bidell TR. Dynamic development of action, thought, and emotion. In: Lerner RM, ed. *Handbook of Child Psychology*. New York, NY: Wiley; 2006:313–399. Theoretical Models of Human Development. 6th ed.; Vol. 1.
335. Osher D, Cantor P, Berg J, Steyer L, Rose T. Drivers of human development: how relationships and context shape learning and development. *Appl Dev Sci.* 2018. https://doi.org/10.1080/10888691.2017.1398650.
336. Strassfeld NM. The future of idea: monitoring disproportionate representation of minority students in special education and intentional discrimination claims. *Case W Res L Rev.* 2017;67(4):1121–1151.
337. Blackwell LS, Trzesniewski KH, Dweck CS. Implicit theories of intelligence predict achievement across an adolescent transition: a longitudinal study and an intervention. *Child Dev.* 2007;78(1):246–263. https://doi.org/10.1111/j.1467-8624.2007.00995.x.
338. Burnette JL, O'Boyle EH, VanEpps EM, Pollack JM, Finkel EJ. Mind-sets matter: a meta-analytic review of implicit theories and self-regulation. *Psychol Bull.* 2013; 139(3):655–701. https://doi.org/10.1037/a0029531.
338a. Burnette JL, Russell MV, Hoyt CL, Orvidas K, Widman L. An online growth mindset intervention in a sample of rural adolescent girls. *British Journal of Educational Psychology.* 2018;88(3):428–445. https://doi.org/10.1111/bjep.12192.
339. Good C, Aronson J, Inzlicht M. Improving adolescents' standardized test performance: an intervention to reduce the effects of stereotype threat. *J Appl Dev Psychol.* 2003; 24(6):645–662. https://doi.org/10.1016/j.appdev.2003.09.002.
340. Penney CG. Rethinking the concept of learning disability. *Canad Psychol.* 2018;59(2):197–202. https://doi.org/10.1037/cap0000128.
341. Kim J, Bryan J. A first step to a conceptual framework of parent empowerment: exploring relationships between parent empowerment and academic performance in a national sample. *J Couns Dev.* 2017;95(2):168–179. https://doi.org/10.1002/jcad.12129.
342. Wingate SE, Postlewaite RR, Mena RM, Neely-Barnes SL, Elswick SE. Parent knowledge of and experiences with response to intervention. *Child Sch.* 2018;40(3): 163–172. https://doi.org/10.1093/cs/cdy010.
343. Riddle S. Ecological congruence and the identification of learning disabilities [Springer US.] *Child Youth Care Forum.* 2017;46(2):161–174. https://doi.org/10.1007/s10566-016-9376-8.

## FURTHER READING

1. Burnette JL, Russell MV, Hoyt CL, Orvidas K, Widman L. An online growth mindset intervention in a sample of rural adolescent girls. *Br J Educ Psychol.* 2017;88(3):428–445. https://doi.org/10.1111/bjep.12192.
2. Davies S, Guppy N. *The Schooled Society: An Introduction to the Sociology of Education.* New York, NY: Oxford University Press; 2010.
3. Farrington DP. Developmental and life-course criminology: key theoretical and empirical issues—the 2002 Sutherland

award address. *Criminology*. 2003;41(2):221–225. https://doi.org/10.1111/j.1745-9125.2003.tb00987.x.
4. Fiske ST, Taylor SE. *Social Cognition: From Brains to Culture*. 2nd ed. Los Angeles, CA: Sage; 2013. https://doi.org/10.4135/9781446286395.
5. Jorge RE, Robinson RG, Moser D, Tateno A, Crespo-Facorro B, Arndt S. Major depression following traumatic brain injury. *Arch Gen Psychiatry*. 2004;61(1):42–50. https://doi.org/10.1001/archpsyc.61.1.42.
6. Kann L, Kinchen S, Shanklin SL, et al. Youth risk behavior surveillance—United States, 2013. *MMWR*. 2014;63(4): 1–168. Retrieved from http://www.jstor.org/stable/24806229.
7. Mikami AY, Griggs MS, Reuland MM, Gregory A. Teacher practices as predictors of children's classroom social preference. *J Sch Psychol*. 2012;50(1):95–111. https://doi.org/10.1016/j.jsp.2011.08.002.
8. Miller BM. *Critical Hours: Afterschool Programs and Educational Success*. Quincy, MA: Nellie Mae Education Foundation; 2003. Retrieved August 31, 2018, from http://www.nmefdn.org/CriticalHours.htm.
9. Nakazawa DJ. *Childhood Disrupted: How Your Biography Becomes Your Biology, and How You Can Heal*. New York, NY: Atria Books National Education Association; 2015 (n.d.). Students affected by achievement gaps. Retrieved from www.nea.org/home/20380.htm.
10. National Center for Education Statistics. *Children and Youth with Disabilities*; 2018. Retrieved from https://nces.ed.gov/programs/coe/indicator_cgg.asp.
11. Nurius PS, Macy RJ. Cognitive-behavioral theory. In: Thyer BA, Sowers KM, Dulmus CN, eds. *Comprehensive Handbook of Social Work and Social Welfare, Volume 2: Human Behavior in the Social Environment*. Hoboken, NJ: John Wiley & Sons Inc; 2008:101–133. https://doi.org/10.1002/9780470373705.chsw002007.
12. Tyrka AR, Ridout KK, Parade SH. Childhood adversity and epigenetic regulation of glucocorticoid signaling genes: associations in children and adults. *Dev Psychopathol*. 2016;28(4pt.2):1319–1331. https://doi.org/10.1017/S0954579416000870.

CHAPTER 9

# Screening Adolescents for ADHD, Oppositional Defiant Disorder, and Conduct Disorder in Primary Care

HEIDI JOSHI, PsyD, MS, BMUS • ROGER APPLE, PhD

## INTRODUCTION

This chapter focuses on screening for attention deficit hyperactivity disorder (AD/HD), oppositional defiant disorder (ODD), and conduct disorder with adolescents in a primary care setting. Primary care settings are arguably, next to schools, one of the most important places to screen for behavioral issues and disorders such as AD/HD, ODD, and conduct disorder.[1,2] Indeed, aside from schools, these behavioral issues are likely to present in this context. This is due, in part, to parents and caregivers looking for answers for worrisome behaviors such as inattention, acting out, and even more severe ones, such as cruelty to others and aggression or violence. Primary care providers also tend to be a primary referral mechanism for getting needed assessment or treatment, and screening measures can assist these providers in determining the patients who need further attention that could lead to a diagnosis.[3]

The chapter will go through important definitions and discuss the specific disorders of AD/HD, ODD, and conduct disorder and the screeners that already exist. The particular issues each disorder presents and, as such, what to do in the absence of specific screening measures will be discussed. The chapter will finally offer ways to augment or expand on what is available for future use by primary care providers.

## SCREENING VERSUS DIAGNOSING

Before diving into the discussion of screening for our three main disorders, it is important to clarify the differences between screening and diagnosis. It is easy to confuse these two concepts, but important to delineate them. Screening measures are those that assess risk factors or symptoms that could, but not necessarily do, lead to a diagnosis. This is due to the fact that screening tends to focus on the healthy population.[4] This is especially true in the medical context. There are many screening opportunities in primary care, for example. Providers screen for breast cancer with mammograms or for HPV that can lead to cervical cancer in women through the routine Pap test; yet, not all of the screenings are diagnostic on their own. A mammogram alone, for example, is not used to diagnose breast cancer. Further tests such as ultrasound and/or biopsy would be administered to confirm the diagnosis of breast cancer and give further information as to the type of tumor and other important diagnostic markers. Similarly, utilizing a pap test to detect HPV is not a diagnosis of cervical cancer. It looks for the correct environment for cervical cancer, and then follow-up tests such as the colposcopy would give more diagnostic information as to whether cervical cancer exists or any other abnormalities warranting attention. Further complicating this discussion is the fact that some screening measures are also used as diagnostic tools depending on the context. This is especially common through the use of screeners in primary care for mental or behavioral disorders. The Vanderbilt, for example, is often used in pediatric settings to screen and diagnose AD/HD.[5] Therefore, screening measures focus primarily on risk factors and individuals who may need further assessment to reach a diagnosis. How does this definition of screening differ from that of diagnosis? In contrast to screening, a diagnosis is making the determination that criteria exist for a particular disorder.[4] Before looking at screening for AD/HD, ODD, and conduct disorder, it is first paramount to understand the diagnostic criteria for those disorders.

Adolescent Health Screening: An Update in the Age of Big Data. https://doi.org/10.1016/B978-0-323-66130-0.00009-0

## DSM-5 CRITERIA

Now that we have looked at the criteria for our three main disorders, let us turn to our discussion of screening measures. As a primary care provider, the goal is to screen (i.e., look for risk factors of conduct disorder, ODD, and AD/HD) and determine whether further evaluation for a diagnosis is justified. One barrier to this process is evident when exploring the literature. It has become apparent that there is much more written regarding *treatment* for AD/HD, ODD, and conduct disorders than is written regarding specific screening measures for those disorders, especially screening measures pertinent to a primary care setting.[7–10] This is likely due to the fact that treating these disorders involves a multilayered approach that includes parents, teachers, and other members of the teen's context.[7,11–14] Treatment of these disorders is not our main focus for this chapter, but it may be worth exploring as primary care providers familiarize themselves further with these disorders.

Another important issue to explore is that of whom to screen. Screening adolescents, for example, is extremely important due to the prevalence of mental health concerns in this population. AD/HD, ODD, and conduct disorder are more prevalent in the child and adolescent population overall as compared to depression, for example.[15] The worldwide prevalence rate of AD/HD is 3.4%, and conduct disorder is 5.7% as compared to 2.6% prevalence of depression.[15] This is also likely due to the fact that these disorders tend to be diagnosed in childhood and adolescence. Therefore, the questions of whom to screen for these diagnoses and how often to screen become paramount. Equally important is the notion of what screeners to use, if any, for the adolescent primary care population. Now that we understand the

TABLE 9.1
ADHD 314.0X (F90.X)

1. **A persistent pattern of inattention and/or hyperactivity–impulsivity that interferes with functioning or development, as characterized by (a) and/or (b):**
   a. Inattention: six (or more) of the following symptoms:
      i. Often fails to give close attention to details
      ii. Often has difficulty sustaining attention in tasks or play activities
      iii. Often does not seem to listen when spoken to directly
      iv. Often does not follow through on instructions and fails to finish schoolwork, chores, or duties in the workplace
      v. Often has difficulty organizing tasks and activities
      vi. Often avoids, dislikes, or is reluctant to engage in tasks that require sustained mental effort
      vii. Often loses things necessary for tasks or activities
      viii. Is often easily distracted by extraneous stimuli
      ix. Is often forgetful in daily activities
   b. Hyperactivity and impulsivity: six (or more) of the following symptoms:
      i. Often fidgets with or taps hands or feet or squirms in the seat
      ii. Often leaves seat in situations when remaining seated is expected
      iii. Often runs about or climbs in situations where it is inappropriate
      iv. Often unable to play or engage in Leisure activities quietly
      v. Is often "on the go," acting as if "driven by a motor"
      vi. Often blurts out an answer before a question has been completed
      vii. Often has difficulty waiting for his or her turn
      viii. Often interrupts or intrudes on others
2. Several inattentive or hyperactive-impulsive symptoms were present before 12 years.
3. Several inattentive or hyperactive-impulsive symptoms are present in two or more settings.
4. There is clear evidence that the symptoms interfere with, or reduce the quality of, social, academic, or occupational functioning.
5. The symptoms do not occur exclusively during the course of schizophrenia or another psychotic disorder and are not better explained by another mental disorder.

*Specify* whether:

**314.01 (F90.2) Combined presentation**

**314.00 (F90.0) Predominantly inattentive presentation**

**314.01 (F90.1) Predominantly hyperactive/impulsive presentation**

Modified and summarized from American Psychiatric Association. Diagnostic and Statistical Manual of Mental Disorders (DSM-5®). American Psychiatric Pub; 2013.

**TABLE 9.2**
**Oppositional Defiant Disorder 313.81 (F91.3)**

1. **A pattern of angry/irritable mood, argumentative/defiant behavior, or vindictiveness lasting at least 6 months as evidenced by at least four symptoms from any of the following categories, and exhibited during interaction with at least one individual who is not a sibling.**

**Angry/Irritable mood**
- Often loses temper
- Is often touchy or easily annoyed
- Is often angry and resentful
- Argumentative/Defiant behavior
- Often argues with authority figures or, for children and adolescents, with adults
- Often actively defies or refuses to comply with requests from authority figures or with rules
- Often deliberately annoys others
- Often blames others for his or her mistakes or misbehavior
- Vindictiveness
- Has been spiteful or vindictive at least twice within the past 6 months

2. **The disturbance in behavior is associated with distress in the individual or others in his or her immediate social context.**
3. **The behaviors do not occur exclusively during the course of a psychotic, substance use, depressive, or bipolar disorder.**

Modified and summarized from American Psychiatric Association. Diagnostic and Statistical Manual of Mental Disorders (DSM-5®). American Psychiatric Pub; 2013.

**TABLE 9.3**
**Conduct Disorder 312.8x (F91.X)**

1. **A repetitive and persistent pattern of behavior in which the basic rights of others or major age appropriate societal norms or rules are violated, as manifested by the presence of at least three of the following 15 criteria in the past 12 months from any of the provided categories, with at least one criterion present in the past 6 months:**
   - Aggression to people and animals
   - Destruction of property
   - Deceitfulness or theft
   - Serious violations of rules
2. **The disturbance in behavior causes clinically significant impairment in social, academic, or occupational functioning.**

**If the individual is age 18 years or older, criteria are not met for antisocial personality disorder**

Modified and summarized from American Psychiatric Association. Diagnostic and Statistical Manual of Mental Disorders (DSM-5®). American Psychiatric Pub; 2013.

prevalence of AD/HD, ODD, and conduct disorder as compared to depression, it is important to realize these disorders are screened for much less often than depression, especially in a primary care setting. Interestingly, schools screen for these disorders regularly using measures such as the BASC. Can primary care take something from the educational environment when it comes to screening the adolescent population for AD/HD, ODD, and conduct disorders?

The following sections discuss available screening tools typically used in primary care to help identify AD/HD, ODD, and conduct disorder. After a discussion of the screening tools, the specific DSM five criteria for each disorder will be listed.

## ATTENTION DEFICIT/HYPERACTIVITY DISORDER

Caregivers often bring their children to primary care physicians asking about the possibility of AD/HD, which is one of the most common behavioral health concerns seen in primary care.[16] Over the course of the last 20 years of our careers, we have seen countless children and adolescents prescribed stimulant medication for AD/HD without any screening done. Fortunately, the last 5–10 years has shown a significant increase in primary care physicians doing more screening and requesting more screening or assessment data before making and prescribing medication for the diagnosis (Table 9.1).

One of the most common screening tools for AD/HD used in primary care for children and young adolescents are the National Initiative for Children's Healthcare Quality (NICHQ) Vanderbilt Assessment Scales for children of 6–12 years old. Although the Vanderbilt Scales do ask questions regarding, not only AD/HD, but also ODD, conduct disorder, and anxiety and depression, clinicians most often are choosing the Vanderbilt Scales to help with identification of AD/HD as the Vanderbilt is a public domain tool that is free and easy to use in primary care.

The Vanderbilt Scales consist of both parent and teacher versions:

- NICHQ Vanderbilt Assessment Scale—Parent Informant
- NICHQ Vanderbilt Assessment Scale—Teacher Informant
- NICHQ Vanderbilt Assessment Follow-up—Parent Informant
- NICHQ Vanderbilt Assessment Follow-up—Teacher Informant

The NICHQ Vanderbilt Assessment Scales were found to not have adequate clinical utility to rule out comorbidities with the exception of the ODD cutoff strategy, which did reach an adequate level of clinical utility. It was suggested that using total sum scores for each subscale may provide the greatest clinical utility. The Vanderbilt Scales have also been found to be a reliable measure of AD/HD[17] with a study by Bard[18] identifying a sensitivity of 80%, specificity of 75%, positive predictive value of 0.19. This makes it seem like a good screening tool but a poor diagnostic tool. However, it can be helpful to use the NICHQ along with a diagnostic interview allowing the provider to ask additional clarifying questions.

The scoring guidelines for the NICHQ are too complex to simply list in a table because there are four tools (Parent, Parent follow-up, Teacher, and Teacher follow-up) with specific scoring criteria for multiple domains. However, the complete first edition of the NICHQ Vanderbilt Assessment Scales and scoring guidelines is available for free download at the National Institute for Children's Health Quality website (www.nichq.org).[19] Table 9.4 lists the domains of the Parent and Teacher scales:

For children and adolescents over the age of 12, many primary care clinics use the Pediatric Symptoms Checklist 17 (PSC-17), which is a shortened version of the Pediatric Symptom Checklist 35 (PSC-35). The normed age range for the PSC-17 is 4–18, making it available to almost all primary care children and adolescents; however, many primary care clinics choose to use the Vanderbilt Scales for the younger children and the PSC-17 for the older adolescents. This could be due to the PSC-17 being more of a general screening tool for a broader range of concerns, while the Vanderbilt Scales are more specific to AD/HD and behavior concerns.

The PSC-17 is a well-validated screening tool used in the pediatric population with adequate to strong validity, reliability, and clinical utility. Studies have shown an acceptable fit with a 3-factor model using confirmatory factor analysis as well as excellent scale level reliabilities and moderate interscale correlations.[20] Primary care physicians can use the PSC-17 to help identify concerns in three broad areas: internalizing, externalizing, and attention with specific questions related to ADHD, anxiety, and mood disorders, conduct disorder, oppositional defiant disorder, and adjustment disorders. It is important when talking with patients to stress that the PSC-17 is not diagnosing these conditions, but rather identifying possible concerns that may need further evaluation. Table 9.5 describes the

**TABLE 9.4**
**NICQH Vanderbilt Parent and Teacher Domains**

| Parent Assessment Scale | Teacher Assessment Scale |
|---|---|
| ADHD Predominantly Inattentive subtype | ADHD Predominantly Inattentive subtype |
| ADHD Predominantly Hyperactive/Impulsive subtype | ADHD Predominantly Hyperactive/Impulsive subtype |
| ADHD Combined Inattention/Hyperactivity | ADHD Combined Inattention/Hyperactivity |
| Oppositional Defiant Disorder Screen | Oppositional Defiant/ Conduct Disorder Screen |
| Conduct Disorder Screen | Anxiety/Depression Screen |
| Anxiety/Depression Screen | |

**TABLE 9.5**
**PSC-17 Cut Off Scores**

| Domain | PSC-17 Score |
|---|---|
| Internalizing | ≥5 |
| Attention | ≥7 |
| Externalizing | ≥7 |
| **Total Score** | **≥15** |

suggested cutoff scores with higher scores indicating a greater chance of a diagnosable behavioral disorder.

As previously mentioned, there are times when, in primary care, we reach a diagnosis with screening measures. One such case is when the Vanderbilt screeners, along with parent report about the occurrence of symptoms, and physician observations are sufficient data to make the diagnosis of AD/HD. However, when more complex presentations occur or when there are possibilities of comorbid diagnoses such as learning disabilities, intellectual impairment, or affective disorders, a more comprehensive psychological evaluation would be appropriate.

Now with technology and electronic health records (EHR), it has never been easier to administer screening tools in primary care; however, many clinics still choose to administer screening tools on paper and then go back and enter the scores in the EHR. This is time consuming and a duplication of work that does not need to be with EHR. The Child Health and Development Interactive System (CHADIS)[21] platform is able to administer over 300 screening tools electronically that patients can complete at home with records sent directly into the EHR. The assessments are specifically designed for use in primary care and are for not only AD/HD but also the following areas: infant and young child, school age, adolescent, teacher data, general health, mental health, sports tools, asthma care, family/environment, clinician tools, and quality monitoring.

## OPPOSITIONAL DEFIANT DISORDER AND CONDUCT DISORDER

We have decided to put our discussion of these two disorders together in the same section given the fact that they fall on the same diagnostic continuum with ODD being considered less severe than conduct disorder. Please see Tables 9.2 and 9.3 for a review of the diagnostic criteria for ODD and conduct disorder.

There are many considerations when thinking about screening for ODD and conduct disorder. One such consideration, some would argue, is gender. Some believe that there is a difference clinically between how males and females present in terms of ODD and conduct disorder.[22] One recent study showed that females, on one hand, tended to have more sexual partners who were also diagnosed with conduct disorder than males. Males, on the other hand, tended to have more substance-related difficulties than females.[22] Therefore, whatever measure is being used, it is important to consider gender during screening.

Another vital consideration, especially with conduct disorder screening, is that of the age of onset. Research illustrates that the younger the onset of the disorder, or its symptoms, the more difficult the disorder is to treat. This has important implications when thinking about screening adolescents with conduct disorder. The research would suggest that screening younger children, given the importance of age of onset, would be extremely critical in managing outcomes for these children. This is not to say that we should not screen adolescents for conduct disorder, but the treatment outcomes are much better if symptoms present in adolescence rather than in younger children.[23]

Another important consideration when taking into account screening measures for adolescents with ODD and conduct disorder is that self-report screening measures are often not effective for this population, as individuals with conduct disorder tend not to attribute their behaviors with anything they are doing wrong.[24] Parents and teachers also have a difficult time attributing disordered behaviors such as aggression and cruelty to conduct disorder specifically.[24] This is likely due to the complex and multilayered nature of the etiology of ODD and conduct disorders.

Indeed, ODD and conduct disorders may be a combination of genetically and environmentally based etiology and may have some connection with maternal depression.[1,24–26] Because of this complicated etiology, it is difficult to attribute specific behaviors to ODD and conduct disorder. As a result, these disorders are difficult to pick up in primary care settings.[24]

Given how complicated ODD and conduct disorder can be to detect in primary care, what can providers do to assist in recognizing young patients with these disorders? One thought is to contemplate using an assessment tool called the BASC Three, or at least portions of this screener.[27] This screener is used as a great deal in school settings when assessing disruptive behaviors in children and adolescents. This assessment system is normed for children, adolescents, and young adults from the ages of 2–25 and has several scales. There is a parent rating scale, a teacher rating scale, a self-report measure of personality, a diagnostic history form, and a form for direct observation by the evaluator.[27] This assessment system looks at behaviors and emotions associated with AD/HD, ODD, and conduct disorder as well as others. The school environment is much more equipped to utilize all of this assessment system, including the observation form, but primary care settings could avail themselves of the parent and teacher rating scales, for example, much like they already do with the Vanderbilt Scales for AD/HD. One reason these scales are not already utilized is likely cost. The Vanderbilt is a free measure, but the BASC costs money and requires the ability to score it on a computer.

Other available assessment tools for conduct disorder and ODD include the DISC,[28] which is highly reliable and has good content validity. As with the other screening tools, the DISC does not address important contextual issues, such as executive functioning deficits, neurodevelopmental issues, etc., that are vital to understanding diagnostic and treatment ramifications.

The pediatric symptom checklist is another screening tool often used in primary care settings for assessing behavioral issues.[29–32] This is a self-report measure commonly used in pediatric primary care settings with 17 questions. These questions assess internalizing and externalizing behaviors with the idea that ODD and conduct disordered patients would exhibit more externalizing behaviors. They believe that their problems are the fault of others and they cannot do much about it.

## CONCLUSIONS

In summary, as previously noted, there is not any one particular screener for AD/HD, ODD, and conduct disorder. As all of the aforementioned diagnoses are comorbid, it is useful to think of a screener for adolescents that incorporate all three diagnoses. An extension of the Vanderbilt for example, that is normed for teens, would be useful. This new screener must also have a place for physicians to note contextual issues such as gender, age, environment, parenting style, prenatal exposure history, and other comorbid diagnoses. Primary care physicians are in a unique position to gather this history given their continuous relationships with patients and their families. Adherent in the primary care provider's role is screening.

Having a screener for these behavioral disorders can also give families the assurance that providers are aware of the potential risk factors for their teens, and that a referral mechanism exists for appropriately treating what can be extremely scary and anxiety provoking for families. Screeners for these disorders may also help minimize the chance of either over referring or under referring these young people for treatment. Screening can also help with appropriate detection in case these disorders were somehow missed in childhood or delayed onset of conduct disorder, for example, exists.

## REFERENCES


1. Hacker KA, Penfold R, Arsenault L, Zhang F, Murphy M, Wissow L. Screening for behavioral health issues in children enrolled in Massachusetts Medicaid. *Pediatrics.* 2014;133(1):46–54.
2. Weitzman C, Wegner L. Promoting optimal development: screening for behavioral and emotional problems. *Pediatrics.* 2015;135(2):384–395.
3. Thornton LC, Frick PJ. *Aggression and Conduct Disorders. Handbook of Childhood Psychopathology and Developmental Disabilities Assessment.* Springer; 2018:245–261.
4. Jeannette N, Denise SC. *Medical Sciences.* Elsevier Health Sciences; 2014.
5. Leslie LK, Weckerly J, Plemmons D, Landsverk J, Eastman S. Implementing the American Academy of Pediatrics attention-deficit/hyperactivity disorder diagnostic guidelines in primary care settings. *Pediatrics.* 2004; 114(1):129–140.
6. Association AP. *Diagnostic and Statistical Manual of Mental Disorders (DSM-5®).* American Psychiatric Pub; 2013.
7. Brahmbhatt K, Hilty DM, Hah M, Han J, Angkustsiri K, Schweitzer JB. Diagnosis and treatment of attention deficit hyperactivity disorder during adolescence in the primary care setting: a concise review. *J Adoles Health.* 2016;59(2): 135–143.
8. Costin J, Chambers SM. Parent management training as a treatment for children with oppositional defiant disorder referred to a mental health clinic. *Clin Child Psychol Psychiatry.* 2007;12(4):511–524.
9. dosReis S, Park A, Ng X, et al. Caregiver treatment preferences for children with a new versus existing attention-deficit/hyperactivity disorder diagnosis. *J Child Adolesc Psychopharmacol.* 2017;27(3):234–242.
10. Ougrin D, Chatterton S, Banarsee R. Attention deficit hyperactivity disorder (ADHD): review for primary care clinicians. *London J Prim Care.* 2010;3(1):45–51.
11. Aalsma MC, White LM, Lau KSL, Perkins A, Monahan P, Grisso T. Behavioral health care needs, detention-based care, and criminal recidivism at community reentry from juvenile detention: a multisite survival curve analysis. *Am J Public Health.* 2015;105(7):1372–1378.
12. McBurnett K, Pfiffner LJ. Treatment of aggressive ADHD in children and adolescents: conceptualization and treatment of comorbid behavior disorders. *Postgraduate Med.* 2009; 121(6):158–165.
13. Weiss B, Han S, Harris V, et al. An independent randomized clinical trial of multisystemic therapy with non-court-referred adolescents with serious conduct problems. *J Consul Clin Psychol.* 2013;81(6):1027–1039.
14. Sultan MA, Pastrana CS, Pajer KA. Shared care models in the treatment of pediatric attention-deficit/hyperactivity disorder (ADHD): are they effective? *Health Serv Res Manag Epidemiol.* 2018;5, 2333392818762886.
15. Polanczyk GV, Salum GA, Sugaya LS, Caye A, Rohde LA. Annual Research Review: a meta-analysis of the worldwide prevalence of mental disorders in children and adolescents. *J Child Psychol Psychiatry.* 2015;56(3):345–365.

16. Shahidullah JD, Carlson JS, Haggerty D, Lancaster BM. Integrated care models for ADHD in children and adolescents: a systematic review. *Fam Syst Health*. 2018;36(2):233.
17. Wolraich ML, Lambert W, Doffing MA, Bickman L, Simmons T, Worley K. Psychometric properties of the Vanderbilt ADHD diagnostic parent rating scale in a referred population. *J Pediatric Psychol*. 2003;28(8):559–568.
18. Bard DE, Wolraich ML, Neas B, Doffing M, Beck L. The psychometric properties of the Vanderbilt attention-deficit hyperactivity disorder diagnostic parent rating scale in a community population. *J Dev Behav Pediatr*. 2013;34(2): 72–82.
19. NICHQ AAoP, McNeil. *National Institue of Children's Health Quality*. Boston, MA: National Institute for Children's Health Quality; 2018. updated 2018.
20. *Pediatric Symptom Checklist-17 Item Version [Internet]*. PsycTESTS American Psychological Association; 2006 [cited October 26, 2018].
21. Total Child Health I. *CHADIS: Evidence-Based Shared Decisions [Website]*. Total Child Health, Inc; 2003-2018 [updated 2018]. Available from: www.info@chadis.com.
22. Brooks Holliday S, Ewing BA, Storholm ED, Parast L, D'Amico EJ. Gender differences in the association between conduct disorder and risky sexual behavior. *J Adolesc*. 2017;56:75–83.
23. Rutter M. Research review: child psychiatric diagnosis and classification: concepts, findings, challenges and potential. *J Child Psychol Psychiatry*. 2011;52(6):647–660.
24. Searight HR, Rottnek F, Abby SL. Conduct disorder: diagnosis and treatment in primary care. *Am Fam Physician*. 2001;63(8):1579–1588.
25. Bener A, Kamal M. Predict attention deficit hyperactivity disorder? Evidence -based medicine. *Glob J Health Sci*. 2013;6(2):47–57.
26. Boden Schlesinger A. In this issue/abstract thinking: primary care providers and ADHD in community settings. *J Am Acad Child Adolesc Psychiatry*. 2008;47(7): 729–730.
27. Altmann RA, Reynolds CR, Kamphaus RW, Vannest KJ. *BASC-3. Encyclopedia of Clinical Neuropsychology*. Springer; 2018:1–7.
28. Algorta GP, Dodd AL, Stringaris A, Youngstrom EA. Diagnostic efficiency of the SDQ for parents to identify ADHD in the UK: a ROC analysis. *Eur Child Adolesc Psychiatry*. 2016;25(9):949–957.
29. Blucker RT, Jackson D, Gillaspy JA, Hale J, Wolraich M, Gillaspy SR. Pediatric behavioral health screening in primary care: a preliminary analysis of the pediatric symptom checklist-17 with functional impairment items. *Clin Pediatrics*. 2014;53(5):449–455.
30. Chaffin M, Campbell C, Whitworth DN, et al. Accuracy of a pediatric behavioral health screener to detect untreated behavioral health problems in primary care settings. *Clin Pediatrics*. 2017;56(5):427–434.
31. Gardner W, Lucas A, Kolko DJ, Campo JV. Comparison of the PSC-17 and alternative mental health screens in an at-risk primary care sample. *J Am Acad Child Adolesc Psychiatry*. 2007;46(5):611–618.
32. Valleley RJ, Romer N, Kupzyk S, Evans JH, Allen KD. Behavioral health screening in pediatric primary care: a pilot study. *J Prim Care Community Health*. 2015;6(3): 199–204.

CHAPTER 10

# Screening for Violent Tendencies in Adolescents

PAUL D. JUAREZ, PhD

National crime arrest statistics reveal that adolescents and young adults in the United States are more likely to perpetrate and be victimized by interpersonal violence than individuals in other age groups. The causes of youth violence perpetration and victimization are multilevel, often have their origins earlier in life, and may overlap significantly with each other.[1] They have been identified as spanning a wide range of factors,[2] including individual factors[3] (high impulsiveness, anger management), family factors[4] (poor supervision, harsh discipline, a violent parent, a young mother, a broken family), peer and social factors[5] (peer delinquency, low socioeconomic status, urban residence, a high-crime neighborhood), community risk factors[6] (concentrated poverty, residential segregation, socially disorganized communities, high rates of violent crime), and situational factors[7] (actions leading to violent events [e.g., alcohol, the escalation of a trivial altercation, arguments]). Outcomes of youth violence include fatal and nonfatal assaults with a blunt instrument, cutting instrument, or firearm; sexual assault; dating/intimate partner violence; family violence; and cyberbullying.[8,9] The focus of this chapter is to provide a description of the range of types of youth violence; a public health perspective of youth violence prevention; risk and preventive factors for preventing youth violence; primary, secondary, and tertiary interventions; a developmental-ecological model; and implications for healthcare providers.

## ADOLESCENCE

The onset of puberty is marked by a sequence of changes to the physical, psychosexual, cognitive, and social growth and development of children and hails the onset of adolescence. Adolescent development is frequently broken down into three levels: early adolescence (ages 12–14 years), mid-adolescence (ages 15–16 years), and late adolescence (ages 17–21 years). Marshall and Tanner[10,11] describe adolescence as five stages of normal pubertal maturation (e.g., the Tanner stages) consisting of predictable changes in secondary sexual characteristics that all girls and boys go through. In contrast, Erickson[12] identified adolescence by the set of major developmental tasks that teens face: (1) personal identity formation, (2) becoming independent, (3) achieving a sense of competency, (4) establishing social status, (5) experiencing intimacy, and (6) determining sexual identity. Bronfrenbrenner[13] describes child and adolescent development as being shaped by the context of roles, norms, and rules of four types of nested ecological systems: the microsystem (family, classroom), mesosystem (interaction of two microsystems), exosystem (external environment), and macrosystem (sociocultural context).

The spike in violence perpetration during adolescence largely parallels the concurrent developmental changes experienced by teens. Developmental growth includes significant increases in height, weight, and internal organ size, as well as changes in skeletal and muscular systems.[14] Although brain size remains relatively unchanged, the prefrontal cortex—an area of the brain that handles executive functions such as planning, reasoning, anticipating consequences, sustaining attention, and making decisions—continues to develop.[15,16] This intense developmental period is marked by rapid changes in the physical, physiologic, sexual, cognitive, socioemotional, and moral development that accompany puberty.

During early adolescence, psychosocial development is characterized by two key developmental tasks: identity formation and the quest for independence. During this period, youths develop the capacity for abstract thought processes; however, the transition to higher levels of cognitive function varies considerably across individuals.[17–19] Young adolescents typically progress from concrete logical operations to acquiring the ability to develop and test hypotheses, analyze

Adolescent Health Screening: An Update in the Age of Big Data. https://doi.org/10.1016/B978-0-323-66130-0.00010-7

and synthesize data, grapple with complex concepts, and think reflectively.[20] During these years, young adolescents seek their own sense of individuality and uniqueness.[21] They may experience an increased awareness of their ethnic identity as well. As young adolescents search for an adult identity and adult acceptance, they strive to maintain peer approval.[14]

Adolescence is the period in which young people are at greatest risk for violence perpetration and victimization. As young adolescents expand their affiliations to include peers, feelings of conflict may arise due to competing allegiances.[22] The search for identity and self-discovery may intensify feelings of vulnerability, as they become attuned to the differences between self and others.[23] Their emotional variability makes young adolescents at risk of making decisions with negative consequences[24] and believing that their experiences, feelings, and problems are unique.[23]

As adolescents develop their sense of personal identity and autonomy during their teenage years, they begin to formulate their own principles of right and wrong. It is not uncommon for teens to see themselves one way when they are with parents and teachers and another way when they are with their peers. Although adults remain essential to their continuing development as caregivers, role models, educators, and mentors, during adolescence the frame of reference of teens expands from family to peers and other adults with whom they increasingly have more contact. The successful transition of teens to adult roles (e.g., work, relationships, parenting) usually reduces involvement in violence and other behaviors that increase the risk for poor health and social outcomes.

Most young people are embedded in four types of communities: family, school, peers, and extracurricular groups (which include faith communities, clubs, and sports leagues, etc.). During adolescence, these communities, composed of parents, siblings, significant others, relatives, peers, coaches, teachers, mentors, and their friends and peers, are the most important people in their lives, yet often fulfill different needs. Although parents tend to provide emotional and instrumental support, other caring adults, such as a teacher, coach, and often counselor, become significant providers of social support to teens, helping them cope with the many issues and choices they face during this transitional period in their lives as they mature and move on toward adulthood. In the absence of support from parents and other caring adults, teens are likely to turn to peers for information, emotional support, and guidance. However, reliance on peer networks can be unhealthy when they reinforce behaviors that are, in themselves, harmful. Although peer support is an essential factor in an adolescent's social network, if peers support harmful behaviors, an adolescent may be more likely to engage in harmful behaviors such as violence.

## YOUTH VIOLENCE

Youth violence is a complex, social, criminal justice and public health issue that requires both a systems approach and a life course perspective to unravel it.[25,26] Interpersonal violence among youths include a number of different categories including homicide, fighting, family violence, dating violence, sexual violence, gang violence, bullying, and cyberbullying. Some risk factors for violence victimization and perpetration are the same, whereas others are unique. For example, childhood physical or sexual victimization is a risk factor for future intimate partner violence perpetration and victimization but not for gang violence or cyberbullying.

Chronic violence exposure is one of the most potent risk factors for an increased propensity to commit subsequent acts of violence. Violence exposure or victimization of school-aged children and adolescents is associated with impaired school functioning and increased anxiety, depression, stress, and hopelessness. Some children, particularly preadolescents and adolescents, develop a diminished perception of risk that can lead to dangerous acting-out behaviors. Particularly worrisome is the fact that many children immersed in violent environments develop a heightened tendency to perceive social interactions as threatening and to view violence and aggression as acceptable ways to resolve conflict.

The Surgeon General's report on youth violence identified two onset trajectories for violence.[27] The first, begins before puberty and is often characterized by sequences of escalating behaviors that lead from early aggression to defiant and antisocial behavior to actual violence. Youths on this trajectory "generally commit more crimes, and more serious crimes, for a longer time." Their violence sometimes continues into adulthood. The second, more common trajectory begins around ages 13 and 14 years and peaks between 16 and 18 years. If youths have not initiated violence by age 20 years, it is highly unlikely they will ever become serious violent offenders.

Current research indicates that the presence of a single risk factor in an individual infrequently, by itself, causes antisocial or violent behavior. Rather, it is now generally believed that multiple factors combine to contribute to and shape behavior over the course of adolescent development. Studies suggest it is the confluence of certain "risk" factors and behaviors that contribute to violent behavior, and the existence of certain "protective" factors that create resiliency. Understanding the complex nature of youth violence and the role of risk and protective factors can lead to improved screening, treatment, and referrals or engagement in community change by physicians and other members of the healthcare team.

## Types of Youth Violence

### Criminal violence

Homicide is the second leading cause of death among persons aged 15–24 years in the United States. The Justice Department reports that the Violent Crime Index offenses arrests for youths aged 10–17 years has steadily declined since 2006, reaching a new low in 2012.[28] In April 2000, the Department of Justice Office of Juvenile Justice and Delinquency Prevention[29] released the results from the Study Group on Serious and Violent Juvenile Offenders, a 2-year initiative that brought together experts to analyze and synthesize current research on the predictors of juvenile criminal violence.[30] This report adds to an extensive body of research that documents the numerous individual, familial, social, and situational factors that place children and youths at elevated risk for violent perpetration.[31] The Study Group Report highlighted the following risk factors for juvenile violence perpetration:

- *Individual factors*: Emotional disorders (such as depression, social withdrawal, nervousness, and anxiety); hyperactivity, concentration problems, and risk-taking; aggressiveness; early initiation of violent behavior; involvement in other forms of antisocial behavior (such as smoking, early sexual behavior, and stealing); beliefs and attitudes favorable to deviant or antisocial behavior; and academic failure, truancy, and dropping out of school.
- *Family factors*: Parental criminality, child maltreatment, poor family management and parenting practices, parental attitudes favorable to substance use and violence, low levels of parental involvement, parent–child separation, delinquent siblings, poor family bonding, and family conflicts.
- *Peer factors*: Delinquent siblings, delinquent peers, and gang membership.
- *Social/neighborhood factors*: Poverty, community disorganization, availability of drugs and firearms, exposure to violence and racial prejudice, neighborhood adults involved in crime, delinquent peers, and gang membership.

### Bullying

School is a key context for the social development of adolescents. In general, the social relations that take place in the school are satisfactory and enriching. Students learn to interact and, by overcoming small conflicts, they forge friendships, some of which will last for many years. However, occasionally some students are involved in dynamics of abuse and maltreatment (bullying) by their peers, which can have a negative impact on their lives.

Bullying refers to a kind of violence among students characterized by intentional attacks, which may take various forms (physical or verbal assaults, theft, destruction, isolation) on a victim by one or more aggressors. These attacks are not isolated but instead continue over time, facilitated by the victim's inferiority and/or isolation, as compared with the aggressors.[32]

Adolescents who bully others tend to exhibit other defiant and delinquent behaviors, have poor school performance, are more likely to drop out of school, and are more likely to bring weapons to school.[33–36] The probability of a student being a bully increases until about age 14 years, when it decreases. Systematic reviews and meta-analyses of longitudinal studies show that being a bully at school is a significant predictor of aggression[37] across the life course. Therefore the prevention and treatment of bullying at school is important not only to optimize students' psychosocial development and learning but also, at the social level, to prevent subsequent criminal behavior.

Risk factors for bullying include impulsivity, hyperactivity, aggressiveness, sensation-seeking, and antisocial behavior. Competitive attitudes, such as a desire for social success[38]; sexist attitudes toward women[39]; and negative attitudes toward homosexuals[40] are also positively associated with being a bully. Helplessness, insecurity, feeling low, moodiness, nervousness, and insomnia, which are internalizing problems, also correlate positively with being a victim and negatively with being a bully.[41] Bullies are more likely to present problems such as hyperactivity and externalizing problems. Empathy, meanwhile, correlates negatively with being a bully.

Exposure to family violence and susceptibility to peer social pressure are also risk factors for being a bully. Being friends of bullies,[42] of delinquents,[43] or with people with antisocial behavior,[44] as well as belonging to gangs,[45] increases one's probability of bullying. The probability of being a bully is higher in students whose teachers have low expectations about their performance in school. Satisfaction with the school and school connectedness are protective factors against being a bully.[46–48] Early identification of children at risk of being bullies in adolescence may serve as a basis for the design of preventive measures and effective treatment.

### Dating violence

Adolescent dating violence is defined as any physically, sexually, or psychologically violent behavior, including stalking, directed toward a current or former dating partner in adolescence.[49] Approximately 9% of high-school students report being hit, slapped, or physically hurt on purpose by their boyfriend or girlfriend in the past year.[50] Teen dating violence rates appear to be even higher among certain populations, such as youths who have a history of exposure to violence.

Peers and the contexts in which peers interact can contribute to their risk for and protection against dating violence. Youths who are victims or perpetrators of peer violence tend to be the same youths at risk for experiencing violence within romantic relationships. Links between youths who bully and youths who perpetrate teen dating violence suggest an overlap in teens who victimize peers and those who victimize dating partners.

Peer risk factors tend to be more strongly associated with dating violence perpetration and victimization in adolescence than with family risk factors. Once teens experience violence in one relationship, they are at significant risk for experiencing violence in another relationship. A few teens seek help from formal sources such as schools, social services, or legal professionals. Instead, male and female teens were most likely to turn to friends for help. Programs and policies aimed at preventing teen dating violence or promoting healthy teen relationships more broadly are likely to be most effective if they take into consideration the potential ways in which peers and peer contexts shape teens' experiences within close relationships.

### Cyberbullying

Cyberbullying has been defined as "willful and repeated harm inflicted" toward another.[9,51,52] What makes cyberbullying distinct is the use of electronic communication technology as the means through which youths threaten, harass, embarrass, or socially exclude others. Cyberbullying can encompass the use of an electronic medium to sexually harass,[53] including distributing unsolicited text or photos of a sexual nature or requesting sexual acts either online or offline.[54] Research has found that cybervictimization predicts worse outcomes than traditional victimization for symptoms of depression, anxiety, self-esteem issues, absenteeism, and physical health[55] and has a stronger relationship with suicidal ideation. Cyberbullying is not just a short-term problem for adolescents but can cause long-term adverse physical and emotional health outcomes.

About 15.5% of high-school students and 24% of middle-school students were cyberbullied in 2015.[56] The percentages of individuals who have experienced cyberbullying at some point in their lifetimes have nearly doubled (18%–34%) from 2007 to 2016.[57] Boys are more likely to be cyberbully perpetrators and girls are more likely to be cyberbully targets.[58]

Students who are perpetrators of cyberbullying are more likely than others to report perpetration of violence toward peers and to use computers for more hours a day. Students who are cyberbullied report feeling sad, anxious, afraid, and unable to concentrate on school[59,60] and may report social difficulties, drug and alcohol use, and eating disorders.[61,62] Victimized youths are more likely to skip school,[62] to have detentions or suspensions, or to take a weapon to school.[63] Youths who cyberbully are likely to engage in rule-breaking and to have problems with aggression.[62] Cyberbullying often occurs in the context of social relationships, which challenges the commonly held assumption that it is anonymous[9,53,64] and is consistent with understanding bullying as a relationship issue.[65] Children who use the Internet in private places at their home (e.g., bedroom) are at higher risk to be victimized than children who used computers in a public space in their home.

### Fighting

Child-on-child violence historically has been regarded as more different in nature than other types of violence, not from empirical evidence, but from moral and philosophic presumptions about young offenders.[66] Compared with peer assaults on older youths, however, very young child victims are actually more likely to be injured and more likely to be hit with an object that could cause injury.[66] Sibling violence is much more likely to occur as a chronic condition than peer violence. Nearly half of the children under the age of 10 years who were hit by a sibling in the previous year experienced five or more such episodes during that year. Younger children are even more likely than older children to experience this chronic sibling violence. For young children, the association between peer violence and trauma symptoms is just as strong as the association for older children.

Sibling violence becomes progressively more atypical with age. Mid-late adolescents who have not yet ceased being physically aggressive with siblings may be at heightened risk for engagement in other forms of physical aggression, such as fighting with nonfamily peers. In this manner, physical fights with siblings could be a marker of risk for physical fighting with peers. Caregiver aggression, substance use, and school failure are routinely cited as risk factors for fighting. Youths who are bullied by siblings are significantly more likely to be bullied at school. Children's violent behavior against their parents reflects failure in the learning of social and emotional skills, which becomes more difficult in contexts of marital violence or child abuse. Juveniles who have charges of parent abuse present more psychologic disorders including higher rates of psychiatric hospitalization and psychotropic medication use than juvenile offenders charged with other crimes. Juveniles who assault their parents often exhibit violence in other environments, such as school, demonstrating antisocial and criminal behaviors. The profile of adolescents who batter their parents has been found to include depressive symptoms, lower self-esteem, and low empathy. In general, parent abuse offenders show more behavior and emotional problems than non–parent abuse offenders or nonoffender adolescents, including higher levels of school maladjustment (school indiscipline, aversion to instruction) and social maladjustment (social aggression). Behavioral symptoms are better predictors of parent abuse than emotional symptoms.

### Sexual violence

The US Centers for Disease Control and Prevention defines *sexual violence* as any attempted or completed sexual act, sexual contact, or noncontact sexual abuse with someone who does not consent or is unable to consent or refuse.[67] Risk factors common to both youth violence, in general, and sexual violence, in particular, include individual level—delinquency/antisocial behavior, general aggression, substance use, and attitudes supportive of violence. Family-level risk factors include child maltreatment/exposure to parental violence and parent–child relationship quality. Common peer-level risk factors include association with delinquent/violent peers and peer norms supportive of violence. Unique risk factors for sexual violence perpetration include belief in rape myths, victim-blaming attitudes, hostility toward women, exposure to sexually explicit media, deviant sexual fantasies, and perceived peer support for forced sex. Other potential risk factors for sexual violence include school disconnectedness, social disorganization/lack of social controls, and availability of drugs/alcohol in community.[68]

### Gang violence

Gang violence accounts for a substantial proportion of homicides among youths in some US cities. From 2002 to 2006, gangs were responsible for approximately 20% of homicides in the 88 largest US cities.[69] Youths may become involved with gangs to gain a sense of control and power over their social situation and to have a sense of camaraderie with others, especially if they lack strong connections with parents, other family members, and peers.[70] Gang-involved youths often become further isolated from more positive social members of society and social, religious, and educational institutions, such as schools, faith-based institutions, and social services.[71] Gang involvement also is a known predictor of violence that contributed to violence risk above and beyond that which comes from being involved with delinquent peers.

During adolescence, several developmentally normative trends emerge that overlap with gang-related behaviors, such as increasing influence of peers,[72] risk-taking activities,[73] antisocial behavior,[74] and co-offending.[75,76] Thus identifying risk factors for gang affiliation is particularly challenging, given that many typically non-gang-affiliated youths may engage in behaviors similar to their gang-affiliated peers.

Gang homicides are unique violent events that require prevention strategies aimed specifically at gang processes.[77] Preventing gang joining and increasing youths' capacity to resolve conflict nonviolently might reduce gang homicides.[78] Rigorous evaluation of gang violence prevention programs is limited; however, many promising programs exist.[79] Secondary and tertiary prevention programs that intervene when youths have been identified at risk or have been injured by gang violence might interrupt the retaliatory nature of gang violence and promote youths leaving gangs.[80] Promising tertiary prevention programs for gang-involved youths include evidence-based programs that provide family therapy or multisystemic therapy (MST) to increase the capacity of youths to resolve conflict.

## PUBLIC HEALTH PERSPECTIVE OF YOUTH VIOLENCE

Historically, youth violence has been thought of as a criminal justice or sociologic problem.[81] However, these traditional approaches do not adequately capture the complexity of the biopsychosocial context and experiences of youths, particularly, young men of color. *Healthy People 2010* spells out a comprehensive set of health objectives for the nation, devoting an entire chapter to injury and violence prevention; some of the initiative's youth-related objectives explicitly address physical fighting and weapon-carrying by adolescents.

In the recent years, youth violence has been identified as a public health issue as evidenced by a wide array of statistics. Homicide is the second leading cause of death among young people between the ages of 10 and 24 years. In 2014, 4300 young people aged 10–24 years were victims of homicide—an average of 12 each day. The Youth Risk Behavior Survey reported that in 2017, 15.7% of youths in the 9th through 12th grades reported carrying a weapon (such as a gun, knife, or club, on at least 1 day during the 30 days before the survey), down from 26.1% in 1991, and 3.8% reported carrying a weapon on school property, down from 11.8% in 1993. About 6% of youths reported they had been threatened or injured with a weapon on school property during the past 12 months, down from 7.3% in 1993, and 8.5% reported having been in a physical fight on school property, down from 16.2% in 1993.[56]

A public health perspective of youth violence prevention is concerned with the well-being of the entire youth population.[27] It goes beyond attention to individual well-being and seeks to address the prevalence of indicators of health in defined populations. Primary prevention aims to prevent disease or injury before it ever occurs. This is done by preventing exposures to hazards that cause disease or injury, altering unhealthy or unsafe behaviors that can lead to disease or injury, and increasing resistance to disease or injury should exposure occur.

Secondary prevention, in contrast, aims to reduce the impact of a disease or injury that has already occurred. This is done by detecting and treating disease or injury as soon as possible to halt or slow its progress, encouraging personal strategies to prevent reinjury or recurrence, and implementing programs to return people to their original health and function to prevent long-term problems. Tertiary prevention, on the other hand, aims to soften the impact of an ongoing illness or injury that has lasting effects. This is done by helping people manage long-term, often-complex health problems and injuries (e.g., chronic diseases, permanent impairments) in order to improve as much as possible their ability to function, their quality of life, and their life expectancy.

The public health perspective seeks to prevent youth violence through combined primary, secondary, and tertiary prevention strategies that aim to decrease risk factors and/or increase protective factors associated with the agent (e.g., vector), host (e.g., victim), and environment (e.g., physical and social).[82] It is important to consider the independent, interactive, and cumulative effects of risk and protective factors to both develop an understanding of the nature of the problem and conceptualize interventions.

Violence prevention experts have identified a number of risk and protective factors that are associated with youth violent perpetration.[83–85] The following is an overview of some of the specific factors that have been linked to youth violence. Given that individuals operate within the context of their surroundings, the section moves from specific factors that relate directly to individual behavior to broader community and environmental factors.

## Risk Factors

Risk factors are defined as scientifically established factors or determinants for which there is strong objective evidence of a causal relationship to a problem.[1,86] These factors can influence the level of risk an individual experiences or can moderate the relationship between the risk and the outcome or behavior.[87] Individual characteristics that have been commonly identified as risk factors for youth violence[74,88,89] include biological and psychologic characteristics identifiable in children at very young ages, which may increase their vulnerability to negative social and environmental influences over the course of development.

A number of studies have found a correlation between youth violent behavior perpetration and hyperactivity, concentration problems, adverse childhood exposures, and risk-taking.[90–92] Aggressive behavior during childhood (from ages 6 to 13 years) appears to consistently predict later violence among men; however, research results for aggressive women are less consistent.[93,94] Early onset of violence and delinquency is also associated with later acts of more serious and chronic violence, as is involvement in other forms of antisocial behavior, such as substance use, stealing, and destruction of property.[95,96] Other research indicates that there is strong evidence for the co-occurrence of mental health disorders, such as depression and posttraumatic stress disorder (PTSD), among children or youths with antisocial or delinquent behavior problems.[97–99]

Poor academic achievement and school failure are other individual-level factors that contribute to risk for youth violence.[84,85] Some research indicates that the relationship between school achievement is stronger for women than for men. Young people who are consistently absent from school during early adolescence (ages 12–14 years) appear to be more likely to engage in violence as adolescents and adults. Leaving school early has also been found to correlate with increased risk for interpersonal violence.

### Family factors

Family factors are related to a youth's position within the family, support system, culture, and functioning that affect behavior.[100–102] Research demonstrates that family dynamics and parental or caregiver involvement are significantly correlated with an individual's propensity to engage in violent behavior. A lack of parental interaction and involvement increases the risk for violence, particularly among men.[103] Failure to set clear expectations, inadequate youth supervision and monitoring, and severe or inconsistent family discipline practices can also contribute to delinquency and violent behavior.[104] Exposure to high levels of marital and family discord or conflict also appears to increase risk, as does antisocial or delinquent behavior by siblings and peers.[105–108] Child abuse and neglect are additional family-level risk factors for violence perpetration. Research evidence suggests that children or youths who have been physically abused or neglected are more likely than others to commit violent crimes later in life.[109,110]

The ways in which children are socialized in their families are strongly tied to positive and negative developmental outcomes.[27,111,112] Children who are raised in families where violence and other forms of antisocial behavior are modeled consistently by siblings or parents are more likely to engage in violence themselves.[112] Exposure to antisocial norms and values held by family members and individuals outside the home may also have a negative effect on children's behavior by presenting violence as acceptable and normalizing the occurrence of violence.[113] Furthermore, poor family management that involves parents' failure to set clear rules for children's behavior, parents' failure to monitor children's social interactions and behavior in developmentally appropriate ways, and parents' use of inconsistent or severe and abusive discipline also increases risk for violence. Alcohol abuse by significant family members, especially by male family members, is a significant predictor of violent behavior.[114] Family management factors have been found to be more influential over youth violence than neighborhood context.[115]

For most adolescents, family support is the most important element in their lives.[116,117] Family-level protective factors include clear boundaries for behavior that enforce structure and rules within the household and reasonable disciplinary actions when rules are violated.[118,119] Family members, especially parents or primary caregivers, can play a significant role in helping protect youths from violence by emphasizing the importance of education and offering support and affection.[120,121] Frequent, in-depth conversations and communication between parents and children help build resilience, as does the existence of a nonkin support network that offers access to a variety of adult viewpoints and experiences. Inadequate support and guidance from parents increases the probability of poor academic performance, inadequate interpersonal skills, and engagement in risk-taking behaviors,[104] all of which have the potential to increase violent behavior.

### Peer factors

There is also an abundant literature demonstrating a positive association between risk-taking behavior of adolescents and that of their peers.[122] One of the strongest predictors of serious violence in adolescence across studies is involvement with delinquent (antisocial) peers.[123] Adolescents appear to be particularly susceptible to peer influence during middle adolescence.[124] Their position within their peer networks provides different opportunities for peer interaction, resulting in varying exposure to delinquent behaviors, communication of delinquent norms, access to information on delinquency opportunities, and opportunities for participation in delinquent behaviors. In addition, teens who struggle with establishing healthy peer relationships frequently have difficulties with romantic relationships, which may increase risk for subsequent dating violence or intimate partner violence.[123]

Although prior research establishes that adolescents are likely to behave in a manner consistent with their friends, it has yet to incorporate the social network structures into empirical models.[125] Geographic information system is increasingly being used to map data, including crime hot spots and locations of friends through social media. Hot spot analysis depicts the crime location, time, and frequency, often at the address level and thus provides opportunities for predicting crime based on location and availability of individuals and similar crime locations. Social network analysis provides an alternative approach for considering social control and differential association, the two dominant theories for studying delinquent behavior. Although the differential association theory focuses on the effects of peer networks and the focus of the social control theory is on adolescents' attachment to friends, neither theory has considered characteristics of the networks themselves.[126] A network perspective of delinquency[122,126–130] and youth violence provides new research opportunities for understanding youth violence.

### Community factors

Although individual, peer, and family dysfunction have been commonly associated with youth violence,[74,88,131,132] research increasingly points to the role of community-level factors as enabling conditions for youth crime and violence.[133] Being exposed to crime and drug selling in a neighborhood, as a consequence of social disorganization, may also increase risk for later violence. Having ready access to drugs may reflect increased opportunities in a neighborhood for deviance and lax norms against antisocial behavior. Exposure to poverty at both the neighborhood and family levels is likely to co-occur with neighborhood disorganization (crime, graffiti, social disorder, disregard for police), also elevating risk for violence.

Community factors include characteristics of the physical environment, available economic and recreational opportunities, existing social supports, and other issues that have an impact on the successful functioning of the residents. Social isolation, lack of social support, unemployment, vacant housing, population loss, percentage of black residents, and percentage of female-headed households are all neighborhood-level characteristics that have been found to be related to the rate of youth violence.[134] Increased concentration of poverty in urban areas has been accompanied by higher levels of violence, stress, and other types of social problems resulting in poorer health outcomes and increasing health disparities for low-income and racial ethnic minority adults and children.[135]

Social factors that have been found to contribute to the risk for youth violence perpetration include weak social bonds,[136] community deterioration or disorganization, lack of social capital,[3] and low levels of neighborhood and organizational collective efficacy.[137–139] The social disorganization theory[140] emphasizes the importance of neighborhood-level factors in understanding youth crime and violence.[133] Social disorganization is defined as the presence of high crime rates, gang activity, poor housing, and general deterioration in a given community. Disorganized communities tend to lack the social capital, resources, and opportunities needed by young people, such as adult mentors, quality schools, safe places, and employment training opportunities and jobs, limiting youths' access to positive and productive developmental experiences. Common characteristics of socially disorganized communities include concentrated poverty, physical deterioration of neighborhoods, residential instability, lack of social control, lack of social capital and collective efficacy, community disconnectedness, and racial/ethnic heterogeneity.[140–142]

Disorganized communities also may have a lack of appropriate institutions and services for young people, such as quality schools and recreational facilities, limiting youths' access to positive and productive developmental experiences. Neighborhoods in which there is a dearth of social capital, supports, and opportunities for youths combined with geographic and economic isolation have been found to be associated with higher rates of youth violence and crime. According to Wilson,[143] youths from disorganized neighborhoods often have lower levels of personal competence, academic success, self-efficacy, social skills, and self-discipline and are not adequately prepared to enter the labor market even when jobs are available. Concentration of poverty and neighborhood disorganization also have been linked to young people having a feeling of hopelessness about ever having legitimate opportunities for success. This lack of hope and opportunities for youths may lead them to accept crime, drug use, and violence as a means of coping with these hardships.[143]

Hirschi[136] found that youths' engagement in delinquent behavior, including violence, occurs when their "social bond" with the society is weak. He described "social bond" as being composed of four elements: (1) attachment, (2) commitment, (3) involvement, and (4) beliefs. Hirschi suggests that a youth who has a strong attachment to family, friends, and traditional community institutions (e.g., school, church, community organization) is more likely to avoid deviant behavior for fear of disappointing valued attachments (e.g., commitment). Hirschi also hypothesized that persons who strongly share social values and norms are less likely to deviate from them, whereas those who question or challenge the norms have a greater propensity to behave in a deviant manner.

Weak social networks, such as those found in neighborhoods with low levels of social capital and collective efficacy and a high concentration of poverty, reduce a community's ability to protect youths from risk-taking behaviors and exposures, supervise their behavior, and provide positive and meaningful opportunities and experiences.[140] In contrast, a strong community infrastructure has been identified as protective against youth violence. This is supported by studies that show that crime is related to certain patterns of neighborhood ties and social interactions and is largely mediated by informal social control and social cohesion.[144,145]

Social capital, a term usually applied to communities, encompasses multiple factors of civic engagement, including citizenship, neighborliness, trust and shared values, community involvement, volunteering, social networks, and civic participation.[146–148] Social capital describes the pattern and intensity of networks among people and the shared values that arise from those networks. There is evidence that youths who live in communities with high levels of social capital are less likely to engage in crime, have better health, and have higher educational achievement. Neighborhood organizations, congregations, and other voluntary groups can create "social capital."[149–151]

The combined and often interrelated social and economic effects of these and other demographic trends such as residential segregation, "white flight," deindustrialization, structural changes in labor demand, and redlining of services have led to increasing concentration rates of poverty in inner-city, predominantly minority, neighborhoods.[143,144,152] Availability of drugs and firearms, community deterioration or disorganization, and lack of access to quality educational and recreational opportunities also have been identified as community-level factors that decrease social capital and increase risk for interpersonal violence among youths.

Other research indicates that exposure to violence in the media, particularly prolonged exposure of children, may contribute to aggressive behavior and desensitization to violence.[153–155] Researchers have found that the prevalence of drugs and firearms in a community predicts a greater likelihood of violent behavior.[156–158] The media also may contribute to the perception of violence as a normative behavior, reinforcing and sensationalizing violence as an appropriate and justifiable problem-solving strategy.[159]

## Protective Factors

Protective factors are factors that potentially decrease the likelihood of engaging in a risky behavior.

### Individual-level protective factors

Bearinger et al.[160] found that most protective factors against youth violence perpetration were positive affect, peer prosocial behavior norms against violence, and parental prosocial behavior norms against violence. Individual-level traits and characteristics that have been identified as protective factors for the prevention of youth violence perpetration include a personal sense of purpose and belief in a positive future, a commitment to education and learning, and the ability to act independently and feel a sense of control over one's environment.[161,162] The ability to be adaptable and flexible and have empathy for and caring toward others is significant, as is the ability to solve problems, plan for the future, and be resourceful in seeking out sources of support.[83] Conflict resolution and critical thinking skills are additional factors that help protect youths from violence, delinquency, and antisocial behavior.[163] Other individual-level protective factors for youth violence perpetration include intolerant attitude toward deviance, high IQ, high grade point average (as an indicator of high academic achievement), high educational aspirations, positive social orientation, popularity acknowledged by peers, highly developed social skills/competencies, highly developed skills for realistic planning, and religiosity.

### Family-level protective factors

A strong connection to parents and other caring adults has been found to be protective factors against a range of risky behaviors including youth violence, gang involvement, teen pregnancy, drug use, and drug dealing.[164–167] Other family-level protective factors include connectedness to family or adults outside the family, ability to discuss problems with parents, perceived parental expectations about school performance, and frequent shared activities with parents.

### Peer-level protective factors

Protective peer factors include possession of affective relationships with those at school that are strong, close, and prosocially oriented; close relationships with nondeviant peers; membership in peer groups that do not condone antisocial behavior; involvement in prosocial activities; exposure to school climates that are characterized by intensive supervision, clear behavior rules, and consistent negative reinforcement of aggression; and engagement of parents and teachers[27,83,89,168–170]

### School-, work-, and community-level protective factors

Greater school connectedness also has been associated in several studies with lower risk for violence perpetration and delinquency among youths.[94,171] Moderate to high levels of connectedness may represent a form of social bonding that serves a protective function for youths, whereas low levels of perceived school connectedness increases the risk for aggressive behavior.

Neighborhood collective efficacy is a community-level protective factor embedded in the social, political, and economic contexts that stratify neighborhoods.[137] Sampson and Laub[172] demonstrated a strong correlation between youth violence rates and level of community cohesion. In their research, they identified a cohort of neighborhoods with characteristics generally associated with high crime rates, such as poverty, unemployment, and single-parent households that actually had low rates of violence. Their findings suggest that a combined measure of informal social control, cohesion, and trust at the neighborhood level is a strong predictor of low rates of violence, a term they described as "neighborhood collective efficacy." According to Sampson et al.,[137] through collective efficacy, neighborhoods can create meaningful opportunities for youths by strengthening social relationships to achieve shared expectations and levels of social capital, defined as the personal relationships that are accumulated when people interact with each other in families, workplaces, neighborhoods, churches, local associations, and a range of informal and formal meeting places.

## IMPLICATIONS FOR HEALTHCARE PROVIDERS

### Developmental-Ecological Model

Youth violence is influenced by the interaction of numerous, multilevel characteristics, and risk and protective factors, including a personal, family, peer, and school history, experiences, and relationships, as well as characteristics of the community and society within which they live and grow up. No one factor, in isolation, leads to the development of youth violence, and the presence of risks does not always mean a young person will perpetrate violence.[173] One way to understand the dynamics between risk and protective factors is to view them within a developmental-ecological framework.[100,174] This approach recognizes that each person functions within a complex network of individual, family, community, environmental, and situational factors that impact their capacity to avoid risk.[175]

A developmental-ecological model provides a frame for considering the complex relationships between risk and protective factors and a life course perspective on factors that increase risk for youth violence perpetration.[176] *The developmental perspective* identifies important tasks, challenges, and milestones at each stage of adolescent development and the opportunities and competencies needed to meet them. Basic developmental needs of adolescents include a sense of safety, guidance from a caring adult, a feeling of social belonging, activities that promote leadership and civic engagement, participation in decision making, and opportunities to establish romantic relationships, earn money, and prepare for future jobs and careers. Successful arrival at adulthood can be determined by a youth's success in fulfilling a series of rites of passage events, such as graduation from high school, entry into the labor market, enrolling in college, marriage and parenthood, etc. Interruptions or failure to complete any one of these developmental benchmarks in a timely manner can have lifelong consequences that increase their risk for violence victimization and/or perpetration. Children and youths who have the resources and opportunities available to successfully accomplish developmental milestones are more apt to avoid risk-taking behaviors and exposures, have a healthy, productive adolescence, and make an easier transition into adult roles.

*The ecological approach* recognizes that each person functions within a complex network of individual, family, peer, school, community, and environmental contexts that impact their capacity to grow, develop, and avoid risk.[177] Instead of focusing solely on the individual characteristics of a youth who is at risk for a negative health event, a developmental-ecological model considers the importance of environment as a critical element in promoting health outcomes. It suggests that youths who reside in socially disorganized communities in which there is a lack of social capital and neighborhood efficacy not only experience a lack of resources, supports, and opportunities for them to successfully negotiate a socially acceptable pathway to adulthood but also frequently experience the presence of unique barriers within their families, neighborhoods, and communities that present obstacles to their progression. The developmental-ecological model suggests that communities that are better organized and have greater levels of social capital and neighborhood efficacy are better equipped to provide a safe and caring environment that supports youth development.

The most effective youth violence prevention interventions are those that use a developmental-ecological framework, which take into account the dynamics and interrelationship of both risk and protective factors. The developmental-ecological approach captures the complexity of youth behavior as the dynamic interaction between a youth's physical, cognitive, social, and psychosexual levels of development and the environmental exposures and contexts that shape the behaviors and relationships a youth has with his or her family, peers, school, neighborhood, community, and the broader society.[4,178–180] Instead of focusing just on the individual who is at risk for, or who engages in, a particular behavior such as violence, this approach considers the individual's relationship to his or her stage of development and the environmental surroundings.

### Primary Prevention

Primary youth violence prevention activities use universal strategies to educate and inform young people and adults and are typically carried out in the home or in a school, clinic, or community setting. Primary prevention interventions provide teens, peers, and/or their parents with information about youth development and the different levels and types of risk factors for youth violence, including individual, family, peer, school, and community levels. The most common primary youth violence prevention interventions seek to promote and enhance youths' knowledge skills, attitudes, and beliefs.[181] They typically include individual education, classroom or group presentations, and the use of mass media and marketing efforts.

Primary youth violence prevention efforts also include those interventions that seek to change the physical and social environments of communities. One of the most powerful protective factors emerging from resiliency studies is the presence of caring, supportive relationships with adults, other than parents. Thus the commitment of resources to programs that support meaningful opportunities for adult/youth interaction will help more adults understand youths' perspectives and behaviors and can contribute to a culture of caring for youths, instead of one that ignores youths or, worse, labels them as deviant or antagonistic. Other community-level protective factors that can be harnessed to help build resiliency and reduce overall risk for violent behavior at the community level include development of effective coalitions[182] and support for public policies that support child- and youth-oriented programs. Efforts to coordinate or expand community assets might serve as health-promoting or protective factors against youth violence. These include activities to enhance the level of social organization, social capital, and neighborhood collective efficacy and the presence of and access to social networks.

Efforts to improve structural and social characteristics that buffer or moderate the effects of risk factors for youth violence include efforts to improve local institutions such as schools (increased school safety, school climate, and mentoring programs), healthcare and social service agencies (trauma-informed systems of care), police (community policing), and policy reforms designed to mitigate the effects of social determinants (low-income housing, increased mental health services, needle exchange programs). Such programs can help adults build a base of understanding and commitment to work with and engage young people.

### Secondary Prevention

Secondary youth violence prevention programs seek to target youths who are at elevated risk for youth violence. The most salient predictors of violence perpetration are previous violence involvement and a history of violence victimization. The predictors include hard drug use, belief that hurting others' property while drunk was acceptable, and high-risk group self-identification.[183] Youths who have experienced physical abuse, experienced sexual abuse by family and/or other persons, witnessed abuse, and experienced household dysfunction caused by family alcohol and/or drug use are also at increased risk of adolescent violence perpetration.[91] Youths who report preteen alcohol use initiation also report involvement in significantly more types of violent behaviors, compared with nondrinkers.[184] Among adolescent inpatients, those who showed symptoms of impulsivity and PTSD were also at increased violence risk.[185]

### Tertiary Prevention

Tertiary prevention interventions can be defined as those focused on youths who have already engaged in violent behavior. Tertiary interventions that have been demonstrated to be effective include delinquency treatment program for early-career juvenile offenders,[186] MST,[187] provision of opportunities for preventing youth gang involvement in children and young people,[78] parenting interventions,[188] and trauma-informed systems of care.[189–191] Other tertiary youth violence prevention interventions that have been identified include community development, increased police presence and penalties, community policing, community and economic development initiatives, expansion of youth development and employment opportunities, school dropout initiatives, and mentoring programs.

## Youth Violence Screening

The complex nature of youth violence means that there is no single instrument or set of questions that will be appropriate as a universal screening tool. Healthcare providers considering incorporation of youth violence prevention strategies should consider the following developmental-ecological dimensions:

1. *Type of violence*: Homicide, fighting, family violence, dating violence, sexual violence, gang violence, bullying, and cyberbullying.
2. *Personal risk factors*: History of exposure to violence, attitudes and beliefs about the use of violence, gender stereotyping, etc.
3. *Purpose*: Primary, secondary, and tertiary prevention.
4. *Stage of youth development*: Early adolescence (ages 12–14 years), mid-adolescence (ages 15–16 years), and late adolescence (ages 17–21 years).
5. *Ecology of the youth's environment*: Family members, peers, school, community, society, and situational factors.

To screen for risk for youth violence perpetration, a combination of individual, family, peer, community, societal, and situational factors that contribute to the risk of a youth becoming a perpetrator of interpersonal violence must be considered. Although this undoubtedly will add to the clinical time needed to allocate to youths, interpersonal violence is the leading cause of death, disability, and injury in teens, particularly black and Latino boys, so the time spent may yield a high return.

Primary youth violence prevention screening tools typically focus on utilizing a positive youth developmental approach that targets the general population of youths, rather than targeting youths who are at risk of or currently engaged in youth violence. Dahlberg et al.[192] has compiled a compendium of primary prevention screening tools used to assess violence-related attitudes, behaviors, and influences among youths (see Table 10.1). These screening tools or individual questions can be used to identify youths at elevated risk for different types of youth violence perpetration.

Strand et al.[210] have identified secondary screening and assessment tools that seek to identify youths who have a history of exposure and/or symptoms arising from exposure to interpersonal violence. They include instruments that seek to assess prior exposure to violence:

**TABLE 10.1**
**Measuring Violence-Related Attitudes, Behaviors, and Influences Among Youths: A Compendium of Assessment Tools**

| |
|---|
| **Aggression/Delinquency** |
| Normative Beliefs About Aggression; 20 items (Huesmann, Guerra, Miller, and Zelli, 1992)[192] |
| Beliefs Supporting Aggression; 6 items (Bandura, 1973)[193] |
| Beliefs About Hitting; 4 items (Orpinas, 1993)[192] |
| Attitude Toward Violence; 6 items (Adapted by Bosworth and Espelage, 1995)[192] |
| Beliefs About Aggression and Alternatives; 12 items (Adapted from Farrell, 2001)[194] |
| Attitude Toward Conflict; 8 items (Lam, 1989)[195] |
| KMPM Questionnaire; 11 items (Adapted by Aber, Brown, Jones, and Samples, 1995)[196] |
| Attitude Toward Interpersonal Peer Violence; 14 items (Slaby, 1989)[192] |
| Beliefs about Conflict—NYC Youth Violence Survey; 9 items (Division of Adolescent and School Health, CDC, 1993)[192] |
| Attitude Toward Delinquency—Pittsburgh Youth Study; 11 items (Loeber, Farrington, Stouthamer-Loeber, and Van Kammen, 1998)[30] |
| Delinquent Beliefs—Rochester Youth Development Study; 8 items (Thornberry, Lizotte, Krohn, Farnworth, and Jang, 1994)[197] |
| Norms for Aggression and Alternatives; 36 items (Adapted from Jackson, 1966 and Sasaki, 1979)[192] |
| **Couple Violence** |
| Acceptance of Couple Violence; 11 items (Foshee, Fothergill, and Stuart, 1992)[198] |
| **Education and School** |
| Attitudes Toward School—Denver Youth Survey; 5 items (Institute of Behavioral Science, 1990)[199] |
| Commitment to School—Seattle Social Development Project; 6 items (Glaser, Van Horn, Arthur, Hawkins, and Catalano, 2005)[200] |
| Commitment to School—Rochester Youth Development Study; 10 items (Thornberry, Lizotte, Krohn, Farnworth, and Jang, 1991)[201] |
| Prosocial Involvement, Opportunities and Rewards—Seattle Social Development Project; 9 items (Arthur, Hawkins, Pollard, Catalano, and Baglioni, 2002)[202] |
| Classroom Climate Scale; 18 items (Adapted from Vessels, 1998)[203] |
| **Employment** |
| Attitudes Toward Employment—Work Opinion Questionnaire; 8 items. (Johnson, Messe, and Crano, 1984)[204] |
| **Gangs** |
| Attitudes Toward Gangs; 9 items (Nadel, Spellmann, Alvarez-Canino, Lausell-Bryant, and Landsberg, 1996)[205] |
| **Gender Roles** |
| Gender Stereotyping; 7 items (Gunter and Wober, 1982)[206] |
| Attitudes Toward Women; 12 items (Galambos, Petersen, Richards, and Gitelson, 1985)[207] |
| **Guns** |
| Attitudes Toward Guns and Violence; 23 items (Applewood Centers, Inc., 1996)[208] |
| **Television** |
| TV Attitudes; 6 items (Huesmann, Eron, Klein, Brice, and Fischer, 1983)[209] |
| **Community Violence** |
| The Children's Exposure to Community Violence Survey[188] |

Second Edition, Attitude and Belief Assessments.[192] https://www.cdc.gov/violenceprevention/pdf/yv-technicalpackage.pdf.

Anatomical Doll Questionnaire (ADQ), Checklist of Sexual Abuse and Related Stressors (C-SARS),[211] and Child Sexual Behavior Inventory (CSBI-I))[211] and Child Trauma Questionnaire (CTQ).[211] A screening tool that assesses for trauma histories that include events beyond maltreatment and family violence is the Traumatic Events Screening Inventory (TESI).[211] Other tools used to assess the impact of exposure to violence are the Childhood PTSD Interview,[212] the Children's PTSD Inventory,[213] When Bad Things Happen Scale (WBTH),[214] and the PTSD Reaction Index.[215] Instruments designed to measure the impact of stressful and traumatic events on children and adolescents, usually in terms of symptom development, include the Adolescent Dissociative Experience Scale (A-DES)[216] and the Child Dissociative Checklist (CDC),[217] the Pediatric Emotional Distress Scale,[211] and the Trauma Symptom Checklist for Children (TSCC).[211]

Tertiary prevention for primary care providers usually falls within the domain of referrals. A primary care provider may be asked to help identify and/or refer a youth who has already been identified as a perpetrator of violence to a program that can help him or her address the underlying issues. In a systematic review of youth violence interventions, Limbos et al.[181] found that youth violence prevention interventions that were tertiary in nature were more likely to report a reduction in violence outcomes than primary or secondary interventions. Tertiary interventions that have been found to have a significant impact in reducing youth violence include

- Tertiary Turning Point: Rethinking Violence (TPRV)[26]
- MST[187]
- Project Back on Track (after-school diversion program)[186]
- Nonrandomized controlled trial multimodal treatment approach with two orientations[218]
- Multifamily counseling program[219]
- Mendota Juvenile Treatment Center program[220]
- Retrospective comparative cohort Family Conflict Resolution program[221]
- Mental health services following adolescents' inpatient hospitalization[222]
- Low- and high-process group interventions for aggressive adolescents[223]
- MST versus individual therapy[224]

### Role of Primary Care Providers

The HEADSS (Home, Education and Employment, Activities, Drugs, Sexuality, Suicide/Depression, and Safety) assessment[225] is a good prevention screening framework for primary care providers and it addresses developmentally appropriate tasks of adolescence that most teens will encounter. Although it offers no differentiation of those youths who may be at risk for violence victimization or perpetration, it provides a good framework for incorporating questions about risk for youth violence perpetration. For instance, under *Home*, questions about relationships with parents and/or siblings can be explored. Under *Education and Employment*, peer relationships can probe for signs of bullying, dating violence, sexual violence, cyberbullying, and gang violence. For *Activities*, a provider can find out if there are other adults who can provide emotional and/or social support and mentoring. *Drugs and Sexuality* provide healthcare provider with an opportunity to identify situational factors, such as partying or drug selling/purchasing behaviors, which may increase the risk for youth violence perpetration. Under *Suicide/Depression*, emotional and psychosocial traits, including anger management and coping skills, can be explored more in depth.

## CONCLUSIONS

Interpersonal violence is the leading cause of death and injury in adolescents. Youths exposed to multiple risks factors and/or who have few protective factors are notably more likely than others to engage in interpersonal violence. The odds of violence in youths exposed to more than five risk factors compared with the odds of violence in youths exposed to fewer than two risk factors at each age were 7 times greater than those at age 10 years, 10 times greater than those at age 14 years, and nearly 11 times greater than those at age 16 years.

Although the overall accuracy in predicting youths who will go on to commit violent acts is limited, there is growing evidence that it is possible to identify youths who possess certain attitudes or behaviors or who are in environments or situations that increase their risk for being a perpetrator of youth violence. Identification of youths who possess certain risk and/or protective factors may increase or decrease the likelihood of youths who are at risk for various types of violence perpetration.[226] Understanding these risk and protective factors may help primary care providers identify various opportunities to incorporate screening questions to identify youths at risk for youth violence perpetration and to identify community resources for referring youths who possess these traits.

## GRANT ACKNOWLEDGMENT

This chapter was developed with support by the Health Resources and Services Administration (HRSA) of the U.S. Department of Health and Human Services (HHS) under grant number UH1HP30348, entitled academic Units for Primary Care Training and Enhancement.

This information or content and conclusions are those of the author and should not be construed as the official position or policy of, nor should any endorsements be inferred by HRSA, HHS or the U.S. Government.

## REFERENCES


1. Dahlberg LL, Krug EG. Violence – a global public health problem. In: Dahlberg LL, Krug EG, eds. *Violence – a Global Public Health Problem*. Geneva, Switzerland: World Health Organization; 2002:1–56.
2. Prevention CfDCa. *Youth Violence: Risk and Protective Factors*; 2018. https://www.cdc.gov/violenceprevention/youthviolence/riskprotectivefactors.html.
3. Sampson RJ, Lauritsen J. Violent victimization and offending: individual-, situational-, and community-level risk factors. In: AJRaJAR, ed. *Understanding and Preventing Violence*. WA DC: National Academy Press; 1994:1–114. Social Influences; Vol. 3.
4. Sheidow AJ, DG-S, Tolan PH, Henry DB. Family and community characteristics: risk factors for violence exposure in inner-city youth. *Am J Community Psychol*. 2001; 29:345–360.
5. Sampson RJ, Morenoff JD, Gannon-Rowley T. Assessing 'neighborhood effects': social processes and new directions in research. *Annu Rev Sociol*. 2002;28:443–478.
6. Sumner SA, Mercy JA, Dahlberg LL, Hillis SD, Klevens J, Houry D. Violence in the United States: status, challenges, and opportunities. *JAMA*. 2015;314(5):478–488.
7. Widom CS, Schuck AM, White HR. An examination of pathways from childhood victimization to violence: the role of early aggression and problematic alcohol use. *Violence Vict*. 2006;21(6):675–690.
8. Organization WH. *Youth Violence Facts*. 2002.
9. Hinduja S, Patchin JW. *Summary of our Cyber Bullying Research From 2005–2010*; 2011. http://cyberbullying.us/research.php.
10. Marshall WA, Tanner JM. Variations in pattern of pubertal changes in girls. *Arch Dis Child*. 1969;44(235):291–303.
11. Marshall WA, Tanner JM. Variations in the pattern of pubertal changes in boys. *Arch Dis Child*. 1970;45(239): 13–23.
12. Erikson EH. *Identity, Youth and Crisis*. New York: W.W. Norton Company; 1968.
13. Bronfrenbrenner U. *The Ecology of Human Development: Experiments by Nature and Design*. Cambridge, MA: Harvard University Press; 1979.
14. Kellough RD, Kellough NG. *Teaching Young Adolescents: Methods and Resources for Middle Grades Teaching*. 5th ed. Upper Saddle River, NJ: Pearson Merrill Prentice Hall; 2008.
15. Blakemore S-J, Choudhury S. Development of the adolescent brain: implications for executive function and social cognition. *J Child Psychol Psychiatry*. 2006;47(3-4): 296–312.
16. Casey BJ, Giedd JN, Thomas KM. Structural and functional brain development and its relation to cognitive development. *Biol Psychol*. 2000;54(1):241–257.
17. Flavell JH, BD, Chinsky JM. Spontaneous verbal rehearsal in a memory task as a function of age. *Child Dev*. 1966; 37(2):283–299.
18. Piaget J. *The Origins of Intelligence in Children*. New York: Int. University Press; 1952.
19. Piaget J. *The Early Growth of Logic in the Child*. London: Routledge and Kegan Paul; 1964.
20. Manning MA, Bear GG, Minke MK. Self-concept and selfesteem. In: Minke GGBKM, ed. *Children's Needs III: Development, Prevention, and Intervention*. Washington DC: National Association of School Psychologists.; 2006.
21. Brown D, Knowles T. *What Every Middle School Teacher Should Know*. 2nd ed. Portsmouth, NH: Heinemann; 2007.
22. Wiles J, Bondi J, Wiles MT. *The Essential Middle School*. 4th ed. Upper Saddle River, NJ: Pearson Prentice Hall; 2006.
23. Scales PC. *Characteristics of Young Adolescents*. Westerville, OH: National Middle School Association; 2010.
24. Milgram S. In: Milgram S, Sabini J, Silver M, eds. *The Individual in a Social World: Essays and Experiments*. New York: McGraw-Hill; 1992.
25. Subcommittee on Youth Violence of the Advisory Committee to the Social BaESD. *Youth Violence: What We Need to Know*. National Science Foundation; 2013.
26. Scott KK, TJ, Frykberg E, et al. Turning point: rethinking violence—evaluation of program efficacy in reducing adolescent violent crime recidivism. *J Trauma*. 2002; 53(21–27).
27. Satcher D. In: (US) OotSGUNCfIPaCUNIoMHUCfMHS, ed. *Youth Violence: A Report of the Surgeon General*. Rockville, MD: Office of the Surgeon General (US); 2001.
28. Online OSBB. *Arrest Estimates Developed by the Bureau of Justice Statistics and Disseminated Through Arrest Data Analysis Tool*. 2017. Online.
29. Prevention OoJJaD. Serious and violent juvenile offenders. In: *Bulletin*. Washington DC: U.S. Department of Justice, Office of Justice Programs, Office of Juvenile Justice and Delinquency Prevention; 1998.
30. Loeber R, Farrington DP. *Serious & Violent Juvenile Offenders: Risk Factors and Successful Interventions*. Thousand Oaks, CA: Sage Publication, Inc; 1998.
31. Loeber R, Farrington DP. Never too early, never too late: risk factors and successful interventions for serious and violent juvenile offenders. In: U.S. Department of Justice OoJP, Office of Juvenile Justice and Delinquency Prevention, ed. *Vol Final Report of the Study Group on Serious and Violent Juvenile Offenders (Grant Number 95-JD-FX-0018)*. Washington DC: U.S. Department of Justice, Office of Justice Programs, Office of Juvenile Justice and Delinquency Prevention.; 1997.
32. Olweus D. Bullying or peer abuse at school: facts and intervention. *Curr Dir Psychol Sci*. 1995;4(6): 196–200.
33. Berthold KA, Hoover JH. Correlates of bullying and victimization among intermediate students in the Midwestern USA. *Sch Psychol Int*. 2000;21(1):65–78.
34. Nansel TR, Overpeck MD, Haynie DL, Ruan W, Scheidt PC. Relationships between bullying and violence

among us youth. *Arch Pediatr Adolesc Med.* 2003;157(4): 348–353.
35. Nansel TR, Craig W, Overpeck MD, Saluja G, Ruan WJ, the Health Behaviour in School-aged Children Bullying Analyses Working G. Cross-national consistency in the relationship between bullying behaviors and psychosocial adjustment. *Arch Pediatr Adolesc Med.* 2004;158(8): 730–736.
36. Sourander A, Helstelä L, Helenius H, Piha J. Persistence of bullying from childhood to adolescence—a longitudinal 8-year follow-up study. *Child Abuse Neglect.* 2000;24(7): 873–881.
37. Ttofi MM, FD, Losel F. School bullying as a predictor of violence later in life: a systematic review and meta-analysis of prospective longitudinal studies. *Aggress Violent Behav.* 2012;17(5).
38. Nocentini A, Menesini E, Salmivalli C. Level and change of bullying behavior during high school: a multilevel growth curve analysis. *J Adolesc.* 2013;36(3):495–505.
39. Ramiro-Sánchez T, Ramiro MT, Bermúdez MP, Buela-Casal G. Sexism and sexual risk behavior in adolescents: gender differences. *Int J Clin Health Psychol.* 2018;18(3): 245–253.
40. Carrera-Fernández M-V, Lameiras-Fernández M, Rodríguez-Castro Y, Vallejo-Medina P. Bullying among Spanish secondary education students: the role of gender traits, sexism, and homophobia. *J Interpers Violence.* 2013; 28(14):2915–2940.
41. Volk AA, Dane AV, Marini ZA, Vaillancourt T. Adolescent bullying, dating, and mating: testing an evolutionary hypothesis. *Evol Psychol.* 2015:1–11.
42. Pepler D, Jiang D, Craig W, Connolly J. Developmental trajectories of bullying and associated factors. *Child Dev.* 2008;79(2):325–338.
43. Espelage DL, Low S, Polanin JR, Brown EC. The impact of a middle school program to reduce aggression, victimization, and sexual violence. *J Adolesc Health.* 2013;53(2):180–186.
44. Volk AA, Camilleri J, Dane AV, Marini ZA. Is adolescent bullying an evolutionary adaptation? *Aggress Behav.* 2012;38:222–238.
45. Bradshaw CP, Waasdorp TE, Goldweber A, et al. Bullies, gangs, drugs, and school: understanding the overlap and the role of ethnicity and urbanicity. *J Youth Adolescence.* 2013;42(220).
46. Simões CM, MG. Offending, victimization, and double involvement: differences and similarities between the three Profiles1. *J Evid Psychother.* 2011;11(1).
47. Shetgiri R, Lin H, Avila RM, Flores G. Parental characteristics associated with bullying perpetration in US children aged 10 to 17 years. *Am J Public Health.* 2012;102(12): 2280–2286.
48. Spriggs AL, Iannotti RJ, Nansel TR, Haynie DL. Adolescent bullying involvement and perceived family, peer and school relations: commonalities and differences across race/ethnicity. *J Adolesc Health.* 2007;41(3): 283–293.
49. CDC. *4 Teen Dating Violence Fact Sheet*; 2014. www.cdc.gov/violenceprevention/pdf/teen-dating-violence-factsheet-a.pdf.
50. Kann L, McManus T, Harris WA, et al. Youth risk behavior surveillance —United States, 2015. *MMWR Surveill Summ.* 2016;65:1–174.
51. Mishna F, Khoury-Kassabri M, Gadalla T, Daciuk J. Risk factors for involvement in cyber bullying: victims, bullies and bully–victims. *Child Youth Serv Rev.* 2012;34(1): 63–70.
52. Englander E, Donnerstein E, Kowalski R, Lin CA, Parti K. Defining cyberbullying. *Pediatrics.* 2017;140(Supplement 2):S148.
53. Shariff S, HD. Cyber bullying: clarifying legal boundaries for school supervision in cyberspace. *Int J Cyber Criminol.* 2007;1(1):76–118.
54. Schrock A. *Boyd Problematic Youth Interaction Online: Solicitation, Harassment, and Cyberbullying.* New York: Peter Lang; 2011.
55. Giumetti GW, Kowalski RM. Cyberbullying matters: examining the incremental impact of cyberbullying on outcomes over and above traditional bullying in north America. In: Navarro R, Yubero S, Larrañaga E, eds. *Cyberbullying Across the Globe: Gender, Family, and Mental Health.* Cham: Springer International Publishing; 2016:117–130.
56. Centers for Disease Control and Prevention DoAaSH. *Trends in the Prevalence of Behaviors that Contribute to Violence National YRBS: 1991–2017.* Youth Risk Behavior Survey; 2018. https://www.cdc.gov/healthyyouth/data/yrbs/pdf/trends/2017_violence_trend_yrbs.pdf.
57. Patchin JW, Hinduja S. *Summary of our Cyberbullying Research (2004–2016)*; 2016. https://cyberbullying.org/summary-of-our-cyberbullying-research.
58. Hamm MP, Newton AS, Chisholm A, et al. Prevalence and effect of cyberbullying on children and young people: a scoping review of social media studies. *JAMA Pediatrics.* 2015;169(8):770–777.
59. Beran T, Qing L. The relationship between cyberbullying and school bullying. *J Student Wellbeing.* 2007;1(2): 15–33.
60. Juvonen J, Gross EF. Extending the school grounds?—bullying experiences in cyberspace. *J Sch Health.* 2008; 78(9):496–505.
61. Dehue F, Bolman C, Völlink T. Cyberbullying: youngsters' experiences and parental perception. *Cyberpsychol Behav.* 2008;11(2):217–223.
62. Ybarra ML, Mitchell K. Prevalence and frequency of internet harassment instigation: implications for adolescent health. *J Adolesc Health.* 2007;41:189–195.
63. Mitchell KJ, Ybarra M, Finkelhor D. The relative importance of online victimization in understanding depression, delinquency, and substance use. *Child Maltreat.* 2007; 12(4):314–324.
64. Kowalski RM, Limber SP. Electronic bullying among middle school students. *J Adolesc Health.* 2007;41(6, Supplement):S22–S30.
65. Craig W, Pepler D, Blais J. *Responding to Bullying what Works?.* Vol 28. 2007.
66. Duncan RD. Peer and sibling aggression:: an investigation of intra- and extra-familial bullying. *J Interpers Violence.* 1999;14(8):871–886.

67. Basile KC, SL. In: Centers for Disease Control and Prevention NCfIPaC, ed. *Sexual Violence Surveillance: Uniform Definitions and Recommended Data Elements*. Atlanta: Centers for Disease Control and Prevention, National Center for Injury Prevention and Control; 2002.
68. DeGue S, Massetti GM, Holt MK, et al. Identifying links between sexual violence and youth violence perpetration: new opportunities for sexual violence prevention. *Psychol Violence*. 2013;3(2):140–150.
69. Pyrooz DC, Decker SH. Motives and methods for leaving the gang: understanding the process of gang desistance. *J Crim Justice*. 2011;39(5):417–425.
70. Howell JC, E G. *Gangs in America's Communities*. Los Angeles: Sage; 2019.
71. Klein MW, M C. *Street Gang Patterns and Policies*. 2006.
72. Labile DJ, Carlo G, Raffaelli M. The differential relations of parent and peer attachment to adolescent adjustment. *J Youth Adolesc*. 2000;29(1):45–59.
73. Steinberg L. A social neuroscience perspective on adolescent risk-taking. *Dev Rev*. 2008;28(1):78–106.
74. Farrington DP. Early predictors of adolescent aggression and adult violence. *Violence Vict*. 1989;4:79–100.
75. Z F. *American Youth Violence*. New York: Oxford University Press; 1998.
76. Piquero AR, Farrington DP, Blumstein A. *Key Issues in Criminal Career Research: New Analyses of the Cambridge Study in Delinquent Development*. Cambridge: Cambridge University Press; 2007.
77. Bishop AS, Hill KG, Gilman AB, Howell JC, Catalano RF, Hawkins JD. Developmental pathways of youth gang membership: a structural test of the social development model. *J Crime Justice*. 2017;40(3):275–296.
78. Fisher H, Montgomery P, Gardner F. Opportunities provision for preventing youth gang involvement for children and young people (7–16). *Cochrane Database Syst Rev*. 2008;2.
79. McDaniel DD. Risk and protective factors associated with gang affiliation among high-risk youth: a public health approach. *Inj Prev*. 2012;18(4):253–258.
80. McDaniel DD, Logan J, Schneiderman J. Supporting gang violence prevention efforts: a public health approach for nurses. *J Issues Nurs*. 2016;19.
81. General US urgeon General's Workshop on Violence and Public Health. *Surgeon General's Workshop on Violence and Public Health; October 27–29, 1985*. 1986. Leesburg VA.
82. Haddon W. On the escape of tigers: an ecologic note. *Am J Public Health Nations Health*. 1970;60(12):2229–2234.
83. Lösel F, Farrington DP. Direct protective and buffering protective factors in the development of youth violence. *Am J Prev Med*. 2012;43(2, Supplement 1):S8–S23.
84. Assink M, van der Put CE, Hoeve M, de Vries SL, Stams GJ, Oort FJ. Risk factors for persistent delinquent behavior among juveniles: a meta-analytic review. *Clin Psychol Rev*. 2015;42:47–61.
85. Bernat DH, Oakes JM, Pettingell SL, Resnick M. Risk and direct protective factors for youth violence: results from the national longitudinal study of adolescent health. *Am J Prev Med*. 2012;43(2, Supplement 1):S57–S66.
86. Greenberg MT, Lippold MA. Promoting healthy outcomes among youth with multiple risks: innovative approaches. *Annu Rev Public Health*. 2013;34:253–270.
87. Carlo G, Mestre MV, McGinley MM, Tur-Porcar A, Samper P, Opal D. The protective role of prosocial behaviors on antisocial behaviors: the mediating effects of deviant peer affiliation. *J Adolesc*. 2014;37(4):359–366.
88. Zingraff M, Leiter J, Myers KA, Johnsen MC. Child maltreatment and youthful problem behavior. *Criminology*. 1993; 31(2):173–202.
89. Lipsey MW, Derzon JH. Predictors of violent or serious delinquency in adolescence and early adulthood. In: Loeber R, Farrington DP, eds. *Serious and Violent Juvenile Offenders: Risk Factors and Successful Interventions*. Thousand Oaks, CA: Sage Publications, Inc; 1998:86–105.
90. Rappaport N, Thomas C. Recent research findings on aggressive and violent behavior in youth: implications for clinical assessment and intervention. *J Adolesc Health*. 2004;35(4):260–277.
91. Duke NN, Pettingell SL, McMorris BJ, Borowsky IW. Adolescent violence perpetration: associations with multiple types of adverse childhood experiences. *Pediatrics*. 2010;125(4):e778–786.
92. Charach A, McLennan JD, Bélanger SA, Nixon MK. Screening for disruptive behaviour problems in preschool children in primary health care settings. *J Can Acad Child Adolesc Psychiatry*. 2017;26(3):172–178.
93. Liu J, Lewis G, Evans L. Understanding aggressive behavior across the life span. *J Psychiatr Ment Health Nurs*. 2013;20(2):156–168.
94. Tolan PH, G-SD. Development of serious and violent offending careers. In: Loeber R, Farrington D, eds. *Serious and Violent Juvenile Offenders: Risk Factors and Successful Interventions*. Thousand Oaks, CA: Sage; 1998:68–85.
95. Jackson CL, Hanson RF, Amstadter AB, Saunders BE, Kilpatrick DG. The longitudinal relation between peer violent victimization and delinquency: results from a national representative sample of U.S. Adolescents. *J Interpers Violence*. 2013;28(8):1596–1616.
96. Brook JS, Lee JY, Finch SJ, Brown EN, Brook DW. Long term consequences of membership in trajectory groups of delinquent behavior in an urban sample: violence, drug use, interpersonal and neighborhood attributes. *Aggress Behav*. 2013;39(6):440–452.
97. Wojciechowski TW. PTSD as a risk factor for the development of violence among juvenile offenders: a group-based trajectory modeling approach. *J Interpers Violence*. 2017. https://doi.org/10.1177/0886260517704231.
98. Tremblay RE, Nagin DS, Séguin JR, et al. Physical aggression during early childhood: trajectories and predictors. *Pediatrics*. 2004;114(1):e43–e50.

99. Reef J, Diamantopoulou S, van Meurs I, Verhulst FC, van der Ende J. Developmental trajectories of child to adolescent externalizing behavior and adult DSM-IV disorder: results of a 24-year longitudinal study. *Soc Psychiatry Psychiatr Epidemiol*. 2011;46(12): 1233–1241.
100. Matjasko JL, Vivolo-Kantor AM, Massetti GM, Holland KM, Holt MK, Dela Cruz J. A systematic meta-review of evaluations of youth violence prevention programs: common and divergent findings from 25 years of meta-analyses and systematic reviews. *Aggress Violent Behav*. 2012;17(6):540–552.
101. Woolfenden S, Williams KJ, Peat J. Family and parenting interventions in children and adolescents with conduct disorder and delinquency aged 10–17. *Cochrane Database Syst Rev*. 2001;(2):CD003015.
102. Cooper WO, Lutenbacher M, Faccia K. Components of effective youth violence prevention programs for 7- to 14-year-olds. *Arch Pediatr Adolesc Med*. 2000;154(11): 1134–1139.
103. Steinberg L. *Youth Violence: Do Parents and Families Make a Difference?* National Institute of Justice Journal: National Institute of Justice; 2000:31–38.
104. Blazei RW, Iacono WG, McGue M. Father-child transmission of antisocial behavior: the moderating role of father's presence in the home. *J Am Acad Child Adolesc Psychiatry*. 2008;47(4):406–415.
105. McKinney CM, Caetano R, Ramisetty-Mikler S, Nelson S. Childhood family violence and perpetration and victimization of intimate partner violence: findings from a national population-based study of couples. *Ann Epidemiol*. 2009;19(1):25–32.
106. Holt S, Buckley H, Whelan S. The impact of exposure to domestic violence on children and young people: a review of the literature. *Child Abuse Neglect*. 2008;32(8): 797–810.
107. Jaffee SR, Moffitt TE, Caspi A, Taylor A, Arseneault L. Influence of adult domestic violence on children's internalizing and externalizing problems: an environmentally informative twin study. *J Am Acad Child Adolesc Psychiatry*. 2002;41(9):1095–1103.
108. Lessard G, Alvarez-Lizotte P. The exposure of children to intimate partner violence: potential bridges between two fields in research and psychosocial intervention: research and interventions often focus on a specific form of violence without considering other forms of victimization. *Child Abuse Neglect*. 2015;48:29–38.
109. Davis KC, Tatiana Masters N, Casey E, Kajumulo KF, Norris J, George WH. How Childhood Maltreatment Profiles of Male Victims Predict Adult Perpetration and Psychosocial Functioning. *J Interpers Violence*. 2018;33(6):915–937. https://doi.org/10.1177/0886260515613345.
110. Leeb RT, Barker LE, Strine TW. The effect of childhood physical and sexual abuse on adolescent weapon carrying. *J Adolesc Health*. 2007;40(6):551–558.
111. Simons DA, Wurtele SK. Relationships between parents' use of corporal punishment and their children's endorsement of spanking and hitting other children. *Child Abuse Neglect*. 2010;34(9):639–646.
112. Withers MC, McWey LM, Lucier-Greer M. Parent–adolescent relationship factors and adolescent outcomes among high-risk families. *Fam Relat*. 2017;65(5): 661–672.
113. Christle C, Nelson C, Jolivette K. *Prevention of Antisocial and Violent Behavior in Youth: A Review of the Literature*. 2005.
114. Sitnik-Warchulska K, IB. Family patterns and suicidal and violent behavior among adolescent girls—genogram analysis. *Int J Environ Res Public Health*. 2018;15(10):2067.
115. Antunes MJL, Ahlin EM. Family management and youth violence: are parents or community more salient? *J Commun Psychol*. 2014;42(3):316–337.
116. Schwarzer R, Leppin A. Social support and health: a theoretical and empirical overview. *J Soc Pers Relat*. 1991;8(1):99–127.
117. Grossman JB, Bulle MJ. Review of what youth programs do to increase the connectedness of youth with adults. *J Adolesc Health*. 2006;39(6):788–799.
118. Parker EM, Lindstrom Johnson SR, Jones VC, Haynie DL, Cheng TL. Discrepant perspectives on conflict situations among urban parent-adolescent dyads. *J Interpers Violence*. 2016;31(6):1007–1025.
119. Pasalich DS, Witkiewitz K, McMahon RJ, Pinderhughes EE. The conduct problems prevention research G. Indirect effects of the fast track intervention on conduct disorder symptoms and callous-unemotional traits: distinct pathways involving discipline and warmth. *J Abnorm Child Psychol*. 2016;44(3):587–597.
120. Raby KL, Lawler JM, Shlafer RJ, Hesemeyer PS, Collins WA, Sroufe LA. The interpersonal antecedents of supportive parenting: a prospective, longitudinal study from infancy to adulthood. *Dev Psychol*. 2015;51(1): 115–123.
121. Culyba AJ, Ginsburg KR, Fein JA, Branas CC, Richmond TS, Wiebe DJ. Protective effects of adolescent–adult connection on male youth in urban environments. *J Adolesc Health*. 2016;58(2):237–240.
122. Haynie DL. Delinquent peers revisited: does network structure matter? *Am J Sociol*. 2001;106:1013–1057.
123. Foshee VA, Benefield TS, Reyes HLM, et al. The peer context and the development of the perpetration of adolescent dating violence. *J Youth Adolesc*. 2013; 42(4). https://doi.org/10.1007/s10964-10013-19915-10967.
124. Dishion TJ, Véronneau M-H, Myers MW. Cascading peer dynamics underlying the progression from problem behavior to violence in early to late adolescence. *Dev Psychopathol*. 2010;22(Special Issue 03):603–619.
125. Juarez P. Social network analysis and youth violence. In: Li G, BSP, eds. *Injury Research: Theories, Methods, and Approaches*. *NY*. 2012.
126. Krohn M. The web of conformity: a network approach to the explanation of delinquent behavior. *Social Problems*. 1986;33:81–93.

127. Baerveldt CS, T. A. B. Influences on and from the segmentation of networks: hypotheses and tests. *Social Networks.* 1994;16:213–232.
128. Snijders TAB, Baeveldt C. A multilevel network study of the effects of delinquent behavior on friendship evolution. *J Math Sociol.* 2003;27:123–151.
129. Tita G, Cohen J, Enberg J. An ecological study of the location of gang set space. *Social Problems.* 2005;52(2): 272–299.
130. Radil SM, Flint C, Tita G. Spatializing social networks: using social network analysis to investigate geographies of gang rivalry, territoriality, and violence in Los Angeles. *Ann Assoc Am Geogr.* 2010;100(2): 307–326.
131. McCord W, McCord J, Zola IK. *Origins of Crime: A New Evaluation of the Cambridge-Somerville Youth Study.* New York: Columbia University Press; 1959.
132. Farrington DP. Predictors, causes, and correlates of male youth violence. *Crime Justice.* 1998;24:421–475.
133. Hawkins JD, HT, Farrington DP, et al. *Predictors of Youth Violence.* OJJDP Juvenile Justice Bulletin; 2000. April 2000.
134. *Neighborhood Poverty: Context and Consequences for Children.* New York: Russell Sage Foundation; 1997.
135. Acevedo-Garcia D. Residential segregation and the epidemiology of infectious diseases. *Social Science and Medicine.* 2000;6(1):45–72.
136. Hirschi T. Causes and prevention of juvenile delinquency. *Sociological Inquiry.* 1977;47:322–341.
137. Sampson RJ, Raudenbush SW, Earls F. Neighborhoods and violent crime: a multilevel study of collective efficacy. *Science.* 1997;277(5328):918–924.
138. Perkins DD, Long DA. Neighborhood sense of community and social capital: a multi-level analysis. In: Fisher A, CS, Bishop B, eds. *Psychological Sense of Community: Research, Applications, and Implications.* New York: Plenum; 2002: 85–110.
139. Perkins DD, Brown BB, Taylor RB. The ecology of empowerment: predicting participation in community organizations. *J Soc Issues.* 1996;52(1):85–110.
140. Sampson R, Groves WB. Community structure and crime: testing social-disorganization theory. *Am J Sociol.* 1989; 94(4):774–802.
141. Bursik Jr RJ. Social disorganization and theories of crime and delinquency. *Criminology.* 1986;26.
142. R K. *Social Sources of Delinquency.* Chicago: University of Chicago Press; 1978.
143. Wilson WJ. *The Truly Disadvantaged.* Chicago: The University of Chicago Press; 1987.
144. Wilson WJ, HD, Simpson RJ, Elliott A, Rankin A. The effects of neighborhood disadvantage on adolescent development. *J Res Crime Delinquen.* 1996;33:389–426.
145. Morenoff J, Sampson RJ, Raudenbush SW. Neighborhood inequality, collective efficacy and the spatial dynamics of homicide. *Criminology.* 2001;39(3):517–560.
146. Putnam RD. *Bowling Alone: The Collapse and Revival of American Community.* New York: Schuster; 2000.
147. Coleman JS. Social capital in the creation of human capital. *Am J Sociol.* 1988;94.
148. Bourdieu P. The forms of capital. In: Richardson JG, ed. *Handbook of Theory and Research for the Sociology of Education.* New York: Greenwood; 1985.
149. Brenner AB, Zimmerman MA, Bauermeister JA, Caldwell CH. Neighborhood context and perceptions of stress over time: an ecological model of neighborhood Stressors and intrapersonal and interpersonal resources. *Am J Community Psychol.* 2013;51(3–4):544–556.
150. Fagan J, Davies G, Carlis A. Race and selective enforcement in public housing. *J Empir Leg Stud.* 2012;9(4): 697–728.
151. Mohnen SM, Völker B, Flap H, Groenewegen PP. Health-related behavior as a mechanism behind the relationship between neighborhood social capital and individual health – a multilevel analysis. *BMC Public Health.* 2012; 12:116.
152. Massey DS, Denton NA. *American Apartheid: Segregation and the Making of the Underclass.* Cambridge, MA: Harvard University Press; 1993.
153. Cassidy T, Inglis G, Wiysonge C, Matzopoulos R. A systematic review of the effects of poverty deconcentration and urban upgrading on youth violence. *Health Place.* 2014;26:78–87.
154. Hair NL, Hanson JL, Wolfe BL, Pollak SD. Association of child poverty, brain development, and academic achievement. *JAMA Pediatrics.* 2015;169(9):822–829.
155. Schulz AJ, Zenk SN, Israel BA, Mentz G, Stokes C, Galea S. Do neighborhood economic characteristics, racial composition, and residential stability predict perceptions of stress associated with the physical and social environment? Findings from a multilevel analysis in detroit. *J Urban Healthl.* 2008;85(5):642–661.
156. Cook PJ, Juarez P, Lee RK, et al. Weapons and minority youth violence. *Public Health Rep.* 1991;106(3):254–258.
157. Bangalore S, Messerli FH. Gun ownership and firearm-related deaths. *Am J Med.* 2013;126(10):873–876.
158. Levine RS, Goldzweig I, Kilbourne B, Juarez P. Firearms, youth homicide, and public health. *J Health Care Poor Underserved.* 2012;23(1):7–19.
159. Rowell Huesmann L, M-T J, Cheryl-Lynn P, Eron LD. Longitudinal relations between children's exposure to TV violence and their aggressive and violent behavior in young adulthood: 1977–1992. *Dev Psychol.* 2003;39(2).
160. Bearinger LH, Pettingell S, Resnick MD, Skay CL, Potthoff SJ, Eichhorn J. Violence perpetration among urban American Indian youth: can protection offset risk? *Arch Pediatr Adolesc Med.* 2005;159(3):270–277.
161. Galla BM, Wood JJ. Trait self-control predicts adolescents' exposure and reactivity to daily stressful events. *J Pers.* 2015;83(1):69–83.
162. Hall JE, Simon TR, Mercy JA, Loeber R, Farrington DP, Lee RD. Centers for disease control and prevention's expert panel on protective factors for youth violence perpetration: background and overview. *Am J Prev Med.* 2012;43(2, Supplement 1):S1–S7.

163. McMahon SD, Todd NR, Martinez A, et al. Aggressive and prosocial behavior: community violence, cognitive, and behavioral predictors among urban African American youth. *Am J Community Psychol.* 2013;51(3–4):407–421.
164. Resnick MD, BP, Blum RW, et al. Protecting adolescents from harm. Findings from the national longitudinal study on adolescent health. *JAMA.* 1997;278(10):823–832.
165. Jang SJ, BR. Neighborhood disorder, individual religiosity, and adolescent use of illicit drugs: a test of multilevel hypotheses. *Criminology.* 2001;39(1):109–144.
166. Blum RR, P. Reducing the risk: connections that make a difference in the lives of youth. In: *Minneapolis: University of Minnesota, Division of General Pediatrics.* Adolescent Health; 1997.
167. Blum R. Healthy youth development as a model for youth health promotion: a review. *J Adolesc Health.* 1998;22:368–375.
168. Mercy J, BA, Farrington D, Cerdá M. Youth violence. In: Krug E, DL, Mercy JA, Zwi AB, Lozano R, eds. *World Report on Violence and Health.* Geneva: World Health Organization; 2002.
169. Resnick MD, Ireland M, Borowsky I. Youth violence perpetration: what protects? what predicts? Findings from the national longitudinal study of adolescent health. *J Adolesc Health.* 2004;35:424. e10.
170. Dubow E, Huesmann LR, Boxer P, Smith C. Direct protective and buffering protective factors in the development of youth violence. *Am J Prev Med.* 2016;43(2):S8–S23.
171. van der Merwe A, DA. Youth violence: a review of risk factors, causal pathways and effective intervention. *J Child Adolesc Ment Health.* 2007;27:95–113.
172. Sampson RJ, Laub JH. Life-course desisters? Trajectories of crime among delinquent boys followed to age 70. *Criminology.* 2003;41:319–339.
173. David-Ferdon C, Vivolo-Kantor AM, Dahlberg LL, Marshall KJ, Rainford N, Hall JE. In: Centers for Disease Control and Prevention NCfIPaC, ed. *A Comprehensive Technical Package for the Prevention of Youth Violence and Associated Risk Behaviors.* Atlanta: Centers for Disease Control & Prevention; 2016.
174. Stokols D, Allen J, Bellingham RL. The social ecology of health promotion: implications for research and practice. *Am J Health Promot.* 1996;10.
175. Stokols D. Translating social ecological theory into guidelines for community health promotion. *Am J Health Promot.* 1996;10(4):282–298.
176. Dahlberg LL. Youth violence developmental pathways and prevention challenges. *Am J Prev Med.* 2001; 20(1 Suppl):3–14.
177. Bronfenbrenner U. *The Ecology of Human Development: Experiments by Nature and Design.* Boston: Harvard University Press; 1979.
178. Juarez P, Schlundt DG, Goldzweig I, Stinson N. A conceptual framework for reducing risky teen driving behaviors among minority youth. *Inj Prev.* 2006; 12(suppl 1):i49–i55.
179. Tolan PH, Guerra NG, Kendall P. Introduction to special section on prediction and prevention of antisocial behavior in children and adolescence. *J Consult Clin Psychol.* 1995;63:515–517.
180. B J. Etiology of child maltreatment: a developmental-ecological analysis. *Psychol Bull.* 1993;114:413–434.
181. Limbos MA, Chan LS, Warf C, et al. Effectiveness of interventions to prevent youth violence: a systematic review. *Am J Prev Med.* 2007;33(1):65–74.
182. Cohen L, BN, Satterwhite P. Developing effective coalitions: an eight step guide. In: Wurzbach ME, ed. *Community Health Education & Promotion: A Guide to Program Design and Evaluation.* 2nd ed. Gaithersburg, MD: Aspen Publishers Inc; 2002:144–161.
183. Sussman S, Skara S, Weiner MD, Dent CW. Prediction of violence perpetration among high-risk youth. *Am J Health Behav.* 2004;28(2):134–144.
184. Swahn MH, BR, SulliventIII EE. Age of alcohol use initiation, suicidal behavior, and peer and dating violence victimization and perpetration among high-risk, seventh-grade Adolescents. *Pediatrics.* 2008;121(2).
185. Fehon DC, Grilo CM, Lipschitz DS. A comparison of adolescent inpatients with and without a history of violence perpetration: impulsivity, PTSD, and violence risk. *J Nerv Ment Dis.* 2005;193(6):405–411.
186. Myers WC, BP, Sanders PD, et al. Project Back-on-Track at 1 year: a delinquency treatment program for early-career juvenile offenders. *J Am Acad Child Adolesc Psychiatry.* 2000;39:1127–1134.
187. Henggeler SW, Clingempeel WG, Brondino MJ, Pickrel SG. Four-year follow-up of multisystemic therapy with substance-abusing and substance-dependent juvenile offenders. *J Am Acad Child Adolesc Psychiatry.* 2002;41(7): 868–874.
188. Woolfenden S, Williams K, Peat J. Family and parenting interventions for conduct disorder and delinquency: a meta-analysis of randomised controlled trials. *Arch Dis Child.* 2002;86(4):251–256.
189. SAMHSA. *SAMHA's Concept of Trauma and Guidance for a Trauma-Informed Approach.* SMA 14-4884. 2014:10.
190. Alpert EJ. A just outcome, or 'just' an outcome? Towards trauma-informed and survivor-focused emergency responses to sexual assault. *Emerg Med J.* 2018;35: 753–754.
191. Reeves E. A synthesis of the literature on trauma-informed care. *Issues Ment Health Nurs.* 2015;36(9): 698–709.
192. Dahlberg LL, TS, Swahn M, Behrens CB. In: Centers for Disease Control and Prevention NCfIPaC, ed. *Measuring Violence-related Attitudes, Behaviors, and Influences Among Youths: A Compendium of Assessment Tools.* 2nd ed. 2005.
193. Bandura A. *Aggression: A Social Learning Analysis.* Englewood Cliffs, NJ: Prentice-Hall; 1973.
194. Farrell AD, MA, Kung EM, Sullivan TN. Development and evaluation of school-based violence prevention programs. *J Clin Child Psychol.* 2001;30:207–220.

195. Lam J. *The Impact of Conflict Resolution Programs on Schools: A Review and Synthesis of the Evidence*. Amherst, MA: National Association for Mediation in Education; 1989.
196. Aber B, Jones & Samples. *Knowledge, Management, & Personal Meaning (KMPM) Questionnaire*. 1995.
197. Jang T. Delinquent peers, beliefs, and delinquent behavior: a longitudinal test of interactional theory. *Criminology*. 1994;32(1):47–83.
198. Foshee VA, Fothergill K, Stuart J. *Results from the Teenage Dating Abuse Study Conducted in Githens Middle School and Southern High Schools*. Chapel Hill, NC: University of North Carolina; 1992.
199. Huizinga D. Denver youth survey waves 1–5, (1988–1992) [Denver, Colorado]. In: *Inter-university Consortium for Political and Social Research [Distributor]*. 2017.
200. Glaser R, Van Horn ML, Arthur MW, Hawkins JD, Catalana RF. Measurement properties of the Communities That Care® youth survey across demographic groups. *J Quant Criminol*. 2005;21(1):73–102.
201. Thornberry L, Krohn, F., & Jang. *Commitment to School*. In. http://www.cdc.gov/ncipc/pub-res/measure.htm1991.
202. Arthur MW, HJ, Pollard JA, Catalano RF, Baglioni Jr AJ. Measuring risk and protective factors for substance use, delinquency, and other adolescent problem behaviors. The Communities that care youth survey. *Eval Rev*. 2002;26(6):575–601.
203. Vessels G. *Character and Community Development: A School Planning and Teacher Training Handbook*. Westport, CT: Praeger; 1998.
204. Johnson C, Messe LA, Crano WD. Predicting job performance of low income workers: the work opinion questionnaire. *Personnel Psychology*. 1984;37(2).
205. Nadel H, SM, Alvarez-Canino T, Lausell-Bryant LL, Landsberg G. The cycle of violence and victimization: a study of the school-based intervention of a multidisciplinary youth violence-prevention program. *Am J Prev Med*. 1996;12(5 Suppl):109–119.
206. Gunter B, WM. Television viewing and perceptions of women's roles on television and in real life. *Curr Psychol Res*. 1982;2:277–288.
207. Galambos N, Petersen AC, Richards M, Gitelson IB. The attitudes toward women scale for adolescents (AWSA): a study of reliability and validity. *Sex Roles*. 1985;13(5/6): 343–356.
208. Shapiro JP, Dorman RL, Burkes WM, Welker CJ, Clough JB. Development and factor analysis of a measure of youth attitudes toward guns and violence. *J Clin Child Psychol*. 1997;26(3):311–320.
209. Huesmann LR, Eron LD, Klein R, Brice P, Fischer P. Mitigating the imitation of aggressive behaviors by changing children's attitudes about media violence. *J Pers Soc Psychol*. 1983;44:899–910.
210. Strand VC, TLS, Pasquale LE. Assessment and screening tools for trauma in children and adolescents a review. *Trauma Violence Abuse*. 2012;6(1):55–78.
211. Strand VC, PL, Sarmiento TL. Child and Adolescent Trauma Measures: A Review, Fordham University.
212. Strand VS, L, Pasquale L. Assessment and screening tools for trauma in children and adolescents. *Trauma Violence Abuse*. 2005;6.
213. Saigh P, Yasik AE, Oberfield RA, et al. The children's PTSD inventory: development and reliability. *J Trauma Stress*. 2000;13.
214. K F. *When Bad Things Happen*. Worcester, MA: U Mass Medical Center; 1992.
215. Pynoos R, RN, Steinberg A, Stuber M, Frederick C. *The UCLA PTSD Reaction Index for DSM IV (Revision 1)1998*. Located at: Los Angeles Trauma Psychiatry Program.
216. Armstrong J, Putnam FW, Carlson E, Libero D, Smith S. Development and validation of a measure of adolescent dissociation: the adolescent dissociative experience scale. *J Nerv Ment Dis*. 1997;185:491–497.
217. Putnam FW, HK. Development, reliability, and validity of a child dissociation scale. *Child Abuse Neglect*. 1993; 17:731–741.
218. C M. A multimodal approach to controlling inpatient assaultiveness among incarcerated juveniles. *J Offender Rehabil*. 1997;25:31–42.
219. Canfield BS, BM, Osmon BC, McCune C. School and family counselors work together to reduce fighting at school. *Professional Sch Counsel*. 2004;8:40–46.
220. Caldwell MF, VRG. Reducing violence in serious juvenile offenders using intensive treatment. *Int Law Psychiatry*. 2005;28:622–636.
221. D BF. The effects of family conflict resolution on children's classroom behavior. *J Instr Psychol*. 2003;30:41–46.
222. Knox MS, CM, Kim WJ, Marciniak T. Treatment and changes in aggressive behavior following adolescents' inpatient hospitalization. *Psychol Serv*. 2004;1:92–99.
223. M MD. A comparison of two group interventions for adolescent aggression: high process versus low process. *Res Social Work Pract*. 2005;15:8–18.
224. Borduin CM, MB, Cone LT, et al. Multisystemic treatment of serious juvenile offenders: long-term prevention of criminality and violence. *J Consult Clin Psychol*. 1995;63:569–578.
225. Cohen E, Mackenzie RG, Yates GL. HEADSS, a psychosocial risk assessment instrument: implications for designing effective intervention programs for runaway youth. *J Adolesc Health*. 1991;12(7):539–544.
226. Services USDoHaH. Youth violence: a report of the surgeon general. In: *Department of Health and Human Services Centers for Disease Control and Prevention NCfIPaCSAaMHSA, Center for Mental Health Services, National Institute of Health, National Institute of Mental Health*. Rockville: USDHHS; 2001.

CHAPTER 11

# Depression and Suicide Screening

GREGORY PLEMMONS, MD, MFA

Major depressive disorder (MDD) is increasingly being recognized among adolescents. Almost one in five teenagers will experience at least one major depressive episode.[1–4] Only half of the adolescents with depression are diagnosed before reaching adulthood.[5] Primary care providers (PCPs) currently fail to identify the majority of youth with depression.[6,7] Screening for depression at adolescent visits has historically been rare.[8] Considering that less than half of young people with a mental disorder seek treatment,[9] PCPs may play a crucial role in identifying youth with depression and providing evaluation, treatment, and linkage with mental health services.

In 2009, the US Preventive Services Task Force (USPSTF) recommended routine screening for MDD in all adolescents aged 12–18 years in primary care settings.[10] This recommendation was reissued in 2016.[11] In 2018, the American Academy of Pediatrics (AAP) issued similar guidelines, recommending that adolescents 12 years and older be screened annually for MDD, with formal self-report screening tools.[12] Both the USPSTF and AAP have found adequate evidence that screening instruments for adolescents can accurately identify MDD in this age group in primary care settings.[12,13]

Nevertheless, despite the endorsement of routine surveillance for depression in adolescents by the USPSTF and AAP, as well as other experts in primary care, nursing, psychology, and child psychiatry,[14] routine screening for depression is not without controversy.[15] Little evidence exists currently to support whether screening for MDD in adolescents in primary care settings leads to improved health outcomes,[16–18] even though treatment of MDD detected through screening has been associated with moderate benefits. Critics have also argued that possible harms from screening, such as overdiagnosis and overtreatment, have not been adequately addressed, and may tax a mental healthcare system already overburdened with caring for those with known mental health disorders.[19–23] Finally, no screening tool has been shown to be perfect, raising the concern many adolescents could be falsely identified as depressed, given normal variations in mood.[24]

Diagnostic criteria for MDD is defined by the Diagnostic and Statistical Manual of Mental Disorders, Fifth Edition (DSM-5) as any period of at least 2 weeks' duration characterized by changes in affect, cognition, mood (adolescents often manifest with irritable rather than depressed mood[25]), as well as neurovegetative symptoms (e.g., sleep, fatigue). Bipolar and related disorders continue to be separate from MDD in the DSM-5.[26] MDD continues to be classified as mild, moderate, and severe, based on the number of symptoms present, the intensity of symptoms, and the level of impairment. Teens with mild MDD, for example, may only show minor functional impairment. Those with severe MDD may include delusions, hallucinations, and suicidal thoughts or behaviors.

Several screening instruments have been studied in adolescents. There is often debate over which tool is the best, as well as how and when to screen. The rapid introduction of electronic screening and self-report instruments, as well as self-monitoring of parameters such as mood, activity, and sleep through technology and even social media would seem to offer promise in not only improving access to screening but also potential interventions, given the increasing demand and continued lack of access to mental healthcare for many individuals.[27] The current tools that exist range from depression-specific questionnaires to broader psychosocial screening tools (such as the Guidelines for Adolescent Preventive Services, or GAPS), which have depression-specific questions embedded within a larger global survey. The many options for depression screening may seem overwhelming. Another question that arises is *whom* to screen—adolescents, their parents or caretakers, or both. Parent checklists are available for several of the tools available but there is limited evidence on the efficacy of screening *only* parents, as mild or moderate degrees of depression in adolescents may be overlooked.[12] Hopefully, the following summary can help to assist with tool selection. For the purpose of this chapter, the tools developed primarily for adolescents will be examined.

Adolescent Health Screening: An Update in the Age of Big Data. https://doi.org/10.1016/B978-0-323-66130-0.00011-9

## SCREENING TOOLS FOR DEPRESSION

Some of the earliest instruments created to assist in the diagnosis and treatment of depression (such as the Hamilton Depression Rating Scale) required interviewers to be specially trained and were time consuming, making them impractical to use in a busy primary care setting. Even early self-report questionnaires (such as the Beck Depression Inventory or the Hopkins Symptom Checklist), first developed in the 1960s and 1970s, were not brief and preceded the current DSM-IV and International Classifications of Diseases (ICD)-10 definitions for depression, rendering them less useful. As diagnostic criteria for MDD based on patterns of symptoms have grown more defined, so has the need for improvement in screening tools. Validity (how accurate a tool is, which may include sensitivity and specificity) and reliability (consistent results obtained when used by different providers) are all important considerations, not to mention ease of implementation and cost when considering a busy practice setting. Tools alone should never be a substitute for interviewing the adolescent. A discussion of several tools that have been studied and published in the medical literature follows later; the list is by no means exhaustive.

## COMMON SCREENING TOOLS FOR DEPRESSION

**PHQ-A, PHQ-9, PHQ-2, and PHQ-9: Modified for Teens.** One of the first screening instruments introduced to improve detection of mental health disorders in a busy setting was the PRIME-MD (an acronym for Primary Care Evaluation of Mental Disorders), developed over 20 years ago.[28] The Patient Health Questionnaire (PHQ) is a 67-item survey and the self-administered version of the PRIME-MD. It was created to assist with the recognition and diagnosis of the most common mental health disorders in primary care patients. The **PHQ-A** (also 67 items) was a version of the PHQ specifically modified for adolescents and was first introduced in 1995. It has been well validated in adolescent patients and is available within the public domain.[29,30] The **PHQ-9** and **PHQ-2** (both derived from the PHQ) consist of a subset of questions that specifically target depression symptoms.

The **PHQ-9** consists of nine questions and scores each of the nine DSM-IV criteria based on the frequency of symptom.[31] First validated in 1999, several follow-up studies have continued to support its validity in outpatient *adult* settings, both as an initial screening tool as well as a follow-up instrument to monitor treatment response.[32–35] To date, however, only one study has validated its use in adolescents; sensitivity and specificity were reported as 89% and 77%, respectively, with a positive predictive value (PPV) of 15% and a negative predictive value (NPV) of 99%.[36] The screen generally takes less than 5 min to administer, is available in several languages, and is currently freely accessible online through Pfizer.[37] One obvious criticism of the tool has been potential conflict of interest, given that increased screening theoretically may lead to false-positive diagnoses for MDD and unnecessary treatment with antidepressants.

The **PHQ-9: Modified for Teens** (often mislabeled as the PHQ-A) was initially developed and introduced as part of a national initiative, TeenScreen, by Columbia University in 2003 to improve mental health and suicide screening of middle and high school students. It was slightly altered to fit adolescent criteria for MDD by including irritability as a symptom as well as including questions regarding suicide. Although it closely resembles the PHQ-9, the exact format was never research validated, different from the PHQ-9.[12] The tool is also copyrighted by Pfizer. It is currently available through the Comprehensive Health and Development Interactive System and can be integrated with many electronic health records (EHRs).[38]

The **PHQ-2**, introduced in 2003, comprises the first two items of the PHQ-9.[39] Similar to the PHQ-9, it has been validated in adults in numerous studies, can be briefly administered, and is easily integrated with many EHRs.[12,40] The stem question is, "Over the last 2 weeks, how often have you been bothered by any of the following problems?" The two items include "little interest or pleasure in doing things" and "feeling down, depressed, or hopeless."[41] Respondents are then asked to report the frequency of symptoms (ranging from 0 = Not at all, to 3 = Nearly Every Day). To date, it has only been validated in one study of adolescents. Richardson et al. found a sensitivity of 74% and a specificity of 82% for detecting youth who met criteria for MDD, using a PHQ-2 score of $>3$; PPV was 42% and NPV was 99%.[42] Using a score of $>2$ in adults may increase sensitivity but also false-positive rates.[43] Comparison between the PHQ-9 and PHQ-2 is limited. Allgaier et al. concluded that the PHQ-9 was superior to the PHQ-2 in adolescents as a screening tool, but the ultrashort format of the PHQ-2 may be a practical compromise when implementing these instruments in a busy practice.[44]

The **Columbia Depression Scale (CDS)** is a self-administered 22-item instrument derived from the National Institute of Mental Health Diagnostic Interview

Scheduled for Children Version IV. First introduced in 2000 by Columbia University as part of the TeenScreen Program, it is available in English and Spanish and has been shown to correlate with the Beck Depression Inventory, one of the oldest validated tools.[45,46] Although not as well studied as the PHQ, it has been shown to be an acceptable tool in an urban Latino practice by providers and patients.[47] Although copyrighted, it is currently freely available online to providers.[48] One criticism of the tool has been that yes–no scoring makes it difficult to assess severity.[12]

The **Center for Epidemiologic Studies Depression Scale (CES-D)**, introduced in 1977 and revised in 2004 as the **CESD-R**, is a 20-item instrument often used in community health settings as well as epidemiologic studies and has been recommended for use for typically underrepresented populations such as the elderly and economically disadvantaged.[49–51] Although it has demonstrated acceptable screening accuracy in primary care settings,[52] it may not be ideal for cross-cultural use.[53] It has been adapted and validated for use in children and adolescents as the **CES-DC**,[54,55] and was included as part of the depression screening toolkit in the first edition of the AAP's *Bright Futures*,[56] although it is no longer recommended by the AAP as the primary screening tool.[57] A shorter 10-item instrument (the **CESDR-10**) has been developed for adolescents, which includes irritability as a symptom.[58] The original CESD-R is free and remains within the public domain.[59]

The **Mood and Feelings Questionnaire (MFQ)**, introduced in 1988, consists of both short and long versions (ranging from 13 to 34 questions) that both parents and children complete.[60,61] It has been shown to correlate with the Children's Depression Inventory and has been studied in large primary care settings.[62–64] The tool demonstrated an 80% sensitivity and 81% specificity when compared to an extended adolescent interview.[62] It is currently free and available online through Duke University.[65] Pros include simple wording which may benefit younger teens and populations with lower literacy levels. Drawbacks include no prescribed cutoff points.[12]

First introduced in 1998 and available in over 30 languages, the World Health Organization's **(WHO) Well-Being Index (WBI-5)** consists of five questions and is one of the most widely used questionnaires worldwide. This 5-item instrument has been well validated as a screening tool for depression in adults, particularly in the fields of gerontology and endocrinology.[66] Although its use in pediatrics is less well studied, it appears to have good sensitivity and specificity. Allgaier et al. reported a sensitivity of 75% and specificity of 92% when a cutoff score of 10 was used[67] and has also been demonstrated to be a reliable and valid instrument for adolescents with diabetes, a group in which depression has an increased prevalence.[68] A free version is currently available through the Dawn2 Study, sponsored by Novo Nordisk.[69]

Several questionnaires currently used in adolescent primary care have a much broader focus than primary screening for depression but warrant mentioning, given their widespread use. Perhaps the best known of these is the **Pediatric Symptom Checklist (PSC)**, available in both long (PSC-35) and short (PSC-17) formats. Both are self-administered and completed by parents or guardians (not teens).[70] The latter is available free of charge. The PSC appears to be fairly sensitive and specific for depression screening but less so for anxiety disorders.[71–74] A mean sensitivity of 72% and a mean specificity of 88% were reported in one systematic review.[74] The **Strengths and Difficulties Questionnaire (SDQ)**, internationally recognized and translated into more than 60 languages, is also freely available online.[75] It requires 5 min to complete, can be administered to teachers as well as parents, and examines five domains (conduct problems, inattention-hyperactivity, emotional symptoms, peer problems, and prosocial behavior). A self-completed version is available for teens. Although the SDQ has not been well studied in American populations, it appears to be reliable for general mental health screening[74,76,77] and has been specifically studied in the U.S. foster care population.[78] One drawback is the tool screens only for "emotional problem" in place of depression.

Specific tools have also been developed for youth entering the juvenile justice system, recognizing that this population has a much higher rate of mental and/or emotional disorders and mental health records are not always immediately or easily accessible. The Massachusetts Youth Screening Instrument **(MAYSI)** was created in the late 1990s to meet this need. The **MAYSI-2**, introduced in 2001, remains the most widely screening tool for this population.[79–82] It is important to note that, like many generalized tools, the MAYSI does not specifically screen for depression but does include questions about suicidal ideation and behavior, which are much more common in detained youth compared to the general population (Table 11.1).

Once a tool is selected, the clinician may still face significant challenges in implementing universal screening for depression in the office setting. In addition to lack of time, other reported barriers to screening have included a lack of mental health referral sites and providers, lack

TABLE 11.1
Depression Screening Tools

| Screening Tools | Year Introduced and/or Validated | Number of Items | Admini stered to: | Available Formats | Time to Perform (min) | Languages | Sensitivity | Specificity | Restrictions | Pros | Cons | Suicide Questions? |
|---|---|---|---|---|---|---|---|---|---|---|---|---|
| **TOOLS SPECIFIC FOR DEPRESSION** | | | | | | | | | | | | |
| CES-DC (Center for Epidemiologic Depression Scale for Children) | 1980 | 12- and 22-item versions available | Teen only | Paper | 8–10 | Available in Spanish | 71%–79%[54] | 53%–62%[54] | Copyrighted but free for use | Included in AAP Bright Futures toolkit | Does not include irritability as a symptom | No |
| MFQ (Moods and Feelings Questionnaire) | 1988 | 13 to 34 | Both teen and parents | Paper | 10 | Only English validated | | | Copyrighted | | May benefit younger teens, lower literacy levels | Yes |
| PHQ-A (Patient Health Questionnaire-Adolescent) | 1995 | 67 | Teen only | Paper, EMR | 5–10 | Available in Spanish | 77%[61] | 73%[61] | Public domain | Also screens for anxiety, drug dependence | Never validated in a primary care setting. Often confused with PHQ-9: Modified For Teens | No |
| WBI-5 (World Health Organization Well Being Index) | 1998 | 5 | Teen only | Paper | 5 | Over 30 | 75%[66] | 92%[66] | Public domain | No suicide questions | Validated in adolescents with diabetes | No |
| PHQ-9 | 1999 | 9 | Teen only | Online MDCalc | 5–10 | Over 50 | 89%[36] | 77%[36] | Copyrighted by Pfizer but free to use | Can help determine severity, response to treatment | Better validated in adults compared to teens | Yes |
| CDS (Columbia Depression Scale) | 2000 | 22 | Both | Paper | 8–10 | Available in Spanish | 85% (cutoff score of 12)[46] | 80% (cutoff score of 12)[46] | Copyrighted but free for use | Simple yes-no scoring | Less able to determine the severity | Yes |
| PHQ-9: Modified For Teens | 2003 | 13 | Teen only | Paper Electronic | 5–10 | Available in Spanish | Not available | Not available | Copyrighted but free for use | Modified to include irritability as a symptom | Not validated | Yes |

| | | | | | | | | | | | | |
|---|---|---|---|---|---|---|---|---|---|---|---|---|
| PHQ-2 | 2003 | 2 | Teen only | Paper Electronic | <5 | Over 50 | 74% (cutoff score $\geq$ 3)[42] | 82% (cutoff score $\geq$ 3)[42] | Copyrighted but free for use | Brief. Useful in two-tiered screening | May miss mild impairment. No suicide questions | No |
| CESD-R (CESD-revised) | 2004 | 20 | Adult only | Paper Online | 5–10 | English, Spanish | 83% (cutoff score $\geq$ 20)[52] | 78% (cutoff score $\geq$ 20)[52] | Public domain | Simple language | May not be useful in cross-cultural populations | Yes |
| CESDR-10 Version for adolescents | 2014 | 10 | Teen | Paper | <5 | English, French | Not available | Not available | Public domain | Includes irritability as a symptom | May be better at assessing severity than screening | Yes |
| **GLOBAL SCREENING INSTRUMENTS** | | | | | | | | | | | | |
| PSC (Pediatric Symptom Checklist) | 1979 | 17- and 35- item versions available | Both | Paper | <5 | Spanish, Chinese | 72%[74] | 88%[74] | Copyrighted but free for use | Well validated across populations and time | No suicide questions | No |
| SDQ (Strengths and Difficulties Questionnaire) | | 25 | Both (including teacher and parent) | Paper | 10 | >60 | Not available | Not available | Copyrighted | Studied in foster care populations | Not well studied in American populations. No suicide questions | No |

of training, and inadequate reimbursement for screening and time required.[83–85] Increasing utilization of web- or app-based tools to augment patient history would seem to offer advantages for the primary care clinician, given current recommendations for screening, as it is estimated that real-time implementation of the current USPSTF recommendations for adolescent screening would require over 2 h of clinician time each day.[86] Early innovations in embedding screening tools into workflow and improving compatibility with EHRs show promise.[87–89] The Guidelines for Adolescent Depression for Primary Care, (GLAD-PC) Toolkit, a 141-page document, recently provided by the AAP[12] is a welcome addition. However, any measure of success at improving the increasing recognition of depression in youth must be commensurate with further investment in child mental health infrastructure to support PCPs and adolescent mental health.

## SUICIDE SCREENING

Suicide is the second leading cause of death among youth ages 10–24 years.[90] According to the most recent CDC national survey of teenagers in high school, almost one in five has considered suicide, almost 15% have made a plan, and over 8% have attempted suicide.[91] After a brief decline in youth suicide from the mid-1900s to the early 2000s, suicide is increasing, along with the rate of self-inflicted injuries.[90,92] Visits to children's hospitals for suicide ideation and self-injurious behavior almost tripled from 2008 to 2015.[93]

In response to numerous suicides that have occurred in medical settings or shortly after discharge over the past two decades, the Joint Commission on Accreditation of Healthcare Organizations issued a sentinel alert in 2010 that called on all medical/surgical units and emergency departments to conduct suicide risk assessments on all patients; this was expanded to *all* healthcare settings in 2016.[94] Assessing suicide risk can be a challenging task for even the highly trained mental health clinician. To date, the clinical interview has remained the gold standard for suicide risk assessment, but is often time- and resource-intensive, demanding a greater need for psychometric instruments to assist with screening. Numerous tools have been developed and continue to be studied in a variety of locations, ranging from healthcare settings to schools and the military. Historically, many of these tools have relied on self-report. Some research suggests that self-report measures can often identify teens at risk for suicidality as well as or better than other methodologies, perhaps because teenagers may more often self-disclose on measures considered "private."[95–98] Other evidence suggests that some adolescents may be motivated to deny or underreport suicidal thoughts for fear of being stigmatized or hospitalized; historically, this has appeared to be particularly true for males as well as certain ethnic groups, such as African-Americans.[99–101]

Often, one barrier to screening that has persisted has been the common misconception that asking about suicide may precipitate suicidal thinking. Research strongly supports that asking about suicide does not increase the likelihood of suicidal ideation in an individual.[102] Most parents of adolescents find screening acceptable in the medical setting.[103–107] Given the variety of tools currently available, the selection of an appropriate tool can be challenging. The specific population being screened, setting, and method of screening (e.g., self-administered vs. clinician-directed) are all important considerations, as well as feasibility and integration with EHRs in busy settings.

Many of the tools currently available for suicide screening were first implemented and studied in emergency departments (ED), given that EDs are frequently the first contact point for persons contemplating suicide. Often, the ED is a primary site for accessing mental healthcare. EDs also play a crucial role in early detection as well as stabilization. Given the reported recent increase in suicide rates across all ages, suicide screening remains an active area of study. As with depression screening, it is important to note that no tool is perfect and should never be a substitute for a full mental health assessment and interview when there is concern about a patient's suicidality. Following is a brief discussion of the tools currently available.

The **Beck Scale for Suicidal Ideation (BSSI)**, originally created as a clinical research instrument in 1979, consists of a 19-item questionnaire that is completed by a clinician based on the patient's answers in a semi-structured interview, making it impractical for rapid screening.[108] The BSSI has not been well validated in U.S. children or adolescents. The **Modified Scale for Suicide Ideation (MSSI)** uses 13 items from the SSI as well as five new items, with improved reliability and validity, but also has limited evidence for use in children or adolescents.

The **Suicidal Behaviors Questionnaire (SBQ)**, introduced in 1981, is a 34-item self-report questionnaire that screens for frequency and severity of suicidal behaviors as well as past and future attempts. Given a large number of items, it has been modified and reduced in several subsequent versions for more general screening; the best known of these is the **SBQ-Revised (SBQ-R).**[109] The most recent version of the SQB-R consists of four items, in which respondents are given several choices for each question. Although the tool has demonstrated good sensitivity and specificity in both high school and college students, one major drawback is it focuses on past behaviors and fails to ask about current suicidality, which makes it impractical for real-time screening.[110]

Brief mention must be given to the **Reasons for Living Questionnaire**, one of the oldest screening tools, first introduced in 1983.[111] The RLQ consists of 48 items that must be answered on a Likert scale from 1 to 6. It has widely been studied in college students, less so in adolescents.[109] Proponents of the RLQ cite its theoretical base as well as its positive wording. Its length precludes its use in busy settings, although a shorter version (the Brief Reasons for Living inventory) is available.

The **Columbia Suicide Screen (CSS)**, introduced in 2004, is a 32-item self-report questionnaire in which 11-items inquiring about mood, previous suicide attempts, and substance abuse are embedded. Responses are entered on a 5-point scale, except for questions on suicide ideation and attempt (answered "yes" or "no"). The CSS was originally created and studied in the high school setting with the intent of providing a validated screening questionnaire for voluntary identification of mental health disorders and suicide risk in middle and high school students.[112] The CSS demonstrated a higher positive predictive value in identifying those at increased risk for suicide, compared to perceptions by school professionals (although teachers, who may be more sensitive to identifying problems, were not included in the group).[113] One criticism of the CSS has been the high false-positive rate.

The **Suicide Risk Screen (SRS)**, introduced in 1999, consists of a series of 20 questions embedded in the High School Questionnaire and was originally validated in at-risk youth (high school dropouts).[114] Although the SRS appears to be a valid tool, when used in a real high school screening setting, its high sensitivity and low NPV may make it unfeasible, given the high number of false-positive results.[115–117]

The **Suicidal Ideation Questionnaire (SIQ)**, first introduced in 1987, is a self-report questionnaire designed for ages 14–17 years. The SIQ was created to address the lack of appropriate screening tools for adolescents[118,119] and has been shown to be moderately to highly sensitive for possible subsequent suicide attempts and broad suicidality (with 98% sensitivity, 37% specificity, and 55% PPV).[120] It contains 30 items, ranging from nonspecific to major thoughts and the respondent is asked to rank the frequency of the statement on a 7-point scale. A junior high version (the SIQ-JR) is also available, which has been validated in an ED setting.[101] It has been used in diverse populations, is available in several languages, and has demonstrated strong validity and reliability, although one recent meta-analysis concluded that it is less than ideal, given its low PPV.[121]

The **Columbia-Suicide Severity Rating Scale (C-SSRS)**, first introduced in 2011, was the first instrument specifically created to help address inconsistencies in nomenclature and improve identification in suicide assessment, as well as to provide a single measure to track severity both acutely and over time.[122] The C-SSRS consists of six "yes" or "no" questions, not all of which may be asked, depending on the respondent's answer. The first two sections determine if the respondent has suicidal ideation; if so, it assesses the severity. The second two sections screen for past suicidal behavior and previous attempts. Administration time may range from 1 to 10 min. There has been substantial momentum to adapt the C-SSRS in healthcare settings because it helps provide further delineation and refinement of terms regarding suicidal behavior and nonsuicidal self-injury (e.g., cutting), which more closely correspond to the CDC's current system of nomenclature. The tool is currently free and online, available in over 100 languages, and can be integrated with many EHRs, including Epic.[123] An electronic form can also be completed using interactive voice response technology.[124] The C-SSRS has demonstrated high sensitivity and specificity[121,122,125] and appears to have some predictive validity in adolescent psychiatric ED patients.[126] The Federal Drug Administration labeled the C-SSRS as the preferred instrument for measuring suicidality in clinical trials in 2012.[127] It has rapidly been adopted for use in many healthcare settings. Despite its widespread use, however, one criticism has been that it has not been rigorously studied in adolescents and young children.[128,129]

Introduced in 2001, the **Risk of Suicide Questionnaire (RSQ)** was originally developed as a tool to assess children at risk for suicide who presented with mental health concerns in ED settings. Consisting of 14 questions, all items are answered "yes," "no," or "no response." The RSQ was shown to be a valid and reliable instrument when the SIQ was used as the criterion standard.[130] Given that four of the original questions in the SIQ identified 98% of adolescents determined to be risk of suicide, a shorter version of the RSQ, the **Ask Suicide-Screening Questions (ASQ)**, was introduced in 2012, in the interest of creating a briefer tool for universal screening of all adolescents who present to ED settings. The ASQ has shown high sensitivity and specificity (97% and 88%, respectively) and has demonstrated to be feasible for screening in busy settings.[131–134] An even shorter version of the ASQ has been developed (the asQ'em, a 2-item tool) for use in busy settings.[135]

Finally, the **Patient Safety Screener-3 (ED-SAFE screener)**, introduced in 2015, assesses depressed mood, active suicidal ideation within the past 2 weeks, and lifetime suicide attempts. Unfortunately, the tool has only been validated in adult patients.[136] (Table 11.2).

Suicide remains unique, compared to the countless other conditions for which adolescents are often screened. The potential outcome of missing a teenager with active suicidal ideation can be considerably more catastrophic (at least immediately) than not detecting someone with elevated cholesterol or hypertension. The most recent practice parameter from the American Academy of Child and Adolescent Psychiatry (AACAP) states that while self-administered suicide scales are useful for screening, they do not have predictive value, their tendency is to be oversensitive and underspecific, and they cannot substitute for clinical assessment (although it must be noted that AACAP recommendations have not been revised since 2001).[137] In general, when selecting a tool for universal screening, choosing one with high sensitivity at the expense of specificity will most likely always be preferred, given that preventing suicide may be valued over falsely labeling someone as suicidal. Universal screening remains controversial in school settings[138] although research shows that such programs have not been shown to create distress or increase suicidal ideation, at least in school-based settings.[139] Unfortunately, it is a given that everyday events in the lives of teenagers, such as being grounded or breaking up with a partner, may occasionally result in a positive screen. Tiered screening approaches may offer a partial solution to improving NPV.

In addition to the issues of variable sensitivity and specificity, another criticism of the screening tools currently available for adolescents and adults is their inability to provide much in the way of predictive validity—that is, correctly identifying those patients most likely to attempt and complete suicide.[140] Research has not been able to offer much guidance on who will most likely act on impulse, given the recognition that in some suicidal individuals, there may be a little history of depression and the impulse to kill oneself is often a transient state.[141–143] Nevertheless, while suicide is a rare event and the current statistical power to predict who will act is low, screening proponents argue that current tools are adequate for detecting youth with suicidal ideation, regardless of the outcome, and can improve linkage to mental health support.[144] one in three adolescents with suicidal ideation will eventually make a plan, and over half of those individuals will attempt suicide, most likely the first year after the onset of suicidal ideation.[145]

In the era of big data, the EHR itself may possess the potential for assistance in screening and detection of those most at risk for suicide. Recent innovations utilizing machine learning with EHRs have demonstrated some accuracy in predicting future suicide risk in adults.[146] Similar efforts with artificial intelligence (AI) surveillance of social media are already occurring.[147] Ironically, at a time when social media and smartphones are increasingly being implicated as the main driver of the recent increase in adolescent depression,[148] Facebook announced in late 2017 that it had partnered with local crisis centers to help dispatch first responders to users suspected of being suicidal.[149] The number of Facebook users who now see support content for suicide prevention has doubled since the company switched on a detection system, which has generated controversy.[150] Despite refinements in AI, however, it appears that the capability of adolescents to generate unique language and hashtags may continue to remain a step ahead of even the best coder. After Instagram recently blocked users from searching for content related to the hashtag #selfharm in an effort to reduce contagion of self-injury, other more ambiguous hashtags were created.[151] Smartphone applications have also been developed to assist with identification of depression and suicide, provide linkage to mental health services, and even alerting designated groups of trusted friends in times of mental health crisis. Despite all these innovations, any efforts to improve depression and suicide screening must be contingent on improving access to quality mental healthcare. Further exploration (and possible solutions) for why depression and suicide are increasing in adolescents is desperately needed. In the era of big data, there are likely more than *13 Reasons Why*. Refinement of current screening tools as well as future research regarding their effectiveness should help to support both clinicians and adolescents in ensuring that mental health remains a priority for all.

TABLE 11.2
Suicide Screening Tools

| Screening Tool | Year Introduced and/or Validated | Number of Items | Self-Report? | Restrictions | Pros | Cons |
|---|---|---|---|---|---|---|
| Beck Scale for Suicidal Ideation (BSSI) | 1979 | 19 | No | Copyrighted | Validated in several cross-cultural populations | Not well validated in adolescents |
| Suicidal Behaviors Questionnaire (SBQ) | 1981 | 30 | Yes | Copyrighted but free | | Not broadly evaluated in the current literature |
| Reasons for Living Questionnaire (RLQ) | 1983 | 48 | Yes | Copyrighted but free | Positivity-oriented questions | Widely studied in college students |
| Modified Scale for Suicide Ideation (MSSI) | 1986 | 18 | No | Copyrighted | | Not well validated in adolescents |
| Suicidal Ideation Questionnaire (SIQ) | 1987 | 30 | Yes | Copyrighted | Specifically created for adolescents | Low PPV |
| Suicide Risk Screen (SRS) | 1999 | 20 | Yes | Copyrighted | | High false-positive rate, low NOV |
| Suicidal Behaviors Questionnaire-Revised (SBQ-R) | 2001 | 4 | Yes | Copyrighted but free | Brief | No questions about active suicidality |
| Risk of Suicide Questionnaire (RSQ) | 2001 | 14 | Yes | Copyrighted | Validated in adolescents | |
| Columbia Suicide Screen (CSS) | 2004 | 11 | Yes | Copyrighted | Designed for screening in the school setting | |
| Columbia-Suicide Severity Rating Scale (C-SSRS) | 2011 | 6 | No | Copyrighted but free | Available in electronic form and embedded in many EHS systems | Not rigorously studied in adolescents |
| Ask Suicide-Screening Questions (ASQ) | 2012 | 4 | Yes | Public domain | Brief. High sensitivity and negative PPV for adolescents | |
| Patient Safety Screener-3 (ED-SAFE Screener) | 2015 | 3 | No | Public domain | Brief | Not validated in adolescents |

## REFERENCES


1. Whitaker A, Johnson J, Shaffer D, et al. Uncommon troubles in young people: prevalence estimates of selected psychiatric disorders in a nonreferred adolescent population. *Arch Gen Psychiatry*. 1996;47:487–496.
2. Lewinsohn PM, Rohde P, Seeley JR. Major depressive disorder in older adolescents: prevalence, risk factors, and clinical implications. *Clin Psychol Rev*. 1998;18:765–794.
3. Kessler RC, Walters MS. Epidemiology of DSM-III-R major depression and minor depression among adolescents and young adults in the national comorbidity survey. *Depress Anxiety*. 1998;7:3–14.
4. Cheung A. Canadian community health survey: major depressive disorder and suicidality in adolescents. *Health Policy*. 2006;2(2):76–89.
5. Kessler RC, Avenevoli S, Ries Merikangas K. Mood disorders in children and adolescents: an epidemiologic perspective. *Biol Psychiatry*. 2001;49:1002–1014.
6. Burns BJ, Costello EJ, Angold A, et al. Children's mental health service use across service sectors. *Health Aff (Millwood)*. 1995;14(3):147–159.
7. Leaf PJ, Alegria M, Cohen P, et al. Mental health service use in the community and schools: results from the four-community MECA study. Methods for the epidemiology of child and adolescent mental disorders study. *J Am Acad Child Adolesc Psychiatry*. 1996;35:889–897.
8. Zenlea IS, Milliren CE, Mednick L, Rhodes ET. Depression screening in adolescents in the United States: a national study of ambulatory, office-based practice. *Acad Pediatr*. 2014;14:186–191.
9. Costello EJ, He JP, Sampson NA, Kessler RC, Merikangas KR. Services for adolescents with psychiatric disorders: 12-month data from the National Comorbidity Survey-Adolescent. *Psychiatr Serv*. 2014;71:81–90.
10. US Preventive Services Task Force. Screening and treatment for major depressive disorder in children and adolescents: US Preventive Services Task Force recommendation statement. *Pediatrics*. 2009;123: 1223–1228.
11. *Final Update Summary: Depression in Children and Adolescents: Screening*. U.S. Preventive Services Task Force; September 2016.
12. Zuckerbrot RA, Cheung A, Jensen PS, Stein REK, Laraque D. Guidelines for adolescent depression in primary care (GLAD-PC): part I. practice preparation, identification, assessment, and initial management. *Pediatrics*. 2018;141(3):e20174081.
13. Forman-Hoffman V, McClure E, McKeeman J, Wood CT, Middleton JC, et al. Screening for major depressive disorder in children and adolescents: a systematic review for the U.S. Preventive Services Task Force. *Ann Intern Med*. 2016;164:342–349.
14. Cheung AH, Zuckerbrot RA, Jensen PS, Stein REK, Laraque D. Expert survey for the management of adolescent depression in primary care. *Pediatrics*. 2008;121(1): e101–e107.
15. Horwitz AV, Wakefield JC. Should screening for depression among children and adolescents be demedicalized? *J Am Acad Child Adolesc Psychiatry*. 2009; 48:683–687.
16. Williams SB, O'Connor EA, Eder M, Whitlock EP. Screening for child and adolescent depression in primary care settings: a systematic evidence review for the U.S. Preventive Services Task Force. *Pediatrics*. 2009;123: e716–e735.
17. Forman-Hoffman V, McClure E, McKeeman J, et al. Screening for major depressive disorder in children and adolescents: a systematic review for the U.S. Preventive Services Task Force. *Ann Intern Med*. 2016;164:342–354.
18. Roseman M, Saadat M, Riehm KE, et al. Depression screening and health outcomes in children and adolescents: a systematic review. *Can J Psychiatry*. 2017;62: 813–817.
19. Thombs BD, Coyne JC, Cuijpers P, et al. Rethinking recommendations for screening for depression in primary care. *CMAJ*. 2012;184:413–418.
20. Thombs BD, Ziegelstein RC. Depression screening in primary care: why the Canadian Task Force of Preventive Health Care did the right thing. *Can J Psychiatry*. 2013; 58:692–696.
21. Thombs BD, Ziegelstein RC. Does depression screening improve depression outcomes in primary care? *BMJ*. 2014;348:g1253.
22. Thombs BD, Ziegelstein RC, Roseman M, Kloda LA, Ioannidis JP. There are no randomized controlled trials that support the United States Preventive Services Task Force guideline on screening for depression in primary care: a systematic review. *BMC Med*. 2014;12:13.
23. Lenzer J. Is the United States Preventive Services Task Force still a voice of caution? *BMJ*. 2017;356:j743.
24. Roseman M, Kloda LA, Saadat N, et al. Accuracy of depression screening tools to detect major depression in children and adolescents: a systematic review. *Can J Psychiatry*. 2016;61:746–757.
25. American Psychiatric Association. *Diagnostic and Statistical Manual of Mental Disorders (DSM-5)*. 5th ed. Washington (DC): American Psychiatric Association; 2013.
26. Black DW, Grant K. *DSM-5@ Guidebook: The Essential Companion to the Diagnostic and Statistical Manual of Mental Disorders*. 5th ed. Washington (DC): American Psychiatric Publishing; 2014.
27. Hollis C, Falconer CJ, Martin JL, et al. Annual research review: digital health interventions for children and young people with mental health problems—a systematic and meta-review. *J Child Psychol Psychiatry*. 2017;58:474–503.
28. Spitzer RL, Williams BJW, Kroenke K, et al. Utility of new procedure for diagnosing mental disorders in primary care: the PRIME-MD 1000 study. *JAMA*. 1994;272: 1749–1756.
29. Spitzer RL, Johnson JG. *The Patient Health Questionnaire, Adolescent Version*. New York: Biometrics Research Unit, New York Psychiatric Institute; 1995.

30. Johnson JG, Harris ES, Spitzer RL, Williams JBW. The patient health questionnaire for adolescents: validation of an instrument for the assessment of mental disorders among adolescent primary care patients. *J Adolesc Health.* 2002;30:196–204.
31. Kroenke K, Spitzer RL, Williams JBW. The PHQ-9: validity of a brief depression severity measure. *J Gen Intern Med.* 2001;16:606–613.
32. Spitzer RL, Kroenke K, Williams JB. Validation and utility of a self-report version of PRIME-MD: the PHQ primary care study. *JAMA.* 1999;282:1737–1744.
33. Lowe B, Spitzer RL, Grafe K, et al. Comparative validity of three screening questionnaires for DSM-IV depressive disorders and physicians's diagnoses. *J Affect Disord.* 2004; 78:131–140.
34. Lowe B, Unutzer J, Callahan CM, Perkins AJ, Kroenke K. Monitoring depression treatment outcomes with the patient health questionnaire-9. *Med Care.* 2004;42: 1194–1201.
35. Kroenke K, Spitzer RL, Williams JBW, Lowe B. The patient health questionnaire somatic, anxiety, and depressive symptoms scales: a systematic review. *Gen Hosp Psych.* 2010;32:345–359.
36. Richardson LP, McCauley E, Grossman DC, et al. Evaluation of the patient health questionnaire-9 Item for detecting major depression among adolescents. *Pediatrics.* 2010;126:1117–1123.
37. *PHQ Screeners*; August 28, 2018. Retrieved from https://www.phqscreeners.com.
38. *PHQ-9-Modified, Comprehensive Health and Development Interactive System*; August 28, 2018. Retrieved from https://www.chadis.com/site/content/patient-health-questionnaire-9-modified-phq-9-m-cts.
39. Kroenke K, Spitzer RL, Williams JB. The patient health questionnaire-2: validity of a two-item depression screener. *Med Care.* 2003;41:1284–1292.
40. Arroll B, Goodyear-Smith F, Crengle S, et al. Validation of PHQ-2 and PHQ-9 to screen for major depression in the primary care population. *Ann Fam Med.* 2010;8: 348–353.
41. Lowe B, Kroenke K, Grafe K. Detecting and monitoring depression with a two-item questionnaire (PHQ-2). *J Psychosom Res.* 2005;58:163–171.
42. Richardson LP, Rockhill C, Russo JE, et al. Evaluation of the PHQ-2 as a brief screen for detecting major depression among adolescents. *Pediatrics.* 2010;125(5): e1097–e1103.
43. Manea L, Gilbody S, Hewitt C, et al. Identifying depression with the PHQ-2: a diagnostic meta-analysis. *J Affect Disord.* 2016;203:382–395.
44. Allgaier A-K, Pietsch K, Fruhe B, Sigl-Glockner J, Schulte-Korne G. Screening for depression in adolescents: validity of the patient health questionnaire in pediatric care. *Depress Anxiety.* 2012;29:906–913.
45. Shaffer D, Fisher P, Lucas CP, Dulcan MK, Schwab-Stone ME. NIMH Diagnostic Interview Schedule for Children Version IV (NIMH DISC-IV): description, differences from previous versions, and reliability of some common diagnoses. *J Am Acad Child Adolesc Psychiatry.* 2000;39:28–38.
46. Zuckerbrot R, Maxon L, Pagar D, Davies M, Fisher PW, Shaffer D. Adolescent depression screening in primary care: feasibility and acceptability. *Pediatrics.* 2007; 119(1):101–108.
47. Rausch J, Hametz P, Zuckerbrot R, Rausch W, Soren K. Screening for depression in urban Latino adolescents. *Clin Pediatr.* 2012;51:964–971.
48. *Community Pediatrics, Columbia Depression Screen Adolescent*; August 28, 2018. Retrieved from: http://www.columbia.edu/itc/hs/medical/residency/peds/new_compeds_site/genpeds_menthealthres_dxandscreening-tools.html.
49. Eaton W, Muntaner C, Smith C, Tien A, Ybarra ML. Center for epidemiologic studies depression scale: review and revision (CESD and CESD-R). In: Maruish ME, ed. *The Use of Psychological Testing for Treatment Planning and Outcomes Assessment.* 3rd ed. Mahwah (NJ): Lawrence Erlbaum; 2004:363–377.
50. Radloff LS. The CES-D scale: a self report depression scale for research in the general population. *Appl Psychol Meas.* 1977;1:385–401.
51. Van Dam NT, Earlywine M. Validation of the center for epidemiologic studies depression scale—revised (CESD-R): pragmatic depression assessment in the general population. *Psychiatry Res.* 2010;186:128–132.
52. Vilagut G, Forero CG, Barbaglia G, Alonso J. Screening for depression in the general population with the Center for Epidemiologic Studies Depression (CES-D): a systematic review with meta-analysis. *PLoS One.* 2016;11(5): e0155431. https://doi.org/10.1371/journal.pone.0155431.
53. Roberts RE, Rhoades HM, Vernon SW. Using the CES-D scale to screen for depression and anxiety: effects of language and ethnic status. *Psychiatry Res.* 1990;31:69–83.
54. Faulstich ME, Carey MP, Ruggiero L, Enyart P, Gresham F. Assessment of depression in childhood and adolescence: an evaluation of the Center for Epidemiologic Studies Depression Scale for Children (CES-DC). *Am J Psychiatry.* 1986;143(8):1024–1027.
55. Fendrich M, Weissman MM, Warner V. Screening for depressive disorder in children and adolescents: validating the Center for Epidemiologic Studies Depression Scale for Children. *Am J Epidemiol.* 1990;131(3): 538–551.
56. Green M, Palfrey JS, eds. *Bright Futures: Guidelines for Health Supervision of Infants, Children, and Adolescents.* 2nd ed. Arlington (VA): National Center for Education in Maternal and Child Health; 2002.
57. Hagan JF, Shaw JS, Duncan PM, eds. *Bright Futures: Guidelines for Health Supervision of Infants, Children, and Adolescents.* 4th ed. Elk Grove Village (IL): American Academy of Pediatrics; 2017.
58. Haroz EE, Ybarra ML, Eaton WW. Psychometric evaluation of a self-report scale to measure adolescent depression: the CESDR-10 in two national adolescent samples in the United States. *J Affect Disord.* 2014;158:154–160.
59. *The Center for Epidemiologic Studies Depression Scale Revised*; August 28, 2018. Retrieved from: http://cesd-r.com/cesdr/.

60. Angold A, Costello EJ, Messer SC, Pickles A, Winder F, Silver D. The development of a short questionnaire for use in epidemiological studies of depression in children and adolescents. *Int J Methods Psychiatr Res*. 1995;5:237–249.
61. Messer SC, Angold A, Costello EJ, Loeber R, Van Kammen W, Stouthammer-Loeber M. Development of a short questionnaire for use in epidemiological studies of depression in children and adolescents: factor composition and structure across development. *Int J Methods Psychiatr Res*. 1995;5:251–262.
62. Katon W, Russo J, Richardson L, McCauley E, Lozano P. Anxiety and depression screening for youth in a primary care population. *Ambul Pediatr*. 2008;8:182–188.
63. Gledhill J, Garralda ME. The short-term outcome of depressive disorder in adolescents attending primary care: a cohort study. *Soc Psychiatry Psychiatr Epidemiol*. 2011;46:993–1002.
64. Gledhill J, Garralda ME. Sub-syndromal depression in adolescents attending primary care: frequency, clinical features and 6 months' outcome. *Soc Psychiatry Psychiatr Epidemiol*. 2013;48:735–744.
65. *Duke University Center for Developmental Epidemiology*; August 28, 2018. Retrieved from: http://devepi.duhs.duke.edu/mfq.html.
66. Topp CW, Ostergaard SD, Sondergaard S, Bech P. The WHO-5 well-being Index: a systematic review of the literature. *Psychother Psychosom*. 2015;84:167–176.
67. Allgaier A-K, Pietsch K, Fruhe B, Prast E, Sigl-Glockner J, Schulte-Korne G. Depression in pediatric care: is the WHO-Five Well-Being inded a valid screening instrument for children and adolescents? *Gen Hosp Psychiatry*. 2012;34:234–241.
68. De Wit M, Pouwer F, Gemke RJBJ, Delemarre-Van de Waal HA, Snoek FJ. Validation of the WHO-5 well-being Index in adolescents with type 1 diabetes. *Diabetes Care*. 2007;30:2003–2007.
69. *Dawn Dialogue Tools*; August 28, 2018. Retrieved from: http://www.dawnstudy.com/tools-and-resources/tools-for-healthcare-professionals/dawn-dialogue-tools.html.
70. Jellinek MS, Murphy JM, Little M, Pagano M, Comer DM, Kelleher KJ. Use of the pediatric symptom checklist to screen for psychosocial problems in pediatric primary care: a national feasibility study. *Arch Pediatr Adolesc Med*. 1999;153:254–260.
71. Wren FJ, Bridge JA, Birmaher B. Screening for childhood anxiety symptoms in primary care: integrating child and parent reports. *J Am Acad Child Adolesc Psychiatry*. 2004;43:1364–1371.
72. Gardner W, Lucas A, Kolko DJ, Campo JV. Comparison of the PSC-17 and alternative mental health screens in an at-risk primary care sample. *J Am Acad Child Adolesc Psychiatry*. 2007;46:611–618.
73. Kamin HS, McCarthy AE, Abel MR, Jellinek MS, Baer L, Murphy JM. Using a brief parent-report measure to track outcomes for children and teens with internalizing disorders. *Child Psychiatry Hum Dev*. 2015;46:851–862.
74. Lavigne JV, Meyers KM, Feldman M. Systematic review: classification accuracy of behavioral screening measures for use in integrated primary care settings. *J Pediatr Psychol*. 2016;41:1091–1109.
75. *Youth in Mind*; August 28, 2018. Retrieved from: http://www.sdqinfo.com/py/sdqinfo/b0.py.
76. Mathai J, Anderson P, Bourne A. Comparing psychiatric diagnoses generated by the strengths and difficulties questionnaire with diagnoses made by clinicians. *Aust N Z J Psychiatry*. 2004;38:639–643.
77. Kovacs S, Sharp C. Criterion validity of the Strenghts and Difficulties Questionnaire (SDQ) with inpatient adolescents. *Psychiatry Res*. 2014;219:651–657.
78. Jee SH, Szilagyi M, Conn A-M, et al. Validating office-based screening for psychosocial strengths and difficulties among youths in foster care. *Pediatrics*. 2011;127:904–910.
79. Grisso T, Barnum R, Fletcher KE, Cauffman E, Peuschold D. Massachussetts youth screening instrument for mental health needs of juvenile justice youths. *J Am Acad Child Adolesc Psychiatry*. 2001;40:541–548.
80. Archer RP, Stredny RV. An examination and replication of the psychometric properties of the Massachusetts youth screening instrument—second edition (MAYSI-2) among adolescents in detention settings. *Assessment*. 2004;11:290–302.
81. Soulier M, McBride A. Mental health screening and assessment of detained youth. *Child Adolesc Psychiatr Clin N Am*. 2016;25:27–39.
82. Russell JD, Marsee MA. Identifying mental health issues in detained youth: testing the structure and invariance of the Massachusetts youth screening inventory—version 2 (MAYSI-2). *Psychol Assess*. 2017;29:720–726.
83. Olson AL, Kelleher KJ, Kemper KJ, Zuckermann BS, Hammond CS, Dietrich AJ. Primary care pediatricians' roles and perceived responsibilities in the identification and management of depression in children and adolescents. *Ambul Pediatr*. 2001;1(2):91–98.
84. Horwitz SM, Helleher KJ, Stein RE, et al. Barriers to the identification and management of psychosocial issues in children and maternal depression. *Pediatrics*. 2007;119:e208–e218.
85. Horwitz SM, Storfer-Isser A, Kerker BD, et al. Barriers to the identification and management of psychosocial problems: changes from 2004 to 2013. *Acad Pediatr*. 2015;15:613–620.
86. Yarnell KSH, Pollak KI, Truls O, Krause KM, Michener L. Primary care: is there enough time for prevention? *Am J Public Health*. 2003;93:635–641.
87. Sudhanthar S, Thakur K, Sigal Y, Turner J. Improving validated depression screen among adolescent population in primary care practice using electronic health records (HER). *BMJ Qual Improv Rep*; 2015;u209517.w3913. https://doi.org/10.1136/bmjquality.u209517.w3913.

88. Aleem S, Torrey WC, Duncan MS, Hort SJ, Mecchella JM. Depression screening optimization in an academic rural setting. *Int J Health Care Qual Assur*. 2015;28:709–725.
89. Iturralde E, Adams RN, Barley RC, et al. Implementation of depression screening and global health assessment in pediatric subspecialty clinics. *J Adolesc Health*. 2017;61: 591–598.
90. QuickStats: suicide rates for teens aged 15–19 years, by sex — United States, 1975–2015. *MMWR Morb Mortal Wkly Rep*. 2017;66:816.
91. Kann L, McManus T, Harris WA, et al. Youth risk behavior surveillance — United States, 2015. *Surveill Summ*. 2016; 65(6):1–174.
92. Mercado MC, Holland K, Leemis RW, Stone DM, Wang J. Trends in emergency department visits for nonfatal self-inflicted injuries among youth aged 10 to 24 years in the United States, 2001–2015. *Letter JAMA*. 2017;318: 1931.
93. Plemmons GS, Hall M, Doupnik S, et al. Hospitalization for suicide ideation or attempt: 2008–2015. *Pediatrics*. 2018;141(6):e20172426.
94. Joint Commission on Accreditation of Healthcare Organizations. *Sentinel Event Alert 56*; August 28, 2018. Retrieved from: www.jointcommission.org.
95. Shain B, Naylor M, Alessi N. Comparison of self-rated and clinician-rated measures of depression in adolescents. *Am J Psychiatry*. 1990;147:793–795.
96. Prinstein M, Nock M, Spirito A, Grapentine W. Multimethod assessment of suicidality in adolescent psychiatric inpatients: preliminary results. *J Am Acad Child Adolesc Psychiatry*. 2001;40:1053–1061.
97. Huth-Bocks AC, Kerr DCR, Ivey AZ, Kramer AC, King CA. Assessment of psychiatrically hospitalized suicidal adolescents: self-report instruments as predictors of suicidal thoughts and behavior. *J Am Acad Child Adolesc Psychiatry*. 2007;46(3):387–395.
98. Connor J, Rueter M. Predicting adolescent suicidality: comparing multiple informants and assessment techniques. *J Adolesc*. 2009;32:619–631.
99. Lewinsohn PM, Rohde P, Seeley JR, Baldwin CL. Gender differences in suicide attempts from adolescence to young adulthood. *J Am Acad Child Adolesc Psychiatry*. 2001;40:427–431.
100. Ward EC, Wiltshire JC, Detry MA, Brown RL. African American men and women's attitude toward mental illness, perceptions of stigma, and preferred coping behaviors. *Nurs Res*. 2013;62:185–194.
101. King CA, Jiang Q, Czyk EK, Kerr DCR. Suicidal ideation of psychiatrically hospitalized adolescents has one-year predictive validity for suicide attempts in girls only. *J Abnorm Child Psychol*. 2014;42:467–477.
102. Maslow GR, Dunlap K, Chung RJ. Depression and suicide in children and adolescents. *Pediatr Review*. 2015;36: 299–310.
103. Williams KR, Ho ML, Grupp-Phelan J. The acceptability of mental health screening in a pediatric emergency department. *Pediatr Emer Care*. 2001;27:611–615.
104. Olfson M, Gameroff MJ, Marcus SC, Greenberg T, Shaffer D. Emergency treatment of young people following deliberate self-harm. *Arch Gen Psychiatry*. 2005;62:1122–1128.
105. King CA, O'Mara RM, Hayward CN, Cunningham RM. Adolescent suicide risk screening in the emergency department. *Acad Emerg Med*. 2009;16:1234–1241.
106. O'Mara RM, Hill RM, Cunningham RM, King CA. Adolescent and parent attitudes toward screening for suicide risk and mental health problems in the pediatric emergency department. *Pediatr Emerg Care*. 2012;28:626–632.
107. Horowitz LH, Ballard E, Teach SJ, Bosk A, Rosenstein DL, et al. Feasibility of screening patients with nonpsychiatric complaints for suicide risk in a pediatric emergency department. *Pediatr Emer Care*. 2010;26:787–792.
108. Beck AT, Kovacs M, Weissman A. Assessment of suicidal intention: the scale for suicide ideation. *J Consult Clin Psychol*. 1979;37:343–352.
109. Osman A, Bagge CL, Gutierrez PM, Konick LC, Kopper BA, Barrios FX. The suicidal behaviors questionnaire—revised (SBQ-R): validation with clinical and nonclinical samples. *Assess*. 2001;8:443–454.
110. Range LM, Knott EC. Twenty suicide assessment instruments: evaluation and recommendations. *Death Studies*. 1997;21(1):25–58.
111. Linehan MM, Goodstein JL, Nielsen SL, Chiles JA. Reasons for staying alive when you are thinking of killing yourself: the reasons for living inventory. *J Consult Clin Psychol*. 1983;51:276–286.
112. Shaffer D, Scott M, Wilcox H, et al. The Columbia suicide screen: validity and reliability of a screen for youth suicide and depression. *J Am Acad Child Adolesc Psychiatry*. 2004;43:71–79.
113. Scott MA, Wilcox HC, Schonfeld IS, et al. School-based screening to identify at-risk students not already known to school professionals: the Columbia suicide screen. *Am J Pub Health*. 2009;99:334–339.
114. Thompson EA, Eggert LL. Using the suicide risk screen to identify suicidal adolescents among potential high school dropouts. *J Am Acad Child Adolesc Psychiatry*. 1999;38:1506–1514.
115. Hallfors D, Brodish PH, Khatapoush S, Sanchez V, Cho H, Steckler A. Feasibility of screening adolescents for suicide risk in "Real-World" high school settings. *Am J Pub Health*. 2006;96:282–287.
116. Peltzer K, Kleintjes S, Van Wyk B, Thompson EA, Mashego TB. Correlates of suicide risk among secondary school students in Cape Town. *Soc Behav Pers*. 2008;36: 493–502.
117. Horowitz LM, Ballard ED, Pao M. Suicide screening in schools, primary care, and emergency departments. *Curr Opin Pediatr*. 2009;21:620–627.
118. Reynolds W. *Suicidal Ideation Questionnaire*. Odessa, Florida: Psychological Assessment Resources; 1987.
119. Reynolds W. *SIQ, Suicidal Ideation Questionnaire: Professional Manual*. Florida: Psychological Assessment Resources; 1998.

120. Huth-Bocks A, Kerr DCR, Ivey AZ, Kramer AC, King CA. Assessment of psychiatrically hospitalized suicidal adolescents: self-report instruments as predictors of suicidal thoughts and behavior. *J Am Acad Child Psy*. 2007;36: 387–395.
121. Erford BT, Jackson J, Bardhoshi G, Duncan K, Zumra A. Selecting suicide ideation assessment instruments: a meta-analytic review. *Meas Eval Couns Dev*. 2018;51: 42–59.
122. Possner K, Brown GK, Stanley B, et al. The columbia-suicide severity rating scale: initial validity and internal consistency findings from three multisite studies with adolescents and adults. *Am J Psychiatry*. 2011;168: 1266–1277.
123. *The Columbia Lighthouse Project*; August 28, 2018. Retrieved from http://cssrs.columbia.edu/.
124. Mundt JC, Greist JH, Jefferson JW, Federico M, Mann JJ, Possner K. Prediction of suicidal behavior in clinical research by lifetime suicidal ideation and behavior ascertained by the electronic columbia-suicide severity rating scale. *J Clin Psychiatry*. 2013;74:e1–e7.
125. Brown GK, Currier GW, Jager-Hyman S, Stanley B. Detection and classification of suicidal behavior and nonsuicidal self-injury behavior in emergency departments. *J Clin Psychiatry*. 2015;76:1397–1403.
126. Gipson PY, Agarwala P, Opperman KJ, Horwitz A, King CA. Columbia-suicide severity rating scale: predictive validity with adolescent psychiatric emergency patients. *Pediatr Emerg Care*. 2015;31(2):88–94.
127. United States Food and Drug Administration, United States Department of Health and Human Services. *Guidance for Industry: Suicidality: Prospective Assessment of Occurrence in Clinical Trials, Draft Guidance*; August 28, 2018. Retrieved from http://www.fda.gov/downloads/Drugs/Guidances/UCM225130.pdfAugust 2012. Revision 1.
128. Chappell P, Feltner DE, Makumi C, Stewart M. Initial validity and reliability data on the columbia-suicide severity rating scale. *Am J Psychiatry*. 2012;169:662–663.
129. Giddens JM, Sheehan KH, Sheehan DV. The Columbia-Suicide Severity Rating Scale (C-SSRS): has the "gold standard" become a liability? *Innov Clin Neurosci*. 2014; 11(9–10):66–80.
130. Horowitz LM, Wang PS, Koocher GP, Burr BH, Smith MF, et al. Detecting suicide risk in a pediatric emergency department: development of a brief screening tool. *Pediatrics*. 2001;107:1133–1137.
131. Horowitz LM, Bridge JA, Teach SJ, et al. Ask Suicide-Screening Questions (ASQ): a brief instrument for the pediatric emergency department. *Arch Pediatr Adolesc Med*. 2012;166:1170–1176.
132. Folse VN, Eich KN, Hall AM, Ruppman JB. Detecting suicide risk in adolescents and adults in an emergency department: a pilot study. *J Psychosocial Nurs*. 2006; 44(3):22–29.
133. Folse VN, Hahn RL. Suicide risk screening in an emergency department: engaging staff nurses in continued testing of a brief instrument. *Clin Nurs Res*. 2009;18: 253–271.
134. Newton AS, Soleimani A, Kirkland SW, Gokiert RJ. A systematic review of instruments to identify mental health and substance use problems among children in the emergency department. *Acad Emerg Med*. 2017;24: 552–568.
135. Horowitz LM, Snyder D, Ludi E, et al. Ask suicide-screening questions to everyone in medical settings: the asQ'em quality improvement project. *Psychosomatics*. 2013;54(3):239–247.
136. Boudreaux ED, Jaques ML, Brady KM, Matson A, Allen MH. The patient safety screener: validation of a brief suicide risk screener for emergency department settings (PERC) – 3. *Arch Suicide Res*. 2015;19:151–160.
137. American Academy of Child and Adolescent Psychiatry. Practice parameter for the assessment and treatment of children and adolescents with suicidal behavior. *J Am Acad Child Adolesc Psychiatry*. 2001;40(suppl 7): S24–S51.
138. Noonan S. *Teen Screen: All or None?* Psychology Today; April 16, 2016. Available from: https://www.psychologytoday.com/us/blog/view-the-mist/201604/teen-screen-all-or-none.
139. Gould MS, Marrocco FA, Kleinman M, et al. Evaluating iatrogenic risk of youth suicide screening programs. *JAMA*. 2005;293:1635–1643.
140. Runeson B, Odeberg J, Pettersson A, Edbom T, Jildevik-Adamsson I, Waern M. Instruments for the assessment of suicide risk: a systematic review evaluating the certainty of the evidence. *PLoS One*. 2017. https://doi.org/10.1371/journal.pone.0180292.
141. Gunn JF, Lester D, Mcswain S. Testing the warning signs of suicidal behavior among suicide ideators using the 2009 National Survey on Drug Abuse and Health. *Int J Emerg Ment Health*. 2011;13:147–154.
142. Klonosky ED, May AM. Differentiating suicide attempters from suicide ideators: a critical frontier for suicidology research. *Suicide Life Threat Behav*. 2014;44:1–5.
143. Alavi N, Reshetukha T, Prost E, Antoniak K, Groll D. Assessing suicide risk: what is commonly missed in the emergency room? *J Psychiatric Practice*. 2017;23(2): 82–91.
144. Horowitz LM, Bridge JA, Pao M, Boudreaux ED. Screening youth for suicide risk in medical settings: time to ask questions. *Am J Prev Med*. 2014;47(3S2): S170–S175.
145. Nock MK, Green JG, Hwang I, et al. Prevalence, correlates, and treatment of lifetime suicidal behavior among adolescents: results from the national comorbidity survey replication adolescent supplement. *JAMA Psychiatry*. 2013;70:300–310.
146. Walsh CG, Ribeiro JD, Franklin JC. Predicting risk of suicide attempts over time through machine learning. *Clin Psychol Sci*. 2017;5:1–13.
147. Won H-H, Myung W, Song G-Y, Lee W-H, Kim J-W, et al. Predicting national suicide numbers with social media data. *PloS One*. 2013;8(4):e61089.
148. Twenge JM. *Have Smartphones Destroyed A Generation?*. Monthly Atlantic; September 2017:58–65. Available

from: https://www.theatlantic.com/magazine/archive/2017/09/has-the-smartphone-destroyed-a-generation/534198/.

149. Kwon D. *Can Facebook's Machine-Learning Algorithms Accurately Predict Suicide?* Scientific American; March 8, 2017. Available from: https://www.scientificamerican.com/article/can-facebooks-machine-learning-algorithms-accurately-predict-suicide/.

150. Novet J. *Facebook Is Using A.I. To Help Predict when Users May Be Suicidal.* CNBC; February 21, 2018. Available from: https://www.cnbc.com/2018/02/21/how-facebook-uses-ai-for-suicide-prevention.html.

151. Moreno MA, Ton A, Selkie E, Evans Y. Secret society 123: understanding the language of self-harm on instagram. *J Adolesc Health.* 2016;58(1):78–84.

CHAPTER 12

# Screening for Body Image Concerns, Eating Disorders, and Sexual Abuse in Adolescents: Concurrent Assessment to Support Early Intervention and Preventative Treatment

SARAH SPINNER, PsyD • BRITTANY D. RUDOLPH, MS

## INTRODUCTION

Adolescents are vulnerable to concerns about their bodies, likely because of the significant psychologic and physiologic changes they experience that may acutely increase awareness of and sensitivity to body image.[1–3] These changes—and the accompanying increased awareness of physical self—may impact adolescents' ability to cope with past or present threats to the well-being and protection of their bodies. In adolescence, body image concerns and eating disorders (EDs) are potential manifestations of an unhealthy relationship with the body. One example of a past or present threat to well-being is childhood abuse. Although childhood abuse has been associated with all types of EDs,[4] the focus here is on the relationship between body image concerns/EDs and one particular form of child abuse, namely, sexual abuse.

The potential connections among body image concerns, EDs, and sexual abuse are complex, requiring a contextual definition of the term *body image*. Body image can be thought of as the "perceptions and attitudes a person holds toward one's own body especially, but not exclusively, their physical appearance."[5(p34)] For adolescents, sociocultural pressure related to physical appearance, in addition to body changes and peer comparison, seem to contribute to increased concern regarding body image.[6] *Body image concerns, negative body image*, or *body dissatisfaction* (often used interchangeably in the literature) can lead to unhealthy behaviors such as frequent mirror checking or avoidance of public situations.[7] Van der kolk[8(p591)] emphasizes this link between one's body—one's "physical reality"—and the ongoing impact of trauma:

> *We have also begun to understand how overwhelming experiences affect our innermost sensations and our relationship to our physical reality—the core of who we are. We have learned that trauma is not just an event that took place sometime in the past; it's also the imprint left by that experience on mind, brain and body. This imprint has ongoing consequences for how the human organism manages to survive in the present.*

As sexual abuse often heightens adolescents' awareness toward their physical integrity (perhaps in part due to what Finkelhor and Browne (1985)[10a] call "traumatic sexualization," which can occur "when certain parts of a child's anatomy are fetishized and given distorted importance and meaning" (p. 531)), it makes sense that it might also send them down a developmental trajectory toward body dissatisfaction and EDs as described later.

Although research increasingly indicates that both biological and genetic factors contribute to the increased risk of EDs during adolescence,[9] body dissatisfaction also is robustly associated with the development of EDs.[10] It is well known that EDs lead to severe psychologic and physical health consequences.[11,12] Subclinical EDs—covering a wide range of disordered eating behaviors—are highly prevalent among adolescents and can similarly lead to serious individual and public health consequences.[13,14] The findings of the study by Hudson et al.,[15] which indicate that EDs are undertreated and often associated with other

Adolescent Health Screening: An Update in the Age of Big Data. https://doi.org/10.1016/B978-0-323-66130-0.00012-0

psychologic disorders, further underscore the significant public health concerns posed by EDs.

Although there are, of course, many factors contributing to the cause of body image concerns/EDs, the high onset rates of both body image concerns and disordered eating in adolescence[14,16] warrant the development of an assessment that measures the interaction between sexual abuse and body image/disordered eating. Detecting the presence of both elements may support preventative treatment outcomes because assessing for aspects of various risk factors, namely, sexual abuse and body image concerns/ED symptoms, could facilitate intervention before the adolescent's symptoms progress to a diagnosable ED.

## PUBERTY, BODY AWARENESS, AND BODY IMAGE CONCERNS IN ADOLESCENTS

While adolescence generally represents the stage of development between childhood and adulthood, it is delineated by culturally and theoretically distinct age spans, depending on context. For this exploration, as defined by the World Health Organization, the term "adolescent" will encompass the ages 10–19 years (World Health Organization, 2012).[16a] Physiologically, adolescence is defined as the period of development between the beginning of puberty and the completion of growth. Puberty is a developmental stage that causes hormonal, physical, behavioral, and psychologic changes impacting many areas of life[1,17] across multiple psychosocial domains, including adult body image.[18]

Profound bodily changes during puberty can contribute to increased concerns about body shape and weight, thereby impacting adolescent body image.[6,19] Puberty appears to be a particularly high-risk period for the development of EDs and symptoms that may accompany EDs, such as body image concern, weight/shape concern, restrictive eating, and binge eating.[2,10]

As puberty entails so many inevitable changes, adolescence, as Voelker et al.[20] characterize it, is a "pivotal stage in the development of positive or negative body image" (p. 149). Various theories have linked sociocultural pressures and body dissatisfaction.[6,21] Sources of these pressures include media,[21–23] peers,[6,21,23,24] and parents.[21,23] Such influences have been found to contribute not only to the development of negative body image but also to eating disturbances.[23]

These concerns are well documented within adolescent populations of Western cultures.[25,26] Researchers, for instance, found that a significant number of adolescents (between the ages of 12 and 18 years, up to 40% in boys and 80% in girls) experience body dissatisfaction[19,27]. In a 10-year longitudinal study examining changes in body dissatisfaction from adolescence to adulthood, Bucchianeri et al.[28] found that body dissatisfaction of male and female participants increased between middle school and high school and increased further during the transition to adulthood. In addition, results from a longitudinal community study of adolescent girls (N = 231) indicated that body image concerns and disordered eating contributed to elevated depression.[29] In a 5-year study, researchers examined and found that body dissatisfaction was a risk factor for depressive symptoms as well as low self-esteem in both girls and boys.[26]

Cash and Smolak[30] point out that the amount of research regarding body image and related concerns has increased considerably, as has the cultural diversity of research participants: "Not long ago, most body image research focused on eating pathology and weight/shape concerns among White female college students. The variety of contexts and populations in which body image is explored has broadened considerably" (p. 7). Despite the increasing diversity among study participants in the area of body image concerns, the majority of studies historically have been conducted among White women.[31,32] There have been limited sample sizes and mixed results from studies examining differences in the type and prevalence of body image concerns and EDs among various ethnic/racial groups.[33] However, results from a 2002 study comparing weight-related concerns and behaviors of male and female adolescents (N = 4746) indicated that while there was some difference between ethnic/racial groups, weight-related concerns and behaviors were prevalent in each group.[25]

These concerns are becoming more pervasive across gender, ethnicity, and culture and have intruded into populations that we might assume are "protected" from such issues. For example, body image concerns are so widespread among women that they could even be considered, according to Olmsted and McFarlane,[34] "statistically 'normal'" (p. 2). Strikingly, results from a representative survey (1995) indicated that almost one-half of North American women experience some form of body dissatisfaction, with White and Hispanic women having more body image concern than African American women.[35]

Research focusing on gender differences related to body dissatisfaction indicates that during adolescence, women experience more body dissatisfaction than men, with men appearing to be underrepresented in the literature.[33,36] In a longitudinal study on the development and cause of body dissatisfaction in adolescent boys and girls (N = 605), Dion et al.[36] found that with regard to adolescents wanting a thinner versus bigger body shape, the proportion of adolescent girls (ages 14–18 years) wanting to be thinner increased with age and the proportion of those wanting to be bigger decreased. Research has found an association not only between desired body shape and severity of ED psychopathologic conditions[37,38] but also between desired weight and severity of ED psychopathologic conditions.[37]

While many studies about body image concerns in adolescence have focused primarily on adolescent girls, given their apparent high risk for EDs, adolescent boys are also afflicted by body image concerns.[39] Girls are more likely to strive for the *thin ideal*,[36,38,40] whereas boys are more likely to alter their behavior in order to obtain muscularity and larger body stature.[39,41] In a review of human and animal studies, Klump[9] found "significant effects of both pubertal status and timing on most eating disorder phenotypes" in girls, with body dissatisfaction being one of the "strongest effects" (p. 404). These results indicated "much more mixed" findings for boys regarding pubertal status and timing of EDs and associated symptoms; however, Klump[9] states, "The lone exception might be body dissatisfaction and weight/shape concerns" (p. 404). Through various forms of media, women regularly face exposure to the thin ideal, which can lead to adverse effects such as body image concerns.[42,43] The negative effects of such pervasive media-messaging and promotion of this "ideal" body type have been found to occur whether women consciously choose to pay attention to such images or not.[44]

## THE RELATIONSHIP BETWEEN BODY IMAGE CONCERNS AND EATING DISORDERS

Body image concerns have been identified as important in understanding the development of EDs and subclinical ED symptoms.[20,45–47] Of course, the origins and consequences of these concerns in any individual are unique. This is partly due to variations in the intensity of these concerns as well as the complexity of the interactions among them. In a literature review covering 2004–14, Madowitz et al.[48] identified and described two pathways that could be influential in causing EDs: the *body perceptions pathway*, which may involve "body dissatisfaction, shame, sexual dysfunction, and fear of future sexual trauma," and the *psychologic difficulties pathway*, which may point to a connection "between EDs and the desire to cope with the failure of the average expected environment, psychologic diagnoses, the need for control, and the regulation of emotions" (p. 281). Research also has shown that psychologic and sociocultural factors such as media and family culture,[49] as well as maternal modeling,[50] can play a role in the development of body image concerns and EDs.

When body dissatisfaction is present in adolescent youths, it can lower self-esteem and increase an individual's vulnerability to psychologic problems.[19] It is well documented that body image concerns are widespread among teens and can lead to psychologic distress,[19] unhealthy behaviors,[7,36,51] and EDs.[45,47,51] Furthermore, body dissatisfaction and low self-esteem have been identified, in and of themselves, as potential precursors to the development of an ED.[19,39,52] For example, it has been estimated that more than one-half of adolescent girls and nearly one-third of adolescent boys engage in harmful behaviors in an attempt to control weight, such as meal-skipping, purging, and smoking cigarettes.[25] Furthermore, adolescents are less likely to participate in self-care practices when they possess a negative view of their own body.[13] Given the relationship between negative body image and unhealthy behaviors, the impact of pervasive body image concerns on public health is significant.[13,14] Identification and intervention concerning the symptomatic expression of body image concerns have been critical in preventing the onset of a disordered eating pattern.

## EATING DISORDER DIAGNOSTIC CRITERIA, CONSEQUENCES, AND PREVALENCE

To further explore the implications of this relationship between body image concerns and EDs, it is useful to summarize the diagnostic criteria for EDs. According to the *Diagnostic and Statistical Manual of Mental Disorders* (Fifth Edition) (*DSM-V*), "Feeding and eating disorders are characterized by a persistent disturbance of eating or eating-related behavior that results in the altered consumption or absorption of food and that significantly impairs physical health or psychosocial functioning."[53] EDs are considered a group of psychologic disorders that cause significant individual distress. Anorexia nervosa (AN) consists of three main diagnostic features: significantly low body weight, intense fear of gaining weight or becoming fat even if underweight, and disturbance in how one's weight or shape is experienced, self-evaluation overly influenced by weight or shape, or denial of the seriousness of one's currently low body weight.[53] Bulimia nervosa (BN) is also characterized by three main diagnostic features: recurrent episodes of binge eating, recurrent inappropriate compensatory behaviors to prevent weight gain, and undue influence of body shape and weight on self-evaluation.[53] Binge episodes and compensatory behaviors must occur at least once per week for 3 months on average, and the diagnosis of BN excludes individuals who meet the criteria for AN.[53] Binge episodes in BN require that the food is consumed in a discrete period and that the amount of food is larger than that most individuals would eat in a similar period under similar circumstances. This excessive food consumption must be accompanied by *loss of control*, the inability to stop eating once started.

The *DSM-V*[53] now recognizes binge eating disorder (BED) as well as newer diagnostic criteria and diagnostic categories for EDs, which, in earlier editions, were considered part of the heterogeneous group Eating Disorders Not Otherwise Specified (EDNOS). EDNOS included but was not limited to subthreshold AN, subthreshold BN, and BED. Some research suggests that BED is as chronic as AN and BN and that it may have a significantly longer lifetime duration than AN and BN.[54]

Accurate data characterizing the prevalence and severity of EDs can be challenging to access, given that those with an ED may hide their symptoms to avoid treatment,[55] which helps to explain the findings that EDs are often undertreated.[15] The data currently available in the United States demonstrates an alarming trend toward disordered eating and a potential public health crisis that demands more intensive focus and preventative measures. In a 2007 nationally representative survey (N = 9282), lifetime prevalence estimates of AN, BN, and BED among women were 0.9%, 1.5%, and 3.5%, respectively, and among men were 0.3%, 0.5%, and 2.0%, respectively.[15] This study also found all three of the examined EDs (AN, BN, and BED) to be comorbid with other *DSM-IV* disorders such as depression, anxiety, and substance use.[15]

According to the National Eating Disorders Association (NEDA), as many as 30 million people in the United States suffer from EDs, and national surveys estimated that 20 million women and 10 million men in the United States will meet the criteria for an ED at some point in their lives. Between 1999 and 2006, the number of hospitalizations due to AN alone increased 17%, while all other ED-related hospitalizations increased 38%, resulting in a 61% increase in ED-related hospital costs (Zhao & Encinosa, 2009).[56a] EDs also have remarkably high correlations with suicidality and mortality,[56–58] and rates of suicidal behavior are higher among those with ED than in individuals suffering from other psychologic disorders. In fact, the mortality rates of AN are the highest of all psychiatric disorders.[59–61] The National Institute of Mental Health estimated that the mortality rate for AN is 10%, a rate that encompasses both the effects of starvation and suicide.[62]

## EATING DISORDERS IN ADOLESCENCE

EDs most often emerge in adolescence[55,63,64]; however, some research indicates that the onset age of AN and BN is decreasing.[63] In a UK study investigating the diagnosis of EDs in primary care settings over a 10-year period, the peak age for AN diagnosis was 10–14 years, while the peak age for BN diagnosis was 15–19 years.[65] The incidence of AN and BN was highest for girls aged 15–19 years and highest for boys aged 10–14 years. In 2010, researchers found that 2.7% of all adolescents fit the criteria for an ED. Not surprisingly, the study indicated that the prevalence rate was twice as high in women as in men.[66] Breaking down the data further, Swanson et al.[14] determined the following lifetime-prevalence estimates for adolescents: 0.3% for AN, 0.9% for BN, and 1.6% for BED. In this study of more than 10,000 adolescents between the ages of 13 and 18 years, Swanson et al.[14] found that 0.3% of youths have at some point been affected by AN, 0.9% by BN, and 1.6% by BED. At the time of this study (2011), the diagnostic domain of EDNOS was used to describe the symptoms of EDs that are considered "subthreshold." Results indicated that EDNOS is the most common ED diagnosis: 0.8% had subthreshold AN and 2.5% had symptoms of subthreshold BED.[14] A 2012 study found EDNOS to be the most common ED diagnosis in both adults and adolescents, and large numbers of both the groups met the criteria for comorbid psychopathologic conditions.[67] Finally, in a Dutch study examining the prevalence and severity of EDs in adolescents within a community cohort (n = 296), AN and BED were found to be the most common among women and BED was found to be the most common among men.[68]

## SEXUAL ABUSE: GENERAL OVERVIEW OF RELEVANT CONSIDERATIONS

Although vulnerability to body image concerns is related to many factors, such as family culture and media,[49] here the examination is narrowed to focus on the relationship between sexual abuse and body image concerns in adolescents. The term *sexual abuse* is widely defined. The definition of *child sexual abuse* provided by the National Child Traumatic Stress Network[69] is both inclusive and concise, in addition to being appropriate for this examination:

> *any interaction between a child and an adult (or another child) in which the child is used for the sexual stimulation of the perpetrator or an observer. Sexual abuse can include both touching and nontouching behaviors. Nontouching behaviors can include voyeurism (trying to look at a child's naked body), exhibitionism, or exposing the child to pornography. Children of all ages, races, ethnicities, and economic backgrounds may experience sexual abuse. Child sexual abuse affects both girls and boys in all kinds of neighborhoods and communities.*

The US Department of Health and Human Services reported that in 2016, Child Protective Services received referrals alleging maltreatment of 7.4 million children; 58% of those referrals became official reports of suspected maltreatment and 676,000 victims were identified.[70] Annual statistics show that this national average is rising each year,[70] indicating a need for more aggressive preventative services and screening measures. In 2011, a study found a global prevalence rate specific to childhood sexual abuse estimated at 11.8%.[71] The study showed significant gender differences in reported childhood sexual abuse, with female prevalence at 18% and male prevalence at 7.6%.[71] Another study found similar results, showing 19.7% prevalence for women and 7.9% prevalence for men.[72] However, the actual rates of sexual abuse are certainly even higher than those found in these and other studies, as some individuals are unwilling to disclose a sexual abuse history because of stigma or shame.[71,73]

The way in which an individual processes trauma will vary, as the underlying physiologic and psychologic systems are complex (Brooke & Mussap, 2012).[74,74a] Many factors contribute to the long-term impact of sexual abuse, such as genetic predispositions, cultural considerations, other experiences of trauma, the age when the sexual abuse occurred, chronicity of the abuse, developmental history, and relationships with caregivers.[8] With respect to cultural considerations associated with childhood sexual abuse, some collectivist cultures may prioritize preserving family structure over disclosing abuse.[71,75] Many studies have shown ethnic differences in the severity of symptom presentation in children who have experienced sexual abuse,[76] demonstrating the variability in how early trauma can affect an individual.

## THE RELATIONSHIP BETWEEN SEXUAL ABUSE AND BODY IMAGE CONCERNS/ED

Sexual abuse is considered a risk factor not only for body image concerns and EDs but also for a variety of mental disorders and symptoms,[77–79] including suicidality[80,81] and nonsuicidal self-injury.[82] An estimated 40%–60% of sexually abused children will develop significant cognitive, emotional, or behavioral symptoms.[76,83] In seeking to distinguish the relationship between psychopathologic conditions and sexual trauma, specifically in comparison to nonsexual trauma (e.g., car accidents, physical attacks, robberies), researchers found that women who had experienced sexual trauma demonstrated a significantly higher prevalence of posttraumatic stress disorder, sexual disorders, and mood disorders.[84] Furthermore, women who had experienced one sexual trauma were 47% more likely to develop EDs than women who had experienced one nonsexual trauma.[84]

As the focus here is on the relationship between sexual abuse and body image concerns/EDs, it is important to note that although sexual abuse does not act as a causal link to body image concerns, EDs, or other psychopathologic conditions, there is evidence to support an increased risk of body image concerns in those who have experienced a sexual trauma.[48,79,85] Indeed, research has indicated that sexual trauma is, as Madowitz et al.[48] put it, "one potential pathway to the development and maintenance of ED." In their review of causative pathways between sexual abuse and EDs, Madowitz et al.[48] presented two relevant theories. In the first causative pathway, the individual's experience of his or her body may change. A negative view of one's body may be the causal link to EDs through "body dissatisfaction, shame, sexual dysfunction, and fear of future sexual trauma".[48(p281)] In the second causative pathway, the individual may try to control aspects of the environment in an attempt to prevent the trauma from reoccurring.[48] These two causative pathways appear somewhat related to the multiple theories cited by Smolak and Murnen[79] about the connection between sexual abuse and EDs (e.g., sexual abuse leading to a dissociative coping style associated with binge eating).

In their meta-analysis of the relationship between childhood sexual abuse and EDs, Smolak and Murnen[79] pointed out that relevant study designs can be inherently challenging, as there are many possible risk factors for the development of body image concerns and EDs as well as many varied definitions of both disordered eating and childhood sexual abuse. Nonetheless, they found evidence of a heterogeneous relationship between the two. Their assessment of the connection between sexual abuse and EDs is supported by many studies,[48,79] such as the study by Sanci et al.,[86] which found that incidence of BN during adolescence was 2.5 times higher among individuals who reported one episode of childhood sexual abuse and 4.9 times higher among those who reported two or more episodes than that in women who reported no episodes of sexual abuse.

## OVERVIEW OF RELEVANT SCREENINGS FOR BODY IMAGE CONCERNS, EATING DISORDERS, AND SEXUAL

Following is a review of relevant screening measures for body image concerns, EDs, and sexual abuse. This list is not exhaustive; rather, it is a review and summary of measures commonly used for assessing each domain. These screening measures have been chosen primarily for applicability to their specific subject, frequency of use, and strength of psychometric review. Regarding the ED screening measures specifically, many of the common assessments are used as diagnostic tools as well as a means for monitoring progress and treatment outcomes. Although a majority of the measures were normed and developed for use in adult populations, many have been administered to adolescents as well.

### Screening for Body Image Concerns

#### *Body attitudes questionnaire*

The Body Attitudes Questionnaire (BAQ) is a 44-item, Likert scale, self-report measure developed to assess women's attitudes toward their bodies. It uses six subscales relating to body experience: *feelings of overall fatness, self-disparagement, strength, salience of weight, feelings of attractiveness,* and *consciousness of lower body fat.*[87] Researchers found the questionnaire to have high split-half reliability, good convergent validity with other body experience measures, and significant discriminative validity, as the responses of a community sample differed significantly from those with documented EDs (Ben-Tovim & Walker)[88, a]. Some measures relating to body image concerns are shown to differentiate between types of EDs. However, as the BAQ subscales are used separately at times, researchers showed that the subscale *strength, disparagement,* and *attractiveness* were not able to differentiate among ED types.[88]

#### *Body attitudes test*

The Body Attitudes Test (BAT) is a 20-item, Likert scale, self-report measure initially developed for female patients with ED and is used to assess the participant's attitude toward his or her body.[89] The measure is divided into three subscales: *negative appreciation of body size, lack of familiarity with one's own body,* and *general dissatisfaction.* The measure was shown to have satisfactory internal reliability, good convergent validity, and significant discriminative validity in both screening and assessing treatment outcomes.[88,89] The BAT also distinguishes ED types. Importantly, the *lack of familiarity with one's own body* was the most significant predictor of treatment outcome and change scores on the Eating Disorder Inventory (EDI)-2.[90] This measure, originally developed in Dutch,[91] has been translated and validated in many languages[89] and has been tested on adult women and adolescents.

#### *Body satisfaction scale*

The Body Satisfaction Scale is a self-report scale that measures an individual's level of satisfaction with specific body parts. Respondents use a Likert scale (1, very satisfied, to 7, very unsatisfied) to determine their level of satisfaction with 16 different body parts.[92] The measure takes 2–3 min to complete and has adequate internal consistency and reliability.[92] In a psychometric review, its comparison groups were composed only of adult women, and it was not initially tested in an adolescent population or in men of any age.[92]

#### *Body shape questionnaire*

The Body Shape Questionnaire (BSQ) is a 34-item, Likert scale, self-report measure that assesses for dissatisfaction and concern with body shape.[93] The questionnaire was created to show the link between body shape concerns and the development of EDs or body image problems, explored in four domains: *body dissatisfaction, fear of gaining weight, feeling of low self-esteem related to appearance,* and *desire to lose weight.* The BSQ can be completed in 10 min or less and was significantly correlated to the total scores on the Eating Attitudes Test (EAT) and the *body dissatisfaction* subscale of the EDI (see later discussion), thus demonstrating concurrent validity.[93] The measure also exhibited high internal consistency, discriminative validity, and good reliability.[93] Women identified as being more concerned with weight and shape produced significantly higher scores than women identified as being unconcerned.[93]

---

[a]Split-half reliability is a measure of consistency. To confirm reliability, the experimenter splits the test in two, administers both tests, and then compares the scores. If the test results are consistent, the experimenter is assured that the tests are most likely measuring the same thing. Split-half reliability is not to be confused with validity. When evaluating validity, the experimenter is interested in whether or not the test measures what it is supposed to measure. With established split-half reliability, experimenters know that the test is consistently measuring something; they just do not necessarily know what that "something" is. For this reason, it is said that reliability sets the ceiling but does not prove validity.

### Contour drawing rating scale

The Contour Drawing Rating Scale, developed by Thompson and Gray,[94] is a rating measure of nine front-view figures (male or female, matching the participant's gender when rating self), with varying silhouettes (1 being the thinnest and 9 being the largest). Participants (college girls who were determined to be at risk for EDs but not diagnosed with ED) were asked to order the drawings from thinnest to largest, to identify any drawings they believed to be "anorexic" or "obese," and to report which of the drawings represented their body size or shape.[94] The measure was reported to have acceptable reliability and validity[94,95] and demonstrated high correlations between selected drawings and body mass index.[94] This measure was tested in early adolescent girls to show adequate validity and correlations between current and ideal body image discrepancies, body dissatisfaction, and restrained eating.[96]

### Rosenberg self-esteem scale

The Rosenberg Self-Esteem Scale (RSES) is a 10-item, Likert scale, self-report measure originally developed to gather information about adolescent feelings of self-esteem and self-worth.[97] It has since become one of the most widely used measures of self-esteem for adult populations.[98] In one study, for example, Johnson and Wardle[52] found that self-esteem, stress, and depression were associated with body dissatisfaction and dietary restraint. The RSES was shown to have strong convergent validity for different genders, ethnicities, and ages.[98] Additionally, the RSES was shown to have high reliability and validity across studies.[98]

### Thought–shape fusion body questionnaire

*Thought–shape fusion* is a term used to describe distorted thoughts relating to body image or shape. In a state of cognitive *fusion*, individuals struggle to view thoughts as independent from themselves, subsequently impacting mood and behavior.[99–101] Researchers sought to assess thought–shape fusion, as it relates to the development and continuance of EDs.[101] The Thought–Shape Fusion Body Questionnaire contains two subscales: *imagination of thin ideals*, which has five items, and *striving for own thin ideals*, which has seven items.[101] Both scales demonstrated good convergent validity and reliability, additionally revealing the ability to appropriately distinguish between individuals with ED and those without ED.[101] It is important to note that the participants of this study were adult women; it was not initially tested in an adolescent sample or in men of any age.[101]

## Screening for Eating Disorders

### Children's eating attitudes test

The Children's Eating Attitudes Test (ChEAT) is a 26-item, self-report, Likert scale measure that collects information related to attitudes and behaviors in children about food and eating.[102] The ChEAT was developed from the EAT that has an identical item content, but the wording in the ChEAT is more appropriate for child participants.[102] Although this measure was specifically normed for child populations (ages 8–13 years), it was found to have both test–retest and internal reliabilities that were comparable to those in adult populations.[102]

### Eating attitudes test

The EAT is also a 26-item, self-report, Likert scale measure that assesses attitudes and behaviors related to eating.[103] Its item content is identical to that of the ChEAT, and the EAT has similarly acceptable psychometric properties normed for an adult population.[103]

### Eating disorder inventory

The EDI-3 is a 91-item, self-report, Likert scale measure developed to assess for the psychologic and behavioral symptoms of various EDs.[104] The EDI-3 takes approximately 20 min to complete and is composed of 11 subscales: *drive for thinness, bulimia, body dissatisfaction, ineffectiveness, perfectionism, interpersonal distrust, interoceptive awareness, maturity fears, asceticism, impulse regulation,* and *social insecurity.* In addition, the EDI-3 contains the EDI Symptom Checklist (EDI-SC), which can be used singularly.[104] The EDI-SC collects information related to current and past eating behaviors and attitudes and takes approximately 10 min to complete.[104] The EDI-3 was found to have clinical utility as a diagnostic measure and as a tool for monitoring treatment progress and outcomes.[104] The EDI-3 was shown to have appropriate content, criterion, and convergent and discriminant validity.[104] The EDI for Children (EDI-C) is a measure derived from the EDI-3 that is to be used specifically in children and adolescents and shows comparable psychometrics to the EDI-3.[105] Additionally, the EDI-3 has been used in male populations[106] and is available in numerous languages.

## Screening for Sexual Abuse

### The childhood trauma questionnaire-short form

The Childhood Trauma Questionnaire-Short Form (CTQ-SF) was derived from the Childhood Trauma Questionnaire, a 70-item, Likert scale questionnaire that measures five subsets: *emotional abuse, physical abuse, sexual abuse, emotional neglect,* and *physical neglect*.[107] Researchers sought to develop an assessment that covered a wide range of abuse while conserving reliability and validity in a 5-min screening measure.[107] They used the following definitions of abuse and neglect in both measures.

> *Sexual abuse was defined as "sexual contact or conduct between a child younger than 18 years of age and an adult or older person." Physical abuse was defined as "bodily assaults on a child by an adult or older person that posed a risk of or resulted in injury." Emotional abuse was defined as "verbal assaults on a child's sense of worth or well-being or any humiliating or demeaning behavior directed toward a child by an adult or older person." Physical neglect was defined as "the failure of caretakers to provide for a child's basic physical needs, including food, shelter, clothing, safety, and health care" (poor parental supervision was also included in this definition if it places children's safety in jeopardy). Emotional neglect was defined as "the failure of caretakers to meet children's basic emotional and psychological needs, including love, belonging, nurturance, and support."*[107(p175)]

The CTQ-SF has demonstrated invariance, as it was measured across four vastly different populations with equivalent responding, while showing criterion-related validity in a subgroup of adolescent psychiatric inpatients in whom independent corroborative data was attained.[107] While comparing adolescent responses on the CTQ-SF with patient history and therapist ratings of abuse and neglect, researchers found that both convergent and discriminative validity were high.[107] Researchers found participants in the adolescent psychiatric population reported the highest level of maltreatment of all four subgroups (adult patients abusing substances, adolescent psychiatric inpatients, adults abusing substances in the community, and normative adults in the community) and were more likely to have experienced more than one type of maltreatment.[107]

#### *Trauma history profile*

The Trauma History Profile (THP) of the University of California at Los Angeles Posttraumatic Stress Disorder Reaction Index[108] is clinician-administered through a clinical interview with the child, caregiver, and other sources. It assesses 19 different types of trauma, loss, and separation. It uses a four-point scale ("yes," "no," "suspected," and "unknown"). The THP holds clinical value by potentially uncovering chronic or multiple types of traumas that are discovered in addition to the initial reason the child is being evaluated.[109] The THP was found to have strong reliability[110] and good to excellent internal consistency across age, sex, and ethnicity.[108]

## DISCUSSION

### Cultural Considerations

Although the screening measures described earlier were found to be more psychometrically sound than others, none of these measures are definitively relevant to all cultural groups. For instance, there is evidence to suggest that the severity of symptoms following sexual abuse varies among racial and ethnic groups.[76,111,112] Historically, the most commonly used measures have been normed to White male populations. While most of the measures cited here were normed to women, it is critical to interpret with caution when considering the assessment of ethnic minorities and nonfemales.

Similarly, the majority of relevant research, as well as testing of relevant screening measures for body image concerns and EDs, has utilized binary gender constructs (i.e., male and female), and within this already limited categorization, the focus has predominantly been narrowed even further to focus on women. One potential explanation for this is that there are higher prevalence and reporting rates for both EDs and sexual abuse in women,[71,72] and therefore the focus of the screening measures has primarily been validated or normed in female populations. Additionally, per the NEDA, men are less likely to seek treatment for EDs, even though in the United States, 10 million men are affected by EDs and one in three people with ED is a man.[113]

### Clinical Implications of Concurrent Assessment

Given their connection to the potential development of EDs, body image concerns and disordered eating behaviors should be identified as early as possible. Moreover, since delayed treatment for EDs is associated with higher relapse rates and poor prognosis, there is considerable need for early identification.[64,114] Given the significant relationship between body image concerns and EDs, the potentially adverse clinical implications of assessing for one without the other are clear. Screening for just one problem may provide an incomplete picture of the symptoms that are current and likely to develop. In other words, assessing for just body image concerns or just EDs might represent inadvertent neglect of the participant's current or future treatment needs. The quality of ED treatment and the efficacy of assessment can be significantly improved if medical and clinical professionals assess for eating concerns, even if the patient did not initially report such concerns.[15]

Furthermore, although there are many questionnaires for adolescents that screen for sexual abuse and many screening measures for adolescents that assess body image concerns/EDs, the connection between sexual abuse and body image concerns/EDs underscores the utility of a screening tool that assesses for both. Given the preponderance of evidence pointing to the relationship between sexual abuse and body image concerns/EDs (called a "reliable relationship" by Smolak and Murnen[79]), assessing for each is an integral part of a comprehensive adolescent screening. Such a concurrent measure would have preventative value in that it could inform relevant treatment and signal the need for preemptive intervention.

## REFERENCES


1. Blakemore SJ, Burnett S, Dahl RE. The role of puberty in the developing adolescent brain. *Hum Brain Mapp*. 2010; 31(6):926–933. https://doi.org/10.1002/hbm.21052.
2. Moore SR, McKone KMP, Mendle J. Recollections of puberty and disordered eating in young women. *J Adolesc*. 2016;53:180–188. https://doi.org/10.1016/j.adolescence.2016.10.011.
3. Turner C, Cadman J. When adolescents feel ugly: cognitive behavioral therapy for body dysmorphic disorder in youth. *J Cogn Psychotherapy*. 2017;31(4):242–254. https://doi.org/10.1891/0889-8391.31.4.242.
4. Molendijk ML, Hoek HW, Brewerton TD, Elzinga BM. Childhood maltreatment and eating disorder pathology: a systematic review and dose-response meta-analysis. *Psychol Med*. 2017;47(8):1402–1416. https://doi.org/10.1017/S0033291716003561.
5. Duarte LS, Steen M, Fujimori E. Adolescence and body image dissatisfaction: increasing awareness of health professionals. *Austr Nurs Midwifery J*. 2017;25(6):34.
6. Ata RN, Ludden AB, Lally MM. The effects of gender and family, friend, and media influences on eating behaviors and body image during adolescence. *J Youth Adoles*. 2007; 36(8):1024–1037. https://doi.org/10.1007/s10964-006-9159-x.
7. Alleva JM, Sheeran P, Webb TL, Martijn C, Miles E. A meta-analytic review of stand-alone interventions to improve body image. *PLoS One*. 2015;10(9):e0139177. https://doi.org/10.1371/journal.pone.0139177.
8. van der Kolk BA. *The Body Keeps the Score: Brain, Mind, and Body in the Healing of Trauma*; 2014 [Kindle version]. Retrieved from: Amazon.com.
9. Klump KL. Puberty as a critical risk period for eating disorders: a review of human and animal studies. *Hormones Behav*. 2013;64(2):399–410. https://doi.org/10.1016/j.yhbeh.2013.02.019.
10. Fornari V, Dancyger IF. Psychosexual development and eating disorders. *Adoles Med*. 2003;14(1):61–75.

10a. Finkelhor D, Browne A. The traumatic impact of child sexual abuse: a conceptualization. In: Chess S, Thomas A, eds. *Annual Progress in Child Psychiatry and Child Development, 1986*. Philadelphia, PA, US: Brunner/Mazel; 1985:632–648.

11. Kärkkäinen U, Mustelin L, Raevuori A, Kaprio J, Keski-Rahkonen A. Do disordered eating behaviours have long-term health-related consequences? *Eur Eat Disord Rev*. 2018;26(1):22–28. https://doi.org/10.1002/erv.2568.
12. Klump KL, Bulik CM, Kaye WH, Treasure J, Tyson E. Academy for eating disorders position paper: eating disorders are serious mental illnesses. *Int J Eat Disord*. 2009;42(2):97–103. https://doi.org/10.1002/eat.20589.
13. Bucchianeri MM, Neumark-Sztainer D. Body dissatisfaction: an overlooked public health concern. *J Public Ment Health*. 2014;13(2):64–69. https://doi.org/10.1108/JPMH-11-2013-0071.
14. Swanson SA, Crow SJ, Le Grange D, Swendsen J, Merikangas KR. Prevalence and correlates of eating disorders in adolescents: results from the national comorbidity survey replication adolescent supplement. *Arch Gen Psychiatry*. 2011;68(7):714–723. https://doi.org/10.1001/archgenpsychiatry.2011.22.
15. Hudson JI, Hiripi E, Pope HG Jr, Kessler RC. The prevalence and correlates of eating disorders in the National Comorbidity Survey replication. *Biol Psychiatry*. 2007; 61(3):348–358. https://doi.org/10.1016/j.biopsych.2006.03.040.
16. Marzilli E, Cerniglia L, Cimino S. A narrative review of binge eating disorder in adolescence: prevalence, impact, and psychological treatment strategies. *Adolescent Health, Medicine And Therapeutics*. 2018;9:17–30. https://doi.org/10.2147/AHMT.S148050.

16a. World Health Organization. *Adolescent Health and Development*; 2019. Retrieved from http://www.searo.who.int/entity/child_adolescent/topics/adolescent_health/en/.

17. Dwyer AA, Phan-Hug F, Hauschild M, Elowe-Gruau E, Pitteloud N. Transition in endocrinology: hypogonadism in adolescence. *Eur J Endocrinol*. 2015;173(1):R15–R24. https://doi.org/10.1530/EJE-14-0947.
18. Friedman LS. Adolescents. In: Feldman MD, Christensen JF, Satterfield JM, Feldman MD, Christensen JF, Satterfield JM, eds. *Behavioral Medicine: A Guide for Clinical Practice*. New York, NY, US: McGraw-Hill; 2014:123–132.
19. Duchesne A, Dion J, Lalande D, et al. Body dissatisfaction and psychological distress in adolescents: is self-esteem a mediator? *J Health Psychol*. 2017;22(12):1563–1569. https://doi.org/10.1177/1359105316631196.
20. Voelker DK, Reel JJ, Greenleaf C. Weight status and body image perceptions in adolescents: current perspectives. *Adolesc Health Med Ther*. 2015;6:149–158. https://doi.org/10.2147/AHMT.S68344.
21. Dittmar H. Vulnerability factors and processes linking sociocultural pressures and body dissatisfaction. *J Soc Clin Psychol*. 2005;24(8):1081–1087.
22. Bell BT, Lawton R, Dittmar H. The impact of thin models in music videos on adolescent girls' body dissatisfaction. *Body Image*. 2007;4(2):137–145. https://doi.org/10.1016/j.bodyim.2007.02.003.

23. van den Berg P, Thompson JK, Obremski-Brandon K, Coovert M. The Tripartite Influence model of body image and eating disturbance: a covariance structure modeling investigation testing the mediational role of appearance comparison. *J Psychosom Res*. 2002;53(5):1007–1020. https://doi.org/10.1016/S0022-3999(02)00499-3.
24. Jones DC, Vigfusdottir TH, Yoonsun L. Body image and the appearance culture among adolescent girls and boys. *J Adoles Res*. 2004;19(3):323–339. https://doi.org/10.1177/0743558403258847.
25. Neumark-Sztainer D, Croll J, Story M, Hannan PJ, French SA, Perry C. Ethnic/racial differences in weight-related concerns and behaviors among adolescent girls and boys: findings from project EAT. *J Psychosomatic Res*. 2002;53(5):963–974.
26. Paxton SJ, Neumark-Sztainer D, Hannan PJ, Eisenberg ME. Body dissatisfaction prospectively predicts depressive mood and low self-esteem in adolescent girls and boys. *J Clin Child Adoles Psychol*. 2006;35(4):539–549.
27. Kostanski M, Gullone E. Adolescent body image dissatisfaction: relationships with self-esteem, anxiety, and depression controlling for body mass. *J Child Psychol Psychiatry*. 1998;39(2):255–262. https://doi.org/10.1017/S0021963097001807.
28. Bucchianeri MM, Arikian AJ, Hannan PJ, Eisenberg ME, Neumark-Sztainer D. Body dissatisfaction from adolescence to young adulthood: findings from a 10-year longitudinal study. *Body Image*. 2013;10(1):1–7. https://doi.org/10.1016/j.bodyim.2012.09.001.
29. Stice E, Bearman SK. Body-image and eating disturbances prospectively predict increases in depressive symptoms in adolescent girls: a growth curve analysis. *Dev Psychol*. 2001;37(5):597–607. https://doi.org/10.1037/0012-1649.37.5.597.
30. Cash TF, Smolak L. Understanding body images: historical and contemporary perspectives. In: Cash TF, Smolak L, Cash TF, Smolak L, eds. *Body Image: A Handbook of Science, Practice, and Prevention*. New York, NY, US: Guilford Press; 2011:3–11.
31. Buckingham-Howes S, Armstrong B, Pejsa-Reitz MC, et al. BMI and disordered eating in urban, African American, adolescent girls: the mediating role of body dissatisfaction. *Eat Behav*. 2018;29:59–63. https://doi.org/10.1016/j.eatbeh.2018.02.006.
32. Grabe S, Hyde JS. Ethnicity and body dissatisfaction among women in the United States: a meta-analysis. *Psychol Bullet*. 2006;132(4):622–640. https://doi.org/10.1037/0033-2909.132.4.622.
33. Eisenberg ME, Neumark-Sztainer D, Paxton SJ. Five-year change in body satisfaction among adolescents. *J Psychos Res*. 2006;61(4):521–527. https://doi.org/10.1016/j.jpsychores.2006.05.007.
34. Olmsted MP, McFarlane T. Body weight and body image. *BMC Women's Health*. 2004;4(suppl 1):S5.
35. Cash TF, Henry PE. Women's body images: the results of a national survey in the U.S.A. *Sex Roles*. 1995;33(1–2):19–28. https://doi.org/10.1007/BF01547933.
36. Dion J, Blackburn M, Auclair J, et al. Development and aetiology of body dissatisfaction in adolescent boys and girls. *Int J Adolesc Youth*. 2015;20(2):151–166. https://doi.org/10.1080/02673843.2014.985320.
37. Boyd HK, Kass AE, Accurso EC, Goldschmidt AB, Wildes JE, Le Grange D. Relationship between desired weight and eating disorder pathology in youth. *Int J Eat Disord*. 2017;50(8):963–969. https://doi.org/10.1002/eat.22720.
38. MacNeill LP, Best LA. Perceived current and ideal body size in female undergraduates. *Eating Behav*. 2015;18:71–75. https://doi.org/10.1016/j.eatbeh.2015.03.004.
39. Bearman SK, Martinez E, Stice E, Presnell K. The skinny on body dissatisfaction: a longitudinal study of adolescent girls and boys. *J Youth Adolesc*. 2006;35(2):217–229. https://doi.org/10.1007/s10964-005-9010-9.
40. Meyers EE. Fashioning worker protections to combat the thin ideal's cost on fashion models and public health. *Vanderbilt J Entertain Technol Law*. 2018;20(4):1219–1257.
41. McCabe MP, Ricciardelli LA. A longitudinal study of pubertal timing and extreme body change behaviors among adolescent boys and girls. *Adolescence*. 2004;39(153):145–166.
42. Levine MP, Harrison K. Media's role in the perpetuation and prevention of negative body image and disordered eating. In: Thompson JK, ed. *Handbook of Eating Disorders and Obesity*. Hoboken, NJ: Wiley; 2004:695–717.
43. Grabe S, Ward LM, Hyde JS. The role of the media in body image concerns among women: a meta-analysis of experimental and correlational studies. *Psychol Bullet*. 2008;134(3):460–476. https://doi.org/10.1037/0033-2909.134.3.460.
44. Bocage-Barthélémy Y, Chatard A, Jaafari N, et al. Automatic social comparison: cognitive load facilitates an increase in negative thought accessibility after thin ideal exposure among women. *PLoS One*. 2018;13(3):e0193200. https://doi.org/10.1371/journal.pone.0193200.
45. Cooley E, Toray T. Body image and personality predictors of eating disorder symptoms during the college years. *Int J Eat Disord*. 2001;30(1):28–36. https://doi.org/10.1002/eat.1051.
46. Rohde P, Stice E, Marti CN. Development and predictive effects of eating disorder risk factors during adolescence: implications for prevention efforts. *Int J Eat Disord*. 2015;48(2):187–198. https://doi.org/10.1002/eat.22270.
47. Stice E, Rohde P, Durant S, Shaw H. A preliminary trial of a prototype Internet dissonance-based eating disorder prevention program for young women with body image concerns. *J Consult Clin Psychol*. 2012;80(5):907–916. https://doi.org/10.1037/a0028016.
48. Madowitz J, Matheson BE, Liang J. The relationship between eating disorders and sexual trauma. *Eat Weight Disord*. 2015;20(3):281–293. https://doi.org/10.1007/s40519-015-0195-y.
49. Radwan H, Hasan HA, Najm L, et al. Eating disorders and body image concerns as influenced by family and media

among university students in Sharjah, UAE. *Asia Pac J Clin Nutr*. 2018;27(3):695–700. https://doi.org/10.6133/apjcn.062017.10.

50. Handford CM, Rapee RM, Fardouly J. The influence of maternal modeling on body image concerns and eating disturbances in preadolescent girls. *Behav Res Therapy*. 2018;100:17–23. https://doi.org/10.1016/j.brat.2017.11.001.
51. Delinsky SS, Wilson GT. Mirror exposure for the treatment of body image disturbance. *Int J Eat Disord*. 2006; 39(2):108–116. https://doi.org/10.1002/eat.20207.
52. Johnson F, Wardle J. Dietary restraint, body dissatisfaction, and psychological distress: a prospective analysis. *J Abnorm Psychol*. 2005;114(1):119–125. https://doi.org/10.1037/0021-843X.114.1.119.
53. American Psychiatric Association. *Diagnostic and Statistical Manual of Mental Disorders*. 5th ed. Arlington, VA: American Psychiatric Publishing; 2013.
54. Pope HG Jr, Lalonde JK, Pindyck LJ, et al. Binge eating disorder: a stable syndrome. *Am J Psychiatry*. 2006; 163(12):2181–2183. https://doi.org/10.1176/appi.ajp.163.12.2181.
55. Smink FR, van Hoeken D, Hoek HW. Epidemiology of eating disorders: incidence, prevalence and mortality rates. *Curr Psychiatry Rep*. 2012;14(4):406–414. https://doi.org/10.1007/s11920-012-0282-y.
56. Fennig S, Hadas A. Suicidal behavior and depression in adolescents with eating disorders. *Nordic J Psychiatry*. 2010;64(1):32–39. https://doi.org/10.3109/08039480903265751.

56a. Zhao Y, Encinosa W. Hospitalizations for eating disorders from 1999 to 2006. *Statistical Brief*. 2006. #70.

57. Fitzsimmons-Craft EE, Karam AM, Wilfley DE. Eating disorders in children and adolescents. In: Butcher JN, Kendall PC, Butcher JN, Kendall PC, eds. *APA Handbook of Psychopathology: Child and Adolescent Psychopathology*. Washington, DC, US: American Psychological Association; 2018:343–368. https://doi.org/10.1037/0000065-016.
58. Patton GC. Mortality in eating disorders. *Psychol Med*. 1988;18(4):947–951. https://doi.org/10.1017/S0033291700009879.
59. Franko DL, Keshaviah A, Eddy KT, et al. A longitudinal investigation of mortality in anorexia nervosa and bulimia nervosa. *Am J Psychiatry*. 2013;170(8):917–925. https://doi.org/10.1176/appi.ajp.2013.12070868.
60. Keel PK, Dorer DJ, Eddy KT, Franko D, Charatan DL, Herzog DB. Predictors of mortality in eating disorders. *Arch Gen Psychiatry*. 2003;60(2):179–183. https://doi.org/10.1001/archpsyc.60.2.179.
61. National Eating Disorders Association. *Statistics & Research on Eating Disorders*; 2018. Retrieved May 27, 2018, from: https://www.nationaleatingdisorders.org/statistics-research-eating-disorders.
62. Insel T. *Spotlight on Eating Disorders*; 2012. Retrieved on August 27, 2018 from: https://www.nimh.nih.gov/about/directors/thomas-insel/blog/2012/spotlight-on-eating-disorders.shtml#i.
63. Favaro A, Caregaro L, Tenconi E, Bosello R, Santonastaso P. Time trends in age at onset of anorexia nervosa and bulimia nervosa. *J Clin Psychiatry*. 2009; 70(12):1715–1721. https://doi.org/10.4088/JCP.09m05176blu.
64. Le Grange D, Loeb KL. Early identification and treatment of eating disorders: prodrome to syndrome. *Early Interv Psychiatry*. 2007;1(1):27–39. https://doi.org/10.1111/j.1751-7893.2007.00007.x.
65. Micali N, Hagberg KW, Petersen I, Treasure JL. The incidence of eating disorders in the UK in 2000-2009: findings from the general practice research database. *BMJ Open*. 2013;3(5). https://doi.org/10.1136/bmjopen-2013-002646.
66. Merikangas KR, He J, Burstein M, et al. Lifetime prevalence of mental disorders in U.S. adolescents: results from the National Comorbidity Survey Replication-Adolescent Supplement (NCS-A). *J Am Acad Child Adoles Psychiatry*. 2010;49(10):980–989. https://doi.org/10.1016/j.jaac.2010.05.017.
67. Le Grange D, Swanson SA, Crow SJ, Merikangas KR. Eating disorder not otherwise specified presentation in the US population. *Int J Eating Disord*. 2012;45(5): 711–718. https://doi.org/10.1002/eat.22006.
68. Smink FR, van Hoeken D, Oldehinkel AJ, Hoek HW. Prevalence and severity of DSM-5 eating disorders in a community cohort of adolescents. *Int J Eat Disord*. 2014;47(6):610–619. https://doi.org/10.1002/eat.22316.
69. The National Child Traumatic Stress Network. *Child Sexual Abuse Fact Sheet*; 2009. www.NCTSN.org.
70. U.S. Department of Health & Human Services. *Administration for Children and Families, Administration on Children, Youth and Families*. Children's Bureau; 2018. Child Maltreatment, 2016. Retrieved from: https://www.acf.hhs.gov/cb/research-data- technology/statistics-research/child-maltreatment.
71. Stoltenborgh M, van Ijzendoorn MH, Euser EM, Bakermans-Kranenburg MJ. A global perspective on child sexual abuse: meta-analysis of prevalence around the world. *Child Maltreat*. 2011;16(2):79–101. https://doi.org/10.1177/1077559511403920.
72. Pereda N, Guilera G, Forns M, Gomez-Benito J. The prevalence of child sexual abuse in community and student samples: a meta-analysis. *Clin Psychol Rev*. 2009;29(4): 328–338. https://doi.org/10.1016/j.cpr.2009.02.007.
73. Kenny MC, McEachern AG. Racial, ethnic, and cultural factors of childhood sexual abuse: a selected review of the literature. *Clin Psychol Rev*. 2000;20(7): 905–922.
74. Ball K, Kenardy J, Lee C. Relationships between disordered eating and unwanted sexual experiences: a review. *Austr Psychol*. 1999;34(3):166–176. https://doi.org/10.1080/00050069908257450.

74a. Brooke L, Mussap AJ. Brief report: maltreatment in childhood and body concerns in adulthood. *J Health Psychol*. 2013;18(5):620–626. https://doi.org/10.1177/1359105312454036.

75. Back SE, Jackson JL, Fitzgerald M, Shaffer A, Salstrom S, Osman MM. Child sexual and physical abuse among college students in Singapore and the United States. *Child Abuse Neglect*. 2003;27(11):1259–1275. https://doi.org/10.1016/j.chiabu.2003.06.001.
76. Clear PJ, Vincent JP, Harris GE. Ethnic differences in symptom presentation of sexually abused girls. *J Child Sexual Abuse*. 2006;15(3):79–98. https://doi.org/10.1300/J070v15n03_05.
77. Dworkin ER, Menon SV, Bystrynski J, Allen NE. Sexual assault victimization and psychopathology: a review and meta-analysis. *Clin Psychol Rev*. 2017;56:65–81. https://doi.org/10.1016/j.cpr.2017.06.002.
78. Egle UT, Franz M, Joraschky P, Lampe A, Seiffge-Krenke I, Cierpka M. Health-related long-term effects of adverse childhood experiences – an update. *Bundesgesundheitsblatt, Gesundheitsforschung, Gesundheitsschutz*. 2016; 59(10):1247–1254. https://doi.org/10.1007/s00103-016-2421-9.
79. Smolak L, Murnen SK. A meta-analytic examination of the relationship between child sexual abuse and eating disorders. *Int J Eat Disord*. 2002;31(2):136–150. https://doi.org/10.1002/eat.10008.
80. Ng QX, Yong BZJ, Ho CYX, Lim DY, Yeo WS. Early life sexual abuse is associated with increased suicide attempts: an update meta-analysis. *J Psychiatric Res*. 2018;99:129–141. https://doi.org/10.1016/j.jpsychires.2018.02.001.
81. Zatti C, Rosa V, Barros A, et al. Childhood trauma and suicide attempt: a meta-analysis of longitudinal studies from the last decade. *Psychiatry Res*. 2017;256:353–358. https://doi.org/10.1016/j.psychres.2017.06.082.
82. Liu RT, Scopelliti KM, Pittman SK, Zamora AS. Childhood maltreatment and non-suicidal self-injury: a systematic review and meta-analysis. *Lancet Psychiatry*. 2018;5(1): 51–64. https://doi.org/10.1016/S2215-0366(17)30469-8.
83. Kendall-Tackett KA, Williams LM, Finkelhor D. Impact of sexual abuse on children: a review and synthesis of recent empirical studies. *Psychol Bullet*. 1993;113(1):164–180. https://doi.org/10.1037/0033-2909.113.1.164.
84. Faravelli C, Giugni A, Salvatori S, Ricca V. Psychopathology after rape. *Am J Psychiatry*. 2004;161(8):1483–1485.
85. Ingram RE, Price JM. *Vulnerability to Psychopathology: Risk across the Lifespan*. 2nd ed. New York, NY, US: Guilford Press; 2010.
86. Sanci L, Coffey C, Olsson C, Reid S, Carlin JB, Patton G. Childhood sexual abuse and eating disorders in females: findings from the Victorian Adolescent Health Cohort Study. *Arch Pediatr Adolesc Med*. 2008;162(3):261–267. https://doi.org/10.1001/archpediatrics.2007.58.
87. Ben-Tovim DI, Walker MK. The development of the Ben-Tovim Walker Body Attitudes Questionnaire (BAQ), a new measure of women's attitudes towards their own bodies. *Psychol Med*. 1991;21(3):775–784.
88. Probst M, Pieters G, Vanderlinden J. Evaluation of body experience questionnaires in eating disorders in female patients (AN/BN) and nonclinical participants. *Int J Eat Disord*. 2008;41(7):657–665. https://doi.org/10.1176/ajp.2006.163.12.2181.
89. Probst M, Vandereycken W, Van Coppenolle H, Vanderlinden J. Body attitude test. *Psyctests*. 1995. https://doi.org/10.1037/t06446-000.
90. Danielsen M, Rø Ø. Changes in body image during inpatient treatment for eating disorders predict outcome. *Eat Disord*. 2012;20(4):261–275. https://doi.org/10.1080/10640266.2012.689205.
91. Vanderlinden J, Vandereycken W, Probst M. Dissociative symptoms in eating disorders: a follow up study. *Eur Eat Disord Rev*. 1995;3(3):174–184.
92. Slade PD, Dewey ME, Newton T, Brodie DA, Kiemle G. Development and preliminary validation of the body satisfaction scale (BSS). *Psychol Health*. 1990;4(3): 213–220. https://doi.org/10.1080/08870449008400391.
93. Cooper PJ, Taylor MJ, Cooper Z, Fairburn CG. The development and validation of the body shape questionnaire. *Int J Eat Disord*. 1987;6(4):485–494. https://doi.org/10.1002/1098-108X(198707)6:4<485::AID-EAT2260060405>3.0.CO;2-O.
94. Thompson MA, Gray JJ. Development and validation of a new body-image assessment scale. *J Pers Assess*. 1995; 64(2):258–269. https://doi.org/10.1207/s15327752jpa6402_6.
95. Gardner RM, Brown DL. Body image assessment: a review of figural drawing scales. *Persona Individ Differ*. 2010;48(2):107–111. https://doi.org/10.1016/j.paid.2009.08.017.
96. Wertheim EH, Paxton SJ, Tilgner L. Test-retest reliability and construct validity of contour drawing rating scale scores in a sample of early adolescent girls. *Body Image*. 2004;1(2):199–205. https://doi.org/10.1016/S1740-1445(03)00024-X.
97. Rosenberg M. Rosenberg self-esteem scale. *Psyctests*. 1965. https://doi.org/10.1037/t01038-000.
98. Robins RW, Hendin HM, Trzesniewski KH. Measuring global self-esteem: construct validation of a single-item measure and the Rosenberg Self-Esteem Scale. *Pers Soc Psychol Rev*. 2001;27(2):151–161. https://doi.org/10.1177/0146167201272002.
99. Hayes SC. Acceptance and commitment therapy, relational frame theory, and the third wave of behavioral and cognitive therapies. *Behav Therapy*. 2004;35(4):639–665. https://doi.org/10.1016/S0005-7894(04)80013-3.
100. Hayes SC, Pankey J. Experiential avoidance, cognitive fusion, and an ACT approach to anorexia nervosa. *Cogn Behav Pract*. 2002;9(3):243–247. https://doi.org/10.1016/S1077-7229(02)80055-4.
101. Wyssen A, Debbeler LJ, Meyer AH, et al. Cognitive distortions associated with imagination of the thin ideal: validation of the Thought-Shape Fusion Body Questionnaire (TSF-B). *Front Psychol*. 2017;8:2194. https://doi.org/10.3389/fpsyg.2017.02194.

102. Maloney MJ, McGuire JB, Daniels SR. Reliability testing of a children's version of the eating attitude test. *J Am Acad Child Adoles Psychiatry*. 1988;27(5):541–543. https://doi.org/10.1097/00004583-198809000-00004.
103. Garner DM, Garfinkel PE. The eating attitudes test: an index of the symptoms of anorexia nervosa. *Psychol Med*. 1979;9(2):273–279. https://doi.org/10.1017/S0033291700030762.
104. Garner DM. *Eating Disorder Inventory-2*. 1991.
105. Thurfjell B, Edlund B, Arinell H, Hägglöf B, Engström I. Psychometric properties of Eating Disorder Inventory for Children (EDI-C) in Swedish girls with and without a known eating disorder. *Eat Weight Disord*. 2003;8(4):296–303. https://doi.org/10.1007/BF0332502.
106. Smith KE, Mason TB, Murray SB, et al. Male clinical norms and sex differences on the Eating Disorder Inventory (EDI) and Eating Disorder Examination Questionnaire (EDE-Q). *Int J Eat Disord*. 2017;50(7):769–775. https://doi.org/10.1002/eat.22716.
107. Bernstein DP, Stein JA, Newcomb MD, et al. Development and validation of a brief screening version of the Childhood Trauma Questionnaire. *Child Abuse Neglect*. 2003;27(2):169–190. https://doi.org/10.1016/S0145-2134(02)00541-0.
108. Steinberg AM, Brymer MJ, Kim S, et al. Psychometric properties of the UCLA PTSD reaction index: part I. *J Trauma Stress*. 2013;26(1):1–9. https://doi.org/10.1002/jts.21780.
109. Pynoos RS, Steinberg AM, Layne CM, et al. Modeling constellations of trauma exposure in the national child traumatic stress network core data set. *Psychol Trauma*. 2014; 6(suppl 1):S9–S17. https://doi.org/10.1037/a0037767.
110. Hodgdon HB, Liebman R, Martin L, et al. The effects of trauma type and executive dysfunction on symptom expression of polyvictimized youth in residential care. *J Traum Stress*. 2018;31(2):255–264. https://doi.org/10.1002/jts.22267.
111. Thompson JL, Kelly M, Kimhy D, et al. Childhood trauma and prodromal symptoms among individuals at clinical high risk for psychosis. *Schizophrenia Res*. 2009; 108(1–3):176–181. https://doi.org/10.1016/j.schres.2008.12.005.
112. Washburn M, Carr LC, Dettlaff AJ. The moderating effects of ethnicity on key predictors of trauma in child welfare involved adolescents. *J Adoles*. 2018;67:179–187. https://doi.org/10.1016/j.adolescence.2018.06.008.
113. National Eating Disorders Association (n.d.). Eating Disorders in Men & Boys. Retrieved August 28, 2018 from: https://www.nationaleatingdisorders.org/learn/general-information/research-on-males.
114. Treasure J, Russell G. The case for early intervention in anorexia nervosa: theoretical exploration of maintaining factors. *Br J Psychiatry*. 2011;199(1):5–7. https://doi.org/10.1192/bjp.bp.110.087585.

CHAPTER 13

# Addressing Substance Use with the Adolescent in Primary Care: the SBIRT Model

ALICIA KOWALCHUK, DO • MARIA MEJIA DE GRUBB, MD, MPH • SANDRA GONZALEZ, MSSW, PhD • ROGER ZOOROB, MD, MPH

## EPIDEMIOLOGY

Substance use is a major public health problem in the United States. Tobacco, alcohol, opioids, or other addictive substances represent a significant health burden and contribute to a growing number of deaths each year. Substance use disorders usually start with recreational or other types of use before the age of 25.[1] Adolescents that initiate substance use before the age of 14 years are at greatest risk for a substance use disorder (SUD) and have a 34% prevalence rate of lifetime substance use.[2] Prevention is essential, and developing strategies for screening and early intervention are key.

### Nicotine

CDC predicts that without change, 5.6 million of today's youth will die from smoking-related illnesses. Tobacco use, as with other drug use, often begins during adolescence, with 90% beginning by age 18. Flavored tobacco products, hookah, and smokeless or e-cigarette types of nicotine delivery are gaining popularity as traditional cigarette use is dropping.[3] In 2014, nearly one-quarter of students in grades 9 through 12 reported using tobacco in some form in the past 30 days and 41% reported having tried cigarettes before.[2] In 2017, 5.6% of middle school and 19.6% of high school students reported current use of tobacco products.[3]

### Alcohol

Underage drinking and binge drinking rates declined between 2002 and 2013 from 28.8% to 22.7% and 19.3% to 14.2, respectively. Still, alcohol is the most used and abused drug by adolescents, with 4300 deaths, and 119,000 emergency department visits associated with youth drinking in 2013 alone. The 2013 Youth Risk Behavior Survey found that "during the last 30 days" 30% drank, 14% binge drank, and 6% drove after drinking. Other associated risks raised by youth drinking include problems with school and social life, legal, sexual, and injury problems, unsafe situations and other drug use, and even death from alcohol poisoning, drunk driving, homicide, and suicide. Furthermore, early drinking is a predictor of adult alcohol use disorder.[4]

### Cannabis

Now is an unprecedented time of cannabis availability, as it becomes legalized in several states. This raises particular concern over expanded access for adolescents and accidental exposures from smokeless products. The CDC High School Youth Risk Behavior Survey found that 38% of high school students report having used marijuana.[5]

The effect of cannabis on cognitive function in adolescents and young adults has been studied. Although small, cross-sectional studies have shown statistically significant negative cognitive effects, a recent systemic review showed nonclinically significant impacts on cognition and no effect on cognitive function in adolescents who have been abstinent for more than 72 hours. Some of the effects noted in previous studies could be due to acute intoxication or withdrawal.[6]

### Opioids

Although the opioid crisis in the United States is gaining attention, surveys have found that 3.6% of adolescents reporting misusing opioids (mostly prescription pills) over the past year. This rises to 7.3% among older adolescents and young adults. Overdose deaths among adolescents are increasing, and the healthcare burden is growing.[7]

Adolescent Health Screening: An Update in the Age of Big Data. https://doi.org/10.1016/B978-0-323-66130-0.00013-2

## Other Drugs

The 2017 Youth Risk Behavior Survey found varying rates for other drugs tried "one or more times during their life," cocaine (4.8%), hallucinogenic drugs (such as LSD, acid, PCP, angel dust, mescaline, or mushrooms) (6.6%), inhalants (sniffed glue, breathed the contents of aerosol spray cans, or inhaled any paints or sprays) (6.2%), ecstasy (4.0%), methamphetamines (2.5), and steroids without a doctor's prescription (2.9).[5]

## Leading Indicators

Adolescents facing social pressure, lacking family and social support, exposed to drugs, drug-use environments, and drug advertising are at greater risk for drug use. Similarly, physical abuse and sexual abuse are leading predictors.[8] Low educational attainment is a common effect and may be a useful indicator. Poly-drug use may also be an important indicator, as alcohol, tobacco, and marijuana tend to be used in some combination by adolescents.[9] For early substance use, males are at greater risk than females, parental substance use disorder is a strong predictor of early initiation, and higher levels of hyperactivity, thought problems, and those with less social skills in kindergarten are at increased risk of early-onset substance use.[10]

Peer experiences can have an influence on substance use and type of substance used in later adolescence. Adolescents who are part of an antisocial peer group demonstrate an increased risk of becoming a polysubstance user, and being bullied as a youth has an increased risk of smoking behavior later in life, whether it be tobacco or cannabis use.[11] Other school factors related to increased regular substance use of smoking, drinking, and cannabis include negative student–teacher relationships and fighting during school.[12]

Other indicators for adolescent substance use continuing into adulthood include problems during adolescence in the home environment such as family conflict, family management, and parental monitoring and punishment and rewards for behavior.[13] In Hispanic adolescents, family and economic stress, acculturation gap, community and gang exposures, and family drug use are all risk factors for multiple substance use behaviors.[14] Additionally, any type of juvenile arrest record increases the risk of substance use.[15]

Screening high-risk adolescents for substance use during primary care appointments is especially needful; with around a third of teens trying alcohol and cannabis, universal screening should be considered.

# SCREENING

## Why Screen for Substance Use in Adolescents

Adolescence is marked by many physical, psychological, and social changes. It is a developmental period, which has been associated with increased risk-taking behaviors, including the initiation of substance use.[16] Substance use is common in adolescence and has been shown to increase significantly between early adolescence and late adolescence, making timely recognition of substance use disorder risk an important part of the clinical assessment.[17] Substance use is associated with the leading causes of morbidity and mortality among adolescents (e.g., motor vehicle and other accidents, suicide, and homicide). Adolescents who engage in heavy drinking (including binge drinking) have been shown to perform poorer on neuropsychological tests assessing attention and executive functioning whereas marijuana use during adolescence has been associated with negative effects on memory.[18]

Routine primary care visits are an ideal setting for early detection of substance and alcohol use by adolescents because they provide a recurrent opportunity to interact with this patient population in a confidential environment. In 2011, rates of attending an annual visit ranged from 43% to 74% among adolescents aged 10–17 years.[19] Several professional societies including NIAAA, NIDA, SAMHSA, and AAP recommend that clinicians screen all adolescents for tobacco, alcohol, or drug use (universal screening) with a formal, validated screening tool (such as CRAFFT, generally the preferred screening tool for adolescents, see Table 13.1) at every preventive healthcare (yearly) visit and appropriate acute care visits in adolescents aged 12–21 years, and respond to screening results with the appropriate brief intervention and referral if indicated (SBIRT).[20–22] However, providers should start asking adolescents about sensitive screening questions, including substance and alcohol use, as soon as the patient is old enough to be interviewed without the parent present.

Most adults with SUD report having started using illicit drugs during adolescence or young adulthood, hence it is key to identify and intervene in drug use as early as possible. SBIRT is a comprehensive and integrated approach to the delivery of early intervention and treatment services through universal screening. Although universal screening might sound overwhelming in a busy primary care practice, several easily implemented and reliable substance use screening tools are available to facilitate identification of adolescents who are at high risk of having or developing a SUD, see Table 13.2. Most adolescents who use substances

**TABLE 13.1**
**The CRAFFT Interview (Version 2.1) – To be Orally Administered by the Clinician**

| Part A: During the PAST 12 MONTHS, on how many days did you: | # of days |
|---|---|
| 1. Drink more than a few sips of beer, wine, or any drink containing alcohol? Put "0" if none | |
| 2. Use any marijuana (weed, oil, or hash by smoking, vaping, or in food) or "synthetic marijuana" (like "K2," "Spice")? Put "0" if none | |
| 3. Use anything else to get high (like other illegal drugs, prescription or over-the-counter medications, and things that you sniff, huff, or vape)? Put "0" if none. | |

| **Did the patient answer "0" for all questions in Part A?** | |
|---|---|
| Yes | No |
| Ask CAR question only, then stop | Ask all six CRAFFT* questions below |

| Part B | | No | Yes |
|---|---|---|---|
| C | Have you ever ridden in a CAR driven by someone (including yourself) who was "high" or had been using alcohol or drugs? | | |
| R | Do you ever use alcohol or drugs to RELAX, feel better about yourself, or fit in? | | |
| A | Do you ever use alcohol or drugs while you are by yourself, or ALONE? | | |
| F | Do you ever FORGET things you did while using alcohol or drugs? | | |
| F | Do your FAMILY or FRIENDS ever tell you that you should cut down on your drinking or drug use? | | |
| T | Have you ever gotten into TROUBLE while you were using alcohol or drugs? | | |

***Two or more YES answers suggest a serious problem and need for further assessment.**

1. Show your patient his/her score on this graph and discuss level of risk for a substance use disorder.

**Percent with a DSM-5 Substance Use Disorder by CRAFFT score***

100%
80%
60%
40%
20%
0%
32%
64%
79%
92%
100%
100%
1
2
3
4
5
6
CRAFFT Score

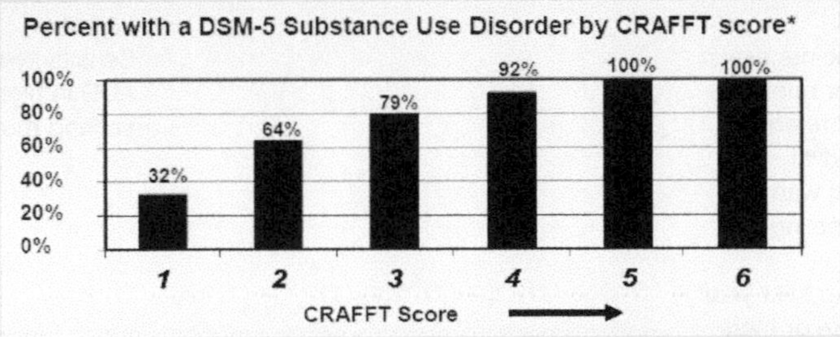

*Data source: Mitchell SG, Kelly SM, Gryczynski J, Myers CP, O'Grady KE, Kirk AS, & Schwartz RP. (2014). The CRAFFT cut-points and DSM-5 criteria for alcohol and other drugs: a reevaluation and reexamination. Substance Abuse, 35(4), 376–80.

2. Use the "5 Rs" talking points for brief counseling: REVIEW, RECOMMEND, RIDING/DRIVING, RESPONSE, REINFORCE

3. Give patient Contract for Life. Available at www.crafft.org/contract

Adapted from the Center for Adolescent Substance Abuse Research (CeASAR), Boston Children's Hospital. Available at www.ceasar.org

Adapted from the Center for Adolescent Substance Abuse Research (CeASAR), Boston Children's Hospital. Available at: www.ceasar.org.

do not have a SUD,[2] and brief counseling in the primary care settings can be effective in helping them decrease or stop using before developing a SUD. A recent national survey of adolescents found a decline in perceived risks of harm from using a number of substances, especially marijuana, suggesting a need to raise awareness of these risks with adolescents.[31]

Adolescents screening positive and thus considered high risk can be followed by more experienced clinicians for brief assessment to determine the appropriate level of care and referral (targeted screening). In 2014, over 2 million adolescents were current users of illicit drugs and thus at increased risk for developing substance use disorders.[2]

TABLE 13.2
Screening Tools Validated for Use With Adolescents

| Description | Length and Time to Administer/ Complete | Statistical Performance |
|---|---|---|
| **S2BI (SCREENING TO BRIEF INTERVENTION)[23]** | | |
| • Single frequency-of-use question per substance<br>• Discriminates between no use, no SUD, moderate SUD, and severe SUD, based on DSM-5 diagnoses | • <2 min<br>• 4 items<br>• Self or provider administered | Sensitivity/specificity 0.90/0.94 for SUD with monthly or more frequent use of any substance. |
| **BSTAD[24](BRIEF SCREENER FOR TOBACCO, ALCOHOL, AND OTHER DRUGS)** | | |
| • Identifies problematic tobacco, alcohol, and marijuana use in pediatric settings | • <2 min<br>• 9 items<br>• Self or provider administered | Optimal cut points for past-year frequency of use: ≥6 days of tobacco use (sensitivity = 0.95; specificity = 0.97); ≥2 days of alcohol use (sensitivity = 0.96; specificity = 0.85); and ≥2 days of marijuana use (sensitivity = 0.80; specificity = 0.93). |
| **NIAAA YOUTH ALCOHOL SCREEN (YOUTH GUIDE)[25]** | | |
| • Two age-specific screening questions about friends' and self-drinking in children and adoles-cents aged ≥9 y<br>• Age-sensitive cutoff points assist in determining whether brief advice, counseling, or referral appropriate. Any report of drinking ≤15 years old warrants brief advice and counseling. For youth ≥16 years old, drinking ≥6 days in the past year is considered moderate or high risk. | • < 2 min<br>• 2 items<br>• Self or provider administered | Sensitivity/specificity 0.89/0/91 for an AUD in middle school age adolescents scoring moderate risk or higher<br>Sensitivity/specificity 0.88/0.81 for an AUD in high school age adolescents scoring moderate risk or higher[26] |
| **CRAFFT (CAR, RELAX, ALONE, FRIENDS/FAMILY, FORGET, TROUBLE)[27]** | | |
| Recommended for quickly identifying problems associated with substance use. | • 5–10 min<br>• 6 items<br>• Self or provider administered | Sensitivity/specificity 0.91/0.93 for detecting any SUD using cut off score >2 |
| **GAIN-SS (GLOBAL APPRAISAL OF INDIVIDUAL NEEDS—SHORT SCREENER)[28]** | | |
| Assesses for both substance use disorders and mental health disorders | • 5 min<br>• 20 items<br>• Self or provider administered | Sensitivity/specificity 0.82/0.95 for detecting any past year SUD using cut off score of 2 |
| **AUDIT (ALCOHOL USE DISORDERS IDENTIFICATION TEST)[29]** | | |
| • Assess quantity, frequency, and consequences of alcohol use only | 2–3 min<br>10 items<br>Self or provider administered | Sensitivity/specificity 0.70/0.94 for AUD<br>Sensitivity/specificity 0.19/0.99 for any past year use<br>Sensitivity/specificity 0.33/0.99 for heavy past year use[30] |

Adapted from: Levy S, Bagley S. Substance use: initial approach in primary care. In: Adam HM, Foy JM, eds. *Signs and Symptoms in Pediatrics*. Elk Grove Village, IL: American Academy of Pediatrics; 2015:887–900

## Incorporating into HEEADSS

Screening for at risk populations can be incorporate as part of the commonly used HEEADSSS (Home environment, Education and employment, Eating, peer-related Activities, Drugs, Sexuality, Suicide/depression, and Safety from injury and violence)[32] assessment to elicit information about substance use (including experimentation) and other risky behaviors. The HEEADSSS interview approach includes a natural transition from expected and less threatening questions to more personal and intrusive questions giving the interviewer an opportunity to establish trust and rapport with the adolescent before asking the most difficult questions in the psychosocial interview. This is a practical, time-tested, complementary strategy that primary care providers can use to build on and incorporate the screening for substance use guidelines into their busy office practices.

Noteworthy, although specific SBIRT screening tools and intervention strategies have well-documented efficacy for adult alcohol use, research of SBIRT efficacy in adolescents is scarce.[33] Based on the limited available data, the 2014 USPSTF recommendation for primary care interventions targeting illicit drug use in children and adolescents is under review as a Grade I, insufficient evidence.[34] The updated USPSTF (2018) recommendation for alcohol misuse concluded that "the current evidence is insufficient to assess the balance of benefits and harms of screening and brief behavioral counseling interventions for alcohol use in primary care settings in adolescents ages 12–17 years."[35]

## Confidentiality

Speaking with the adolescent alone for the screening process is key to ensuring an accurate assessment as most adolescents who are using substances will not readily disclose their use with a parent or guardian present.[36] Developing a standard script and process for excusing the parent or guardian from a portion of the healthcare visit can be helpful. Asking the accompanying adult to leave the room when it is time for the physical exam portion of the healthcare visit addresses the developmental need of the adolescent for physical privacy and allows for the provider and teen to confidentially discuss substance use and sexual health topics during this portion of the encounter.

It is also needful to address issues of confidentiality up front with the adolescent who may have concerns about conversation shared during this private part of the encounter being subsequently disclosed to the parent or guardian at the close of the encounter. Again, a standard script that invites discussion of questions or concerns, such as "What we discuss is confidential unless there is immediate risk of injury to yourself or someone else. Do you have any questions about that?" can be helpful. Adolescents are legally entitled to privacy around substance use treatment per federal and state privacy laws, with state law taking precedent.[36]

## Parental Requests for Drug Testing

Due to the transient nature of substance detection in urine, and its detection of substance use at a single point in time rather than patterns and consequences of use, urine drug testing is a poor method of screening for substance use disorders. Parental request for drug testing of the adolescent should be handled by discussing the request with parents, hearing out their concerns, and sharing the limited utility of drug testing in identifying substance use disorders that are defined by patterns and consequences of use, not use or abstinence at a single point in time. This should be followed by a similar discussion with the adolescent alone. If the adolescent agrees to drug testing, a plan for disclosure of results should be mutually agreed upon before proceeding to testing. Although parents have the legal right to demand testing of a nonemancipated minor, if the adolescent refuses, drug testing is rarely worth the ensuing damage to the patient–provider relationship.[36]

## Evidence-Based Screens

Prescreening is completed with three evidence-based questions that can be asked during the clinical encounter or completed as part of a preencounter health questionnaire.[37]

*In the past 12 months, did you:*

1. *Drink any alcohol (more than a few sips)?*
2. *Smoke any marijuana or hashish?*
3. *Use anything else to get high? ("Anything else" includes illegal drugs, over the counter and prescription drugs, and things that you sniff or "huff.")*

Adolescents who answer NO to all questions (complete abstinence) should be commended and reassured of the good choices they are making. Those with any positive answer should be screened with a more comprehensive evidence-based tool.

The CRAFFT 2.1 (updated version) is a short evidence-based screening tool developed to screen adolescents aged 12–18 years old for high-risk alcohol and other drug use disorders simultaneously.[38] CRAFFT stands for the key words of the six questions—**C**ar, **R**elax, **A**lone, **F**orget, **F**riends, **T**rouble. This revised version enhances sensitivity to identify adolescents with substance use, and includes new recommended clinician talking points (https://ceasar.childrenshospital.org/wp-content/uploads/2018/04/CRAFFT-2.1_Clinician-Interview_2018-04-23.pdf).[38,39] In addition, the time-efficient self-administered version (https://ceasar.childrenshospital.org/wp-content/uploads/2018/04/CRAFFT-2.1_Selfadministered_2018-04-23.pdf) is recommended as there is evidence that adolescents prefer paper forms and computerized questionnaires over interviews with physicians or nurses and are more likely to be truthful when answering questions related to substance use.[39]

The CRAFFT 2.1 screening tool begins with past-12-month frequency items, rather than the previous "yes/no" initial screening questions stated earlier.

The first step is to tell adolescents their CRAFFT "score" and to show where that score falls on the bar chart based on the percentage of adolescents meeting criteria for a DSM-5 SUD.[27] The next step is to have a brief motivational enhancement discussion with the adolescent using the recommended "5 Rs" Talking Points for brief counseling: (1) REVIEW screening results; (2) RECOMMEND not to use; (3) RIDING/DRIVING risk counseling; (4) RESPONSE: elicit self-motivational statements; and (5) REINFORCE self-efficacy. Finally, the clinician should provide each patient with the "Contract for Life" that asks adolescents to agree never to accept a ride from a driver who has been drinking alcohol or using other drugs and to always wear a seat belt (available at https://ceasar.childrenshospital.org/contract-for-life/).

For additional evidence-based screening tools for adolescent substance use, see Table 13.2.

### Anticipatory Guidance

Primary care providers should reinforce the "nonuse" message through culturally sensitive, nonstigmatizing, and consistent information to patients, parents, and other family members while developing and maintaining a trusting patient-care relationship.[40]

For adolescents who screen negative, positive reinforcement for making this smart decision and related healthy choices is key to maintain a trustworthy patient-provider relationship. Counseling regarding the health effects of drug use, such as "science has shown that your brain continues to grow into at least your 20s, and alcohol and other recreational drug use poison developing brain cells," may benefit this at-risk population.

Research has shown that the NIAAA youth alcohol screening question about friends' drinking is a strong predictor of current and future alcohol problems in elementary (ages 9–11) and middle school (ages 11–14) patients.[25] If the patient reports their friends drink, providers should explore the patient's views about this, ask about their plans to stay alcohol-free, and rescreen at next visit. If friends do not drink, the provider should praise the choice of nondrinking friends, elicit and affirm reasons for staying alcohol-free, and rescreen in 1 year.

Anticipatory guidance includes screening for family and environmental issues that could have an impact on the adolescent and is often done as part of the frequently used HEEADSSS assessment. Providers should counsel parents about the risks of substance use in adolescents and address concerns about misconceptions on potential protective factors. For example, some parents may perceive a permissive home environment, such as allowing supervised adolescent alcohol consumption in the home, as a means to help protect their children from alcohol problems later in life. However, research indicates that the opposite is the case. Adolescents allowed to drink in the home are more likely than other teens to drink outside the home, drink more often, and consume higher quantities of alcohol[25,41] Parents have a strong influence over their childrens decisions whether to engage in risky behaviors even through high school and the transition to college. Providers should also offer resources for learning about high-risk behaviors (e.g., substance use, underage drinking) and encourage parents to discuss the realities and consequences with their kids.

## BRIEF INTERVENTIONS

After sharing a positive screening result, asking the adolescent their thoughts on the result with an open-ended question such as "what do you think about that?," shows the provider's curiosity and willingness to listen rather than to judge and lecture. Following that dialogue with permission to continue the conversation sets the stage for a motivationally enhancing brief intervention that respects the adolescent's autonomy. If the adolescent shuts down and does not want to engage in further discussion, a brief statement of provider concern about their use and offer to talk at future visits is warranted. Continuing the conversation, despite the adolescent's reluctance to engage, negates their autonomy and is not likely to yield positive behavior change.[25]

In integrated clinical settings, the primary care provider may conduct substance use screening with the adolescent or evaluate and respond to screening completed by the adolescent as part of the rooming process, give brief feedback, and then transition the adolescent to the behaviorist to complete the brief intervention as needed.[42]

### Motivational Interviewing Basis of Models

Adolescents who screen positive should receive an additional assessment to determine whether they have developed a SUD. Adolescents who are using alcohol or drugs but not meeting criteria for a SUD may benefit from a brief intervention. A brief intervention is an evidence-based practice that can assist individuals in making behavioral changes by raising awareness of the effects of their use. Brief interventions can be delivered by a primary care provider and are grounded in motivational interviewing techniques. Motivational interviewing (MI) is a therapeutic approach that addresses an individual's ambivalence about making a behavior change and utilizes techniques to engage patients and evoke motivation to make positive changes.[43] At the heart of MI-based brief interventions is the philosophy that motivation for change must come from the patient rather than the clinician, an approach that has been shown to resonate with adolescent populations.[44] To date, research has yielded small, yet statistically significant, decreases in substance use among adolescents following the receipt of a brief intervention.[45,46] Previous studies have shown reductions in alcohol use[47] and marijuana use among high-risk teens[48] and adolescents under the age of 18[49] following receipt of an MI intervention in primary care settings. There are several models of brief intervention that are currently used by primary care clinicians. Two of these approaches, the Brief Negotiated Interview and FRAMES, are described in this chapter.

### Brief Negotiated Interview

The Brief Negotiated Interview (BNI) is a brief intervention that is used in medical settings to assist healthcare providers in exploring substance use and willingness to change with their patients.[50] The BNI uses an algorithm and scripts to guide the provider through the intervention and is intended to be delivered in a limited time period, usually 5–15 min. The BNI involves the following four steps: (1) Raise the subject of alcohol or drug use; (2) Provide feedback about the results of the screening instrument and review risk guidelines; (3) Enhance motivation to cut back or quit using; (4) Negotiate a plan for change. The BNI has been recommended by the American Academy of Pediatrics for adolescents who screen positive but who are not in immediate need of specialized substance use disorder treatment.[51] The intent of the BNI in lower risk adolescents is to encourage abstinence or reduce risks associated with current use.[52]

### FRAMES

The FRAMES model is an approach to brief interventions that emphasizes a core set of principles: F = Feedback, R = Responsibility, A = Advice, M = Menu of Options, E = Empathy, and S = Self-efficacy. In short, the FRAMES acronym serves as a guideline for exploring motivation to change and begins with tailored feedback that may include providing results from a validated screening instrument such as the CRAFFT. Other elements include promoting a sense of personal responsibility (i.e., the patient has a choice when it comes to their use of substances), providing clear advice about the risks of continued use, and working with the patient to identify strategies to cut down or stop. As a provider, it is important to use an empathic (warm, nonjudgmental) style that highlights the patient's ability to achieve their stated goals.[53]

## REFERRAL TO TREATMENT

### Identifying Treatment Resources

Referral to specialized treatment is indicated for teens screening positive for a substance use disorder. Primary care providers and families can use the Substance Abuse and Mental Health Services Administration (SAMHSA) online treatment locator at https://www.findtreatment.samhsa.gov/or the SAMHSA National Helpline 1-800-662-HELP (4357) to begin the search for appropriate, evidence-based treatment programs and providers serving adolescents in their local or regional community. Before implementing SBIRT into clinical practice, it can be helpful to develop a list of local treatment options to make the referral to treatment process more standardized and less time consuming. In an integrated practice setting, the behaviorist may be the person to do treatment planning with families and make needed referrals, as they frequently already have knowledge and experience with community providers.[42]

In selecting appropriate treatment providers, it is important to ask what evidence-based programs they offer as well as their successful treatment completion rates. Table 13.3 lists behavioral, family-based, and recovery support approaches that have proven efficacy with adolescent SUD. No medications for SUD treatment are currently FDA approved for adolescents, and medications are rarely used in the treatment of adolescent SUD. Family-based approaches may be more effective than other individual and group treatments for adolescents because they are often living with and getting significant support from their families. Adolescents with SUD are typically treated in the specialized outpatient setting, with more intensive residential treatment

**TABLE 13.3**
**Evidence-Based Adolescent SUD Treatment and Recovery Support Resources**

| Behavioral | Family–Based | Recovery Support |
|---|---|---|
| Adolescent Community Reinforcement Approach (A-CRA) | Brief Strategic Family Therapy (BSFT) | Assertive Continuing Care (ACC) |
| Cognitive-Behavioral Therapy (CBT) | Family Behavior Therapy (FBT) | Mutual Help Groups -e.g., 12-step programs: Alcoholics Anonymous (AA), Narcotics Anonymous (NA), etc. |
| Contingency Management (CM) | Functional Family Therapy (FFT) | Peer Recovery Support Services |
| Motivational Enhancement Therapy (MET) | Multidimensional Family Therapy (MDFT) | Recovery High Schools |
| Twelve-Step Facilitation Therapy (TSF) | Multisystemic Therapy (MST) | |

Developed from: NIDA. Principles of Adolescent Substance Use Disorder Treatment: A Research-Based Guide. National Institute on Drug Abuse website. https://www.drugabuse.gov/publications/principles-adolescent-substance-use-disorder-treatment-research-based-guide/principles-adolescent-substance-use-disorder-treatment. January 14, 2014. Accessed 30.08.2018.

programs reserved for those teens lacking sober, safe, supportive home environments, with recurrent relapses, or complex co-occurring mental health needs.[54]

### Involving Parents/Guardians in the Treatment Referral Process

Although adolescents can consent to SUD treatment on their own (with state age-of-consent statutes taking precedent over federal),[36] parents frequently remain involved in the referral and treatment processes. Asking the adolescent's preference on discussing the need for SUD treatment with their parents with either the adolescent or the provider initiating the conversation supports the adolescent's autonomy and may reduce resistance to disclosure. When the adolescent is resistant to treatment referral or to acknowledging their problematic use of substances, referring parents to community family support resources, such as Community Reinforcement and Family Training (CRAFT), can be helpful. CRAFT teaches families to support the individual with a substance use disorder in a positive way that reinforces teen's actions toward abstaining and engaging treatment services while avoiding inadvertently reinforcing behaviors associated with ongoing substance use. CRAFT has been shown to help the adolescent enter treatment sooner and even cut back on use prior to treatment entry.[55]

## PRIMARY CARE FOLLOW-UP AND MANAGEMENT OF THE ADOLESCENT WITH SUD

### Preventive Health Care and Screenings

Primary care providers should ensure their adolescent patients with SUDs are up to date on immunizations and recommended routine health screenings such as for obesity, depression, and chlamydia and gonorrhea infection in sexually active female teens.[56] Additionally, adolescents with SUD should be screened for syphilis, Hepatitis C, tuberculosis, interpersonal violence, and trauma history, given their higher risk for these conditions.[57,58] Depending on substance or substances used and route of administration, additional assessments for skin infections, valvular and other heart diseases (in injection drug users), bronchial dysfunction (inhalants), and memory or thought disorders (hallucinogens) may be warranted. Female adolescents with SUDs are at high risk of unintended pregnancy, and effective contraceptive methods particularly long-acting options such as the intrauterine device (IUD), implants, and depot injections may be preferred.[59] Additionally adolescents with opioid use disorder (OUD) and their families should be offered opioid overdose prevention training including naloxone.[60]

### Treating Adolescents With Tobacco Use Disorders in Primary Care

Tobacco is among the substances most commonly used by youth and it can be a gateway to the use of other drugs.[61] Primary care clinicians should talk with children and adolescents about the harms of smoking and other reasons not to start smoking and advise all families to make their homes and cars smoke-free.[62] Any use of tobacco/nicotine in the past 30 days in adolescents is considered risky use (positive screening). Brief intervention should include information about the harmful effects of tobacco use: "You've probably heard that tobacco causes heart disease and cancer and a lot of other health problems. Quitting now will help you stay healthy. Also, tobacco is one of the most addictive substances. Quitting now will be much easier than quitting later, when you are addicted."[63] Currently, there are no medications approved by the US Food and Drug Administration for tobacco cessation in children and adolescents.

### Treating Adolescents With Alcohol and Opioid Use Disorders in Primary Care

None of the medications FDA approved to treat alcohol use disorder (AUD) in adults are approved to treat adolescents, and adolescent AUD is rarely treated with medication. Although medication-assisted treatment for OUD is standard of care for adults, methadone maintenance is only approved and available in some states for adolescents of ages 16–18 years old who have relapsed after several prior medication unassisted treatment episodes, and methadone cannot legally be prescribed for OUD outside of a licensed methadone clinic precluding its use in the primary care setting. Buprenorphine is not approved for use in the pediatric population, and safety data on patients under the age of 16 years old are lacking.[64] Currently, some primary care providers are using buprenorphine maintenance treatment in older adolescents, that is, age 16 years and older, in light of the ongoing severity of the opioid epidemic and several studies suggesting efficacy in this age group, but this is not yet a widespread practice.[65,66]

### Treating Adolescents With Other Substance Use Disorders in Primary Care

There are currently no FDA-approved medication-assisted treatments for other SUDs such as cannabis in adults or adolescents.[54]

## SPECIAL POPULATIONS

### Identifying and Supporting Adolescents With Parental Substance Use Disorder

Recent data show that roughly one in eight children (8.7 million) lives with at least one parent who has a SUD.[67] Parental substance use is associated with many short- and long-term negative effects, including disruptions in attachment, maltreatment (e.g., physical or sexual abuse, neglect), and troubles during adolescent development.[68,69] As a whole, children who are reared in homes where a parent is misusing substances are at greater risk for emotional, behavioral, and social problems. That risk increases when both parents have a substance use disorder or when the parent has a co-occurring mental health disorder.[70] Adolescents may believe that they caused their parent or caregivers' substance use disorder. They are also at high risk of developing their own substance use disorder, as they may begin using substances as a coping mechanism. Screening for parental substance use is an important component of the adolescent clinical encounter. Adolescent patients should be offered a confidential space to respond to questions regarding concerns they may have about a parent or caregiver who is using substances. Parents who are abusing substances may need to be referred to their own primary care provider for further assessment. Adolescents can be encouraged to reach out to trusted adults (e.g., teachers, coaches, or clergy) or to participate in a self-help group such as Alateen (https://al-anon.org/for-members/group-resources/alateen/).

### LGBTQ Adolescents and Substance Use

Lesbian, gay, bisexual, transgender, and questioning (LGBTQ) report higher rates of substance use compared to their youth heterosexual peers.[71] LGBTQ adolescents face a number of issues that place them at risk for substance use, including bullying, developmental challenges related to sexual and gender identity formation, parental rejection, and experiences of discrimination.[72,73] Among a nationally representative sample of US students in grades 9–12, researchers found higher prevalence rates for lesbian, gay, and bisexual youth (LGB) across several domains of current substance use, including cigarettes, cigars, or smokeless tobacco (25.7% of LGB students compared to 17.5% of heterosexual students), alcohol (40.5% of LGB students compared to 32.1% of heterosexual students), and marijuana (32.0% compared to 20.7% of heterosexual students). LGB youth were also more than twice as likely to have ever used cocaine, ecstasy, and hallucinogenic drugs and four times as likely to have used methamphetamines.[74] Routine screening should include questions about sexual orientation and gender identity. However, it is important to recognize that sexual orientation is a multidimensional construct involving behavioral, affective, and cognitive realms.[75] Female youth who are sexually active, regardless of sexual identity, should be asked about sexual behaviors and use of substances and counseled regarding their reproductive health, including the use of contraception. Providers must be sensitive to issues affecting LGBTQ adolescents and refer to affirming treatment providers.

### Pregnancy and Substance Use in Adolescence

In 2017, approximately 29% of high school students reported that they are sexually active and, of those, 13.8% reported that they did not use any contraception method to prevent pregnancy, and nearly one in five reported that they used alcohol or drugs before sexual intercourse.[76] Given that three out of four adolescent pregnancies are unintended,[77] screening for risky sexual behavior and substance use is a particular target for prevention efforts because of the risks for substance-exposed pregnancy. Substance use during pregnancy has been associated with an increased risk of harmful birth outcomes including low birth weight, stillbirth, fetal alcohol spectrum disorders (FASD), and neonatal abstinence syndrome.[78] Substance use significantly increases the risk of pregnancy in adolescents. Pregnant adolescents should be screened for substance use and offered intervention and treatment resources as needed.[57,59]

## Adolescents with Co-occurring Disorders

Co-occurring disorders, the presence of both mental health and substance use disorder, are common among adolescents. It is estimated that up to three-fourths of adolescents with a substance use disorder also meet criteria for a mental health condition.[79] When compared to adolescents with substance use disorders alone, teens with co-occurring disorders begin using substances at an earlier age, use substances more frequently and for a longer period of time, and have increased rates of family, school, and legal problems.[80] In adolescents, co-occurring disorders are typically categorized as either internalizing (e.g., anxiety, depression, low self-esteem) or externalizing (e.g., aggression, attention difficulties, impulsivity) disorders. The relationship between comorbid depression and substance use in adolescents and suicide risk is well established.[79] Primary care clinicians should utilize formal assessment methods that screen for the presence of *both* mental health and substance use disorders and refer to treatment providers that can treat the conditions concurrently.

## Adolescents with Fetal Alcohol Spectrum Disorders and Substance Use

Adolescents with an FASD or suspected FASD may experience secondary disabilities resulting from in utero exposure to alcohol, including problems with drug and alcohol use.[81] It is estimated that over one-third of individuals living with an FASD have a comorbid substance use disorder. Adolescents with an FASD may begin using substances in order to mitigate difficulties with socialization (i.e., establish belonging in a peer group) or cope with stressors. Poor judgment and poor impulse control make decision-making and refusal more difficult for adolescents with an FASD compared to their peers.[82] Adolescents with an FASD are also more likely to be victimized or taken advantage of by others who may encourage them to engage in substance use or participate in criminal behavior associated with alcohol or illicit drugs.

## REFERENCES


1. Peiper NC, et al. Overview on prevalence and recent trends in adolescent substance use and abuse. *Child Adolesc Psychiatr Clin N Am*. 2016;25(3):349–365.
2. Center for Behavioral Health Statistics and Quality. *Behavioral Health Trends in the United States: Results from the 2014 National Survey on Drug Use and Health*; 2015. HHS Publication No. SMA 15-4927, NSDUH Series H-50. Avaliable from: http://www.samhsa.gov/data/.
3. Smoking and Tobacco Use; Fact Sheet; Youth and Tobacco Use. Smoking and Tobacco Use. http://www.cdc.gov/tobacco/data_statistics/fact_sheets/youth_data/tobacco_use/. Published July 2, 2018. Accessed 16.08.2018.
4. CDC – Fact Sheets-Underage Drinking – Alcohol. https://www.cdc.gov/alcohol/fact-sheets/underage-drinking.htm. Published August 2, 2018. Accessed 16.08.2018.
5. Trends in the Prevalence of Marijuana, Cocaine, and Other Illegal Drug Use National YRBS: 1991–2017. https://www.cdc.gov/healthyyouth/data/yrbs/pdf/trends/2017_us_drug_trend_yrbs.pdf. Accessed 16.08.2018.
6. Scott JC, Slomiak ST, Jones JD, Rosen AFG, Moore TM, Gur RC. Association of cannabis with cognitive functioning in adolescents and young adults: a systematic review and meta-analysis. *JAMA Psychiatry*. 2018;75(6):585–595. https://doi.org/10.1001/jamapsychiatry.2018.0335.
7. Opioids and Adolescents. HHS.gov. https://www.hhs.gov/ash/oah/adolescent-development/substance-use/drugs/opioids/index.html. Published November 29, 2017. Accessed 16.08.2018.
8. Shin SH, Hong HG, Hazen AL. Childhood sexual abuse and adolescent substance use: a latent class analysis. *Drug Alcohol Depend*. 2010;109(1–3):226–235. https://doi.org/10.1016/j.drugalcdep.2010.01.013.
9. Moss HB, Chen CM, Yi H-Y. Early adolescent patterns of alcohol, cigarettes, and marijuana polysubstance use and young adult substance use outcomes in a nationally representative sample. *Drug Alcohol Depend*. 2014;136:51–62.
10. Kaplow JB, et al. Child, parent, and peer predictors of early-onset substance use: a multisite longitudinal study. *J Abnorm Child Psychol*. 2002;30(3):199–216.
11. Lamont AE, Woodlief D, Malone PS. Predicting high-risk versus higher-risk substance use during late adolescence from early adolescent risk factors using latent class analysis. *Addict Res Theory*. 2014;22(1):78–89.
12. Perra O, Fletcher A, Bonell C, Higgins K, McCrystal P. School-related predictors of smoking, drinking and drug use: evidence from the belfast youth development study. *J Adolesc Health*. 2012;35(2):315–324.

13. Herrenkohl TI, Olivia Jungeun L, Kosterman R, Hawkins JD. Family influences related to adult substance use and mental health problems: a developmental analysis of child and adolescent predictors. *J Adolesc Health*. 2012; 51(2):129–135.
14. Cardoso JB, Goldbach JT, Cervantes RC, Swank P. Stress and multiple substance use behaviors among hispanic adolescents. *Prev Sci*. 2016;17(2):208–217. https://doi.org/10.1007/s11121-015-0603-6.
15. Tolou-Shams M, Brown LK, Gordon G, Fernandez I, Project SSG. Arrest history as an indicator of adolescent/young adult substance use and HIV risk. *Drug Alcohol Depend*. 2007;88(1):87–90.
16. Hardin MG, Ernst M. Functional brain imaging of development-related risk and vulnerability for substance use in adolescents. *J Addict Med*. 2009;3(2):47–54.
17. SAMHSA. *National Survey on Drug Use and Health*. 2016.
18. Thoma RJ, Monnig MA, Lysne PA, et al. Adolescent substance abuse: the effects of alcohol and marijuana on neuropsychological performance. *Alcohol Clin Exp Res*. 2010; 35(1):39–46.
19. Adams SH, Park MJ, Irwin Jr CE. Adolescent and young adult preventive care: comparing national survey rates. *Am J Prev Med*. 2015;49(2):238–247.
20. Bright Futures/American Academy of Pediatrics. *Recommendations for Preventive Pediatric Health Care (Periodicity Schedule)*. 4th ed.; February 15, 2017. https://www.aap.org/en-us/Documents/periodicity_schedule.pdf. Accessed 30.07.18.
21. Committee on Substance Use and Prevention. Substance use screening, brief intervention, and referral to treatment. *Pediatrics*. 2016;138(1).
22. Substance Abuse and Mental Health Services Administration. About Screening, Brief Intervention, and Referral to Treatment (SBIRT). Last updated 9/20/2017. Available at: www.samhsa.gov/sbirt/about. Accessed 23.07.2018.
23. Levy S, Weiss R, Sherritt L, et al. An electronic screen for triaging adolescent substance use by risk levels. *JAMA Pediatrics*. 2014;168(9):822–828.
24. Kelly SM, Gryczynski J, Mitchell SG, Kirk A, O'Grady KE, Schwartz RP. Validity of brief screening instrument for adolescent tobacco, alcohol, and drug use. *Pediatrics*. 2014;133(5):819–826.
25. National Institute on Alcohol Abuse and Alcoholism. Alcohol Screening and Brief Intervention for Youth. A practicioner's guide. https://pubs.niaaa.nih.gov/publications/Practitioner/YouthGuide/YouthGuide.pdf. Accessed 7.8.2018.
26. Spirito A, Bromberg JR, Casper TC, et al. Network Reliability and validity of a two-question alcohol screen in the pediatric emergency department. *Pediatrics*. 2016; 138(6). https://doi.org/10.1542/peds.2016-0691. e2016 0691.
27. Mitchell SG, Kelly SM, Gryczynski J, et al. The CRAFFT cutpoints and DSM-5 criteria for alcohol and other drugs: a reevaluation and reexamination. *Subst Abus*. 2014;35(4): 376–380.
28. Smith DC, Bennett KM, Dennis ML, Funk RR. Sensitivity and specificity of the GAIN Short-Screener for prediction substance use disorders in a large national sample of emerging adults. *Addict Behav*. 2017;68:14–17.
29. Babor T, de la Fuente J, Saunders J, Grant M. *AUDIT, The Alcohol Use Disorders Identification Test: Guidelines for Use in Primary Health Care*. Geneva: Switzerland World Health Organization; 1992.
30. D'Amico EJ, Parast L, Meredith LS, Ewing BA, Shadel WG, Stein BC. Screening in primary care: what is the best way to identify at-risk youth for substance use? *Pediatrics*. 2016; 138(6). http://pediatrics.aappublications.org/content/138/6/e20161717.
31. Miech RA, Schulenberg JE, Johnston LD, Bachman JG, O'Malley PM, Patrick ME. *National Adolescent Drug Trends in 2017: Findings Released*; December 14, 2017. Monitoring the Future: Ann Arbor, MI. Available from: http://www.monitoringthefuture.org.
32. Reif CJ, Elster AB. Adolescent preventive services. *Primary Care: Clinics in Office Practice*. March 1998;Vol. 25(No. 1). WB Saunders: Philadelphia, PA; Goldenring JM, Cohen E. Getting into adolescent heads. *Contemp Pediatr*. 1988; 5(7):75–90.
33. O'Connor EA, Perdue LA, Senger CA, et al. *Screening and Behavioral Counseling Interventions in Primary Care to Reduce Unhealthy Alcohol Use in Adolescents and Adults: Updated Systematic Review for the U.S. Preventive Services Task Force*. Evidence Synthesis No. 171. AHRQ Publication No. 18-05242-EF-1. Rockville, MD: Agency for Healthcare Research and Quality; 2018.
34. *Draft Recommendation Statement: Unhealthy Alcohol Use in Adolescents and Adults: Screening and Behavioral Counseling Interventions*. U.S. Preventive Services Task Force; June 2018. https://www.uspreventiveservicestaskforce.org/Page/Document/draft-recommendation-statement/unhealthy-alcohol-use-in-adolescents-and-adults-screening-and-behavioral-counseling-interventions.
35. *Draft Update Summary: Illicit and Nonmedical Prescription Drug Use in Children and Adolescents: Interventions*. U.S. Preventive Services Task Force; May 2018. https://www.uspreventiveservicestaskforce.org/Page/Document/UpdateSummaryDraft/illicit-and-nonmedical-prescription-drug-use-in-children-and-adolescents-interventions.
36. Weddle M, Kokotailo PK. Confidentiality and consent in adolescent substance abuse: an update. *Virtual Mentor*. 2005;7(3):239–243. https://doi.org/10.1001/virtualmentor.2005.7.3.pfor1-0503.
37. Cavacuiti C. Screening and brief intervention for adolescents. In: Cavacuiti C, ed. *Principles of Addiction Medicine: The Essentials*. Philadelphia, PA: Lippincott Williams & Wilkins; 2011.
38. The CRAFFT. The center for adolescent substance abuse research. In: *Children's Hospital Boston*. Available at: https://ceasar.childrenshospital.org/crafft/.
39. Harris SK, Knight Jr JR, Van Hook S, et al. Adolescent substance use screening in primary care: validity of computer self-administered versus clinician-administered screening. *Subst Abus*. 2016;37(1):197–203.

40. Kulig JW, American Academy of Pediatrics, Committee on Substance Abuse. Tobacco, alcohol, and other drugs: the role of the pediatrician in prevention, identification, and management of substance abuse. *Pediatrics*. 2005;115(3): 816–821.
41. McMorris BJ, Catalano RF, Kim MJ, Toumbourou JW, Hemphill SA. Influence of family factors and supervised alcohol use on adolescent alcohol use and harms: similarities between youth in different alcohol policy contexts. *J Stud Alcohol Drugs*. 2011;72(3):418–428.
42. Rahm AK, Boggs JM, Martin C, Price DW, Beck A, Backer TE, Dearing JW. Facilitators and barriers to implementing screening, brief intervention, and referral to treatment (SBIRT) in primary care in integrated health care settings. DOI: 10.1080/08897077.2014.951140.
43. Miller WR, Rollnick S. *Motivational Interviewing: Helping People Change*. Guilford press; 2012.
44. Naar S, Suarez M. *Motivational Interviewing with Adolescents and Young Adults*. Guilford Press; 2011.
45. Tait RJ, Hulse GK. A systematic review of the effectiveness of brief interventions with substance using adolescents by type of drug. *Drug Alcohol Rev*. 2003;22(3):337–346.
46. Jensen CD, Cushing CC, Aylward BS, Craig JT, Sorell DM, Steele RG. Effectiveness of motivational interviewing interventions for adolescent substance use behavior change: a meta analytic review. *J Consult Clin Psychol*. 2011;79(4): 433–440.
47. Spirito A, Monti PM, Barnett NP, et al. A randomized clinical trial of a brief motivational intervention for alcohol-positive adolescents treated in an emergency department. *J Pediatr*. 2004;145(3):396–402.
48. D'Amico EJ, Miles JNV, Stern SA, Meredith LS. Brief motivational interviewing for teens at risk of substance use consequences: a randomized pilot study in a primary care clinic. *J Subst Abus Treat*. 2008;35(1):53–61.
49. Laporte C, Vaillant-Roussel H, Pereira B, et al. Cannabis and young users—a brief intervention to reduce their consumption (CANABIC): a cluster randomized controlled trial in primary care. *Ann Fam Med*. 2017;15(2):131–139.
50. D'Onofrio G, Pantalon MV, Degutis LC, Fiellin DA, O'Connor PG. Development and implementation of an emergency practitioner–performed brief intervention for hazardous and harmful drinkers in the emergency department. *Acad Emerg Med*. 2005;12(3):249–256.
51. Committee on Substance Abuse, Levy SJ, Kokotailo PK. Substance use screening, brief intervention, and referral to treatment for pediatricians. *Pediatrics*. 2011;128(5): e1330–e1340.
52. Pilowsky DJ, Wu L-T. Screening instruments for substance use and brief interventions targeting adolescents in primary care: a literature review. *Addict Behav*. 2013;38(5): 2146–2153.
53. Henry-Edwards S, Humeniuk R, Ali R, Monteiro M, Poznyak V. *Brief Intervention for Substance Use: A Manual for Use in Primary Care*. Geneva: World Health Organization; 2003.
54. NIDA. *Principles of Adolescent Substance Use Disorder Treatment: A Research-Based Guide*. National Institute on Drug Abuse website; January 14, 2014. https://www.drugabuse.gov/publications/principles-adolsecent-substance-use-disorder treatment-research-based-guide. Accessed 30.08.2018.
55. Kirby KC, Versek B, Kerwin ME, et al. Developing community reinforcement and family training (CRAFT) for parents of treatment-resistant adolescents. *J Child Adoles Subst Abuse*. 2015;24(3):155–165. https://doi.org/10.1080/1067828X.2013.777379.
56. USPSTF A and B Recommendations. *U.S. Preventive Services Task Force*; August 2018. https://www.uspreventiveservicestaskforce.org/Page/Name/uspstf-a-and-b-recommendations/. Accessed 28.08.18.
57. Clayton HB, Lowry R, August E, Jones SE. Nonmedical use of prescription drugs and sexual risk behaviors. *Pediatrics*. 2016;137(1). e20152480.
58. Cavazos-Rehg PA, Krauss MJ, Spitznagel EL, Schootman M, Cottler LB, Bierut LJ. Number of sexual partners and associations with initiation and intensity of substance use. *AIDS Behav*. 2011;15(4):869–874.
59. Cavazos-Rehg PA, Krauss MJ, Spitznagel EL, Schootman M, Cottler LB, Bierut LJ. Brief report: pregnant by age 15 years and substance use initiation among US adolescent girls. *J Adolesc*. 2012;35(5):1393–1397.
60. Substance Abuse and Mental Health Services Administration. *SAMHSA Opioid Overdose Prevention Toolkit*. HHS Publication No. (SMA) 16-4742. Rockville, MD: Substance Abuse and Mental Health Services Administration; 2016. Available at: https://store.samhsa.gov/shin/content//SMA16-4742/SMA16-4742.pdf.
61. Sims TH. From the American Academy of Pediatrics: technical report—tobacco as a substance of abuse. *Pediatrics*. 2009;124:e1045–e1053.
62. *Final Recommendation Statement: Tobacco Use in Children and Adolescents: Primary Care Interventions*. U.S. Preventive Services Task Force; December 2016. https://www.uspreventiveservicestaskforce.org/Page/Document/RecommendationStatementFinal/tobacco-use-in-children-and-adolescents-primary-care-interventions.
63. American Academy of Pediatrics. *Substance Use Screening and Intervention Implementation Guide*. https://www.aap.org/en-us/Documents/substance_use_screening_implementation.pdf. Accessed 7.08.2018.
64. Woody GE, Poole SA, Subramaniam G, et al. Extended vs short-term buprenorphine-naloxone for treatment of opioid-addicted youth: a randomized trial. *JAMA*. 2008; 300(17):2003–2011. *Erratum in Journal of the American Medical Association*. 2009;301(8):830.
65. Marsch LA, Bickel WK, Badger GJ, et al. Comparison of pharmacological treatments for opioid-dependent adolescents: a randomized controlled trial. *Arch Gen Psychiatry*. 2005;62(10):1157–1164.
66. Levy S, Mountain-Ray S, Reynolds J, Mendes SJ, Bromberg J. A novel approach to treating adolescents with opioid use disorder in pediatric primary care. *Substance Abuse*. 2018. https://doi.org/10.1080/08897077.2018.1455165.

67. Lipari RN, Van Horn SL. Children living with parents who have a substance use disorder. In: *The CBHSQ Report. Rockville (MD)*. 2013:1–7.
68. Lander L, Howsare J, Byrne M. The impact of substance use disorders on families and children: from theory to practice. *Soc Work Public Health*. 2013;28(0):194–205.
69. Calhoun S, Conner E, Miller M, Messina N. Improving the outcomes of children affected by parental substance abuse: a review of randomized controlled trials. *Subst Abuse Rehabil*. 2015;6:15–24.
70. Solis JM, Shadur JM, Burns AR, Hussong AM. Understanding the diverse needs of children whose parents abuse substances. *Curr Drug Abuse Rev*. 2012;5(2):135–147.
71. Marshal MP, Friedman MS, Stall R, et al. Sexual orientation and adolescent substance use: a meta-analysis and methodological review. *Addiction*. 2008;103(4):546–556.
72. Reisner SL, Greytak EA, Parsons JT, Ybarra M. Gender minority social stress in adolescence: disparities in adolescent bullying and substance use by gender identity. *J Sex Res*. 2015;52(3):243–256.
73. Ryan C, Russell ST, Huebner D, Diaz R, Sanchez J. Family acceptance in adolescence and the health of LGBT young adults. *J Child Adolesc Psychiat Nurs*. 2010;23(4):205–213.
74. Kann L, Olsen EO, McManus T, et al. Sexual identity, sex of sexual contacts, and health-related behaviors among students in grades 9-12-United States and selected sites, 2015. *MMWR Surveill Summ*. 2016;65(9). Centers for Disease Control and Prevention.
75. Mohr JJ, Kendra MS. Revision and extension of a multidimensional measure of sexual minority identity: The Lesbian, Gay, and Bisexual Identity Scale. *J Couns Psychol*. 2011;58(2):234.
76. Kann L, McManus T, Harris WA, et al. Youth risk behavior surveillance – United States, 2017. *MMWR Surveill Summ*. 2018;67(8):1–114.
77. Finer LB, Zolna MR. Declines in unintended pregnancy in the United States, 2008–2011. *N Engl J Med*. 2016;374(9): 843–852.
78. Forray A. Substance use during pregnancy. *F1000Res*. 2016;5. F1000 Faculty Rev-1887.
79. Lichtenstein DP, Spirito A, Zimmermann RP. Assessing and treating Co-occurring disorders in adolescents: examining typical practice of community-based mental health and substance use treatment providers. *Community Ment Health J*. 2010;46(3):252–257.
80. Hills H. *Treating Adolescents with Co-occurring Disorders*. 2007.
81. Streissguth A, Barr H, Kogan J, Bookstein F. *Understanding the Occurrence of Secondary Disabilities in Clients with Fetal Alcohol Syndrome (FAS) and Fetal Alcohol Effects (FAE)*. Final Report to the Centers for Disease Control and Prevention (CDC). 1996, 96-06.
82. Rasmussen C, Wyper K. Decision making, executive functioning and risky behaviors in adolescents with prenatal alcohol exposure. *Int J Disabil Hum Dev*. 2007;6:405.

CHAPTER 14

# Screening for Leading Indicators of Juvenile Delinquency

VINCENT MORELLI, MD

## INTRODUCTION

There is considerable overlap between the risk factors for juvenile criminality/recidivism and the risk factors for adolescent violence, obesity, depression, behavioral and emotional problems, and educational shortcomings. (See chapters devoted to these topics.) For example, adverse childhood experiences (ACEs) are risk factors for poor physical and mental health, obesity, depression, criminality, risky behavior, behavioral problems, and educational underachievement.

The idea behind looking at these "crossover" risk factors through the lens of criminal justice is the hope that screening with criminality in mind will highlight some of the more *immediate* dangers to adolescent health and well-being, thus add a sense of urgency to intervention. In other words, if we do not address these risk factors *now*, this adolescent will engage in risky behavior and end up in the criminal justice system with considerable loss of potential and all of the associated societal costs. This is quite different from saying: If we do not address these risk factors, this child will be obese or will die prematurely from heart disease and other stress-related maladies.

Thus, we feel that looking at juvenile crime and recidivism in a book on adolescent health screening is justified. If risk factors for criminality are uncovered, this may lead the practitioner to intervene more urgently and may help prevent both crime and other physical, behavioral, and mental health issues. Moreover, if such intervention can take place quickly and effectively, the adolescent's behavior, educational achievement, mental state, and physical health might be improved and the path to adult actualization made more accessible.

The juvenile justice system (JJS) assesses risk factors for criminality and recidivism in the following manner. First, they stratify youth into low, medium, or high risk for recidivism categories via a brief risk assessment. Following this relatively brief screening, those who screen at moderate or high risk usually undergo a more extensive needs assessment—a more in-depth evaluation of an individual's vulnerabilities, needs, and strengths. Such a needs assessment examines not only the *individual* factors at play, but also the family, community, and societal factors that may contribute to future criminality. The literature exploring these two screening tools—risk assessment and the needs assessment—will be the emphasis of this chapter. A penultimate brief section on the effective types of treatment (intervention) will follow. Finally, a brief concluding note on prevention programs has been added to help the practitioner to see the bigger picture.

Overall, this chapter is written with the intent of making the PCP aware of the risk factors leading to criminality—some of the same risk factors can lead to suboptimal mental, physical health, and spiritual health. Our aim is to help the practitioner gain knowledge of screening and intervening to prevent criminality, prevent recidivism, promote rehabilitation, and enhance "adolescent thriving." This chapter is a truncated version of a more in-depth review and analysis. Please contact the author if a full detailed literature review is desired.

## PART I—RISK ASSESSMENT

The risk assessment estimates a youth's likelihood to reoffend. As only 5%–6% will go on to be "life persistent offenders,"[33] and only 1%–9% will go on to be serious, violent, or chronic offenders (SVCs), identifying these youth early provides both optimal public

Adolescent Health Screening: An Update in the Age of Big Data. https://doi.org/10.1016/B978-0-323-66130-0.00014-4

safety and affords more prompt and focused rehabilitation efforts.

**Risk assessment tools** are of two basic varieties: actuarial assessments (surveys without subjective components) and professional judgment-based tools. Studies seem to indicate that a combination of the two methods may be best. Various states and private companies have formulated risk assessment surveys with varying degrees of effectiveness. An ideal risk assessment tool:

- includes risk factors that exhibit a significant association with recidivism
- includes both static and (some) dynamic risk factors[a]
- is properly weighted so that more impacting risk factors are given greater consequence
- accounts for individual strengths and protective attributes
- includes relevant family, school, and community factors
- combines all of these components into an efficient, effective risk-screening tool.

This is a tall order, especially for PCPs who have limited time and who may not yet realize the importance of screening in this manner.

## The Risk Factors Associated With Juvenile Recidivism

Based on several reviews (Gendreau, 1996),[12,16,3,10,9,31 (p3),40,48,49,57] the risk factors associated with recidivism are generally divided into the following categories: individual, family and peer, school and work, and community factors.

### Individual Risk Factors

Examples of individual factors are as follows:

- Genetic/neurologic: learning disabilities, emotional disturbances, etc.
- Attitudes/values: antisocial thinking, rejection of the law, tolerance of criminal behavior
- Behavioral: aggression, restlessness, antisocial behavior (e.g., arrests for vandalism, gang involvement), anger, impulsiveness, ADHD, callousness, early sexual experiences
- Alcohol and drug use
- Criminal history: number of prior arrests, type of crime, etc.
- Poor use of leisure time
- Mental health issues: depression, anxiety, etc.
- Skills deficits: poor coping skills, problem solving, communication, impulse control, etc.
- Poor psychosocial functioning and/or executive functioning
- Low education, low IQ, special education status
- Few employment skills and low social achievement

The most impacting individual risk factors in a 2001 meta-analysis[8] were in descending order: age at first confinement, age at first contact with the law, stress/anxiety and nonsevere mental health issues, conduct problems, poor use of leisure time, delinquent peers, length of first incarceration, out of home placements, number of prior confinements, type of crime (e.g., auto theft, assault) low standardized and verbal IQ (but not school reported academic performance or school attendance), substance abuse, and low socioeconomic status (SES).

Other later studies have corroborated these findings[58] and have added to the list: low social capacity, poor social networks, aggression, antisocial behavior, axis I psychopathology, and lack of empathy and conscience.[35,b] Interestingly, neither race nor ethnicity has been significantly associated with recidivism once SES is removed. Similarly, neither substance *use* nor prior psychological treatment has been associated with recidivism—though substance *abuse* has been.[8]

Researchers have documented that individual risk factors are amplified if they occur at a young age, if exposure occurs over a prolonged period,[19] and that the tie between risk factors and recidivism generally

[a]Note: Dynamic risk factors are attributes that are malleable—can be improved or changed—such as the youth's friends or academic standing. Static factors are those that cannot be changed, such as a history of physical abuse. It is recommended that static factors be emphasized in the initial risk assessment because extensive surveying of dynamic risk at this stage takes too long, tries to capture too much information, and does not focus adequately on stratification. The assessment of dynamic risk factors, on the other hand, are more appropriately screened in a needs assessment then considered more strongly in intervention programming.

[b]Some of the risk factors mentioned earlier (e.g., substance abuse, poor use of leisure time, etc.) are dynamic factors—theoretically more of a focus of the *needs* assessments. However, some dynamic factors are mentioned here because some jurisdictions screen for them in their initial risk assessment while others use a combined risk/needs assessment as their initial assessment tool.

decreases with age. The correlation between risk factors and recidivism drops roughly 40% as the child ages from 12 to 17, with much of the drop (25%) occurring shortly after age 12 or 13.[50] Thus, individual risk factors are more impacting in younger juveniles and risk assessment tools are considered more accurate and useful in younger age groups.

### Family/Peer Risk Factors

Several family and social risk factors are significant predictors of criminality and recidivism. Such factors include physical, emotional, or sexual abuse, number of out-of-home placements, family instability, inconsistent discipline, poor relationships between members, household violence or substance abuse, low educational level of parents, sibling antisocial behavior, incarceration of family member, sibling arrests, poor use of leisure time, and delinquent peers. Interestingly, neglect, especially ongoing neglect, has been documented as especially significant in terms of reoffense.[8,43]

**Individual and Family Risk,** the first two domains, are the ones most strongly associated with recidivism[8] with age-related influence declining as noted earlier. In addition, risk factors are known to have varying impacts on different age groups. As juveniles age from 12 to 17, the impact of family factors becomes less significant,[50] and the influence of peers and social relationship factors increase. The most impacting risk factors in those under 12 or 13 are individual attitude, aggression, and family factors. The most impacting factors for older juveniles are the use of free time, attitudes, school factors, and peer/adult relationships.

With this in mind, intervention programs should likely focus on individual attitude, aggression, and family factors in the younger age groups and attitudes, free time, substance abuse, school factors, and peers relationships in the older age groups. Risk-assessment results should be viewed through an age-adjusted lens and that intervention should be programmed accordingly.

### School/Workplace Risk Factors

Risk factors for criminality and recidivism at school or work include low achievement, negative attitude about school/work, disciplinary actions at work and school, suboptimal school environment such as tolerance for bullying or violence, poor teacher attitudes, low teacher pay, poor physical plant/facilities, and values at work or school.

### Community Risk Factors

Although less studied and less sought in risk assessment tools,[c] some important community contributors to recidivism are the prevalence of poverty, crime, drugs/alcohol, guns, gangs, low rates of home ownership, low physical attachment to community, and a country's and community's set of values.

### Cumulative and Grouping of Risk Factors

Some combination of the factors mentioned earlier is incorporated into all risk assessment tools, and while each factor reflects a certain risk of recidivism, research has shown that it is the *cumulative number* of factors that is the most accurate predictor of recidivism, especially if risk factors span more than one of the domains listed earlier (i.e., individual, family, and community).[8,19,30(p133),41]

In addition, researchers have recently begun examining *groupings* of risk factors in search for illuminating keys. For example, one study looked at school problems, mental health issues, and substance abuse. They found that 55%–75% of juveniles with deficits in two of the three of these areas ended up as chronic serious offenders.[22] This and other "grouping studies" are slowly beginning to be incorporated into risk assessment tools.

There is a caveat, however. When applied to an individual case, each risk factor should be looked at through a cultural lens. For example, "increased contact with law enforcement," a strong risk factor for recidivism, is much more common in minority communities, and thus may not as strongly predict risk. However, it may unfairly stratify minority youth into a high-risk grouping, which in turn may unfairly mandate incarceration or intervention (and may contribute to the racial disparities in youth incarceration). Thus, contact with law enforcement and prior offenses may not be as reliable an indicator of recidivism in minority communities.[37]

### The Flip Side: Screening for Protective Factors in the Risk Assessment

The OJJDP notes factors protective against recidivism in three realms:

- Individual characteristics, including dispositional attributes, such as easy temperament, positive

[c]Some risk assessment tools superficially survey community and environmental factors. For example, the Childhood and Adolescent Needs and Strengths (CANS) inquires into community safety and environmental issues. However, how contributory this information is, and how it should be used in risk stratification, is unclear.

orientation, intelligence, self-esteem, autonomy, and sociability;

- Family characteristics, such as secure attachments, lack of conflict and supportive family interactions that provide emotional sustenance and affection;
- External support at school, work, church, or community that strengthens individuals and families factors and help provide a sense of control, belonging, and meaning (Mihalic, 2004).[59]

Several reviews[6,14] and studies[17,34,36,51,44] have substantiated the importance of these three categories of protective factors. Researchers have noted that, in the individual realm, intellectual ability, self-esteem, academic achievement, self-regulation, social competence, problem-solving skills, autonomy, positive temperament, acceptance of responsibility for behavior, respect for rules, meaningful participation in activities, sense of purpose, and future orientation were all *associated* with resiliency and reduced recidivism. In the family realm, caring and supportive relationships, and high expectations again were *associated* with enhanced resiliency. All of these factors are thought to promote good decision making, thus preventing recidivism, promoting resilience, and moving the individual toward a more productive life.

Despite these associations; however, research in the "protective factor domain" is sorely lacking (We could only find 34 articles on the Psyche Info Database when we searched protective factors AND recidivism AND juvenile.) and no "protective factor risk-screening tools" have yet proven effective.[4] Still, some risk assessment tools screen for these factors with the idea that their presence may lessen an offender's likelihood of criminality and recidivism, and that the possession of certain strengths may place an otherwise high-risk juvenile into a lower risk category thus obviating the need for detrimental incarceration. In some jurisdictions, protective factors are being considered when designing intervention programs as well—with the *hope* (no data yet) that enhancing strengths may not only steel an adolescent against reoffending but also may aid in general resiliency and lead toward more empowered lives.[53]

Future research in this area is needed, as it is not known which strengths might be "most protective", which are most important in adolescent development, which grouping of factors might be synergistic, or even *if* protective factors *can* be enhanced by intervention to prevent recidivism.

## Which Risk Assessment Tool Is Best?

A recent 2013 review of 10 risk assessment tools[5] found only three to be effective in predicting future recidivism: the Virginia Youth Assessment and Screening Instrument (YASI), the Solano County Juvenile Sanctions Center (JSC), and the Oregon Juvenile Crime Prevention (JCP) assessment. The other seven tools[d] could not be validated as effective in predicting recidivism.[e]

The YASI's utility in the previous review was initially based on favorable short-term results and incomplete implementation of YASI in Virginia—results that far exceed YASI results elsewhere. Since this time, the YASI has been evaluated *somewhat* more favorably in more than 7000 youth in New York and Illinois, albeit by nonpeer-reviewed company-sponsored studies. These studies noted a mild-to-moderate predictive capability of the YASI.[38,39] A later 2016 company-sponsored study (and therefore subject to design, outcome, and editorial bias)[23] found the YASI to be highly predictive of recidivism[f] in Canadian male juvenile offenders over an 18-month follow-up period.

---

[d]Note: The *ineffective* tools studied earlier included: The Positive Achievement Change Tool (PACT), the Youth Assessment and Screening Instrument (YASI), the Youth Level of Service/ Case Management Inventory (YLS/CMI), the Comprehensive Risk and Needs Assessment (CRN, a derivative of Correctional Offender Management Profiling and Alternative Sanctions (COMPAS), the Girls Link risk assessment instrument, the Arizona Administrative Office of the Courts risk assessment instrument, and the Arizona Department of Juvenile Correction Dynamic Risk Instrument (DRI). The JSC and Girls Link are public-domain instruments; the others are designed and sold by private organizations. Three tools that are not included in this study were the Ohio Youth Assessment Survey (OYAS), the Washington State Juvenile Court Assessment Instrument (WSJCA), and the North Carolina Assessment of Risk (NCAR). The NCAR, one of the 14 tools on which the JSC was modeled, has been validated as highly effective and the WSJCA as moderately predictive.[5,21]

[e]Note: the NCAR, (North Carolina), OYAS (Ohio), and WSJCA (Washington State) were not included in the previous study but have since been validated and are widely used.

[f]Note: The statistical metric used to measure effect size in the previous YASI studies was the "area under the curve" (AUC) measurements. Theoretically, AUCs can range from 0 to 1. 00, with 0.50 signaling chance level accuracy. According to Rice Harris criteria,[42] 0.56–0.63 correspond to small effect sizes, 0.64 and 0.70 to medium effect sizes, and 0.71 and above to large effect sizes. The 2016 company study noted earlier found an AUC of 0.79 for the YASIs reoffense predictive ability.

Despite YASI being less than ideal and despite being validated *only* by company studies, YASI is currently one of the most widely used risk assessment tools—used in over 70 juvenile justice agencies in the United States.[52] The reasons for this are unclear, possibly due to lack of an ideal alternative, possibly due to YASI's incorporation of strength-based items and attempts at "factor weighting" or possibly due to the company's marketing and ongoing research and teacher training efforts.[g]

The JSC, another widely used risk assessment tool in the court system, is a composite survey amalgamated from the strongest, most common risk factors found in 14 different well-validated actuarial risk instruments. The JSC was tested in Florida and Georgia, where it was proven to be more effective than the risk tools in use at the time in both states.[5] The tool has been validated in different demographic and geographic regions, has been adopted by the National Council of Juvenile and Family Court Judges, and is now used by more than a dozen jurisdictions across the United States.[56] It consists of just 10 items—four static factors and six dynamic factors: age at first encounter with the courts, number of times referred to juvenile court, number of referrals for violent offenses, number of out-of-home placements, school discipline or attendance issues, substance abuse, peer relationships, prior abuse or neglect, parenteral supervision, and parent or sibling criminality. It is said to be available in the public domain; however, despite our best efforts (including contacting Solano County by phone), we could not procure a copy of the instrument.[h]

### Limitations of Risk Assessment Tools

Finally, it should be emphasized that risk assessment tools are far from perfect. Two things are important to keep in mind. First, many jurisdictions use combined risk/needs assessment tools which, for reasons stated earlier, limit predictive accuracy; second, even with the most effective risk assessment tools, 20% of low-risk individuals, 40% of moderate-risk individuals, and "only" 60% of high-risk individuals will reoffend in the following year.[5] The search for more accurate assessment tools and a more comprehensive understanding of these tools is ongoing.

## SPECIAL ASSESSMENTS

There are also several "special assessments" done by most jurisdictions that deserve mention. Such special screenings are usually done after the initial risk assessment when more time is available and an offending juvenile's needs are more fully known. These special screenings include violence and SVCs screening, ACEs screening, sexual screening, mental health screening, intellectual disabilities screening, suicide screening, and substance abuse screening.

Each of these will be discussed in depth in their respective chapters in this publication as they impact adolescent health. If the reader wishes a full-text document evaluating each of these special assessment screenings with reference to juvenile delinquency, please contact the author of this chapter.

## PART II—THE NEEDS ASSESSMENT

Once offending youth are stratified into low, moderate, or high-risk categories by the risk assessment, those falling in the moderate- or high-risk groups should then receive a more extensive needs assessment. This assessment more closely examines the individual, family, peer, school, and community deficits that interfere with youth functioning and contribute to recidivism. Dynamic factors (those amenable to change) receive special attention here, as these factors will be the focus of an individual's "matched" intervention program (see later). In addition, at this stage, a more in-depth look at special screenings is often undertaken (e.g., mental health, suicide, violence risk, substance abuse, sexual screening), with highlighted needs being taken into consideration when formulating individualized intervention/redirection programs.[47] As the needs assessment requires greater insight and is more comprehensive, it is ideally administrated by more highly trained workers who are more qualified to make placement/intervention decisions.

There are several problems with the current needs assessment tools in use today. Many tools are not validated by rigorous research. Others take excessive time to administer or are administered by poorly trained staff. Howell, Lipsey, and Wilson, in their *Juvenile Justice Handbook,* recommend that staff workers be trained to

[g]Note: The YASI training consists of 2 days of staff training in how to administer and score the tool followed a few months later by 2 days of training in how to incorporate scores into intervention programs. It is unknown/unstudied as to how effective test administrators are able to adhere to the proper implementation of administration and scoring methods in the "real world."

[h]Note: I could find no PDF of the JSC tool on line. When I contacted Solano County in California, where the tool was initially developed, I was told that they used the YLS/CMI—a suboptimal tool according to strict academic criteria.

do the initial risk assessment and, perhaps, a brief, superficial needs assessment, then leave the more in-depth needs assessment to trained specialists.[20] Still, other tools lack an "age appropriate interpretation" treating all offenders the same. There can also be confusion on a "systems level" when assessment tools are duplicated by various agencies (e.g., juvenile courts, child protective agencies) or by similar questions being asked on several different forms during the risk and needs assessment. Such a lack of coordination leaves parents and juveniles unsure of agency roles and suspicious of careless survey construction. To compound this lack of confidence in the system, agencies often fail to share information with each other creating even more confusion. Other administrative shortcomings exist. Many jurisdictions, in the interest of time and cost, use a combination risk/needs assessment tool. This is a suboptimal practice as discussed earlier, with insufficient time devoted for a quality needs assessment to be generated.[i] Another common flaw is that many facilities do not *repeat* the needs assessment during a youth's interaction with the JJS, thus resulting in suboptimal evaluation of youth progress and intervention program effectiveness.

The lack of clarity on exactly how to process information from the needs assessment has led to confusion and inconsistency across the JJS. In fact, studies have documented problems in survey use and interpretation, noting that only *one-half* of court professionals use tools consistently in their decision making.[45] Instead, without clear, evidence-based guidelines, many assessors will alter their risk and needs scoring to fit their subjective judgments.[32]

Although the above-mentioned problems with needs assessment tools are significant, the most glaring hurdle facing the needs assessment is this: the information gleaned from needs assessments have not yet proven to be useful in directing intervention programs! Research in this area is critically lacking and due to this deficit, intervention programs are often forced to integrate "assessed needs" into their programs without data substantiating the efficacy of *addressing* those needs. This is especially problematic because programs addressing *misidentified* needs or providing unsubstantiated methods of intervention will waste resources and can be potentially harmful.[15,29]

Despite all of these shortcomings, we can still offer some insights on what an optimal approach to adolescent needs might entail. For example, when conducting a needs assessment, professionals should not simply compile scores, but instead closely examine the factors involved. Offenders who are at high risk for violent reoffense should be screened to see the specific needs that are contributory—e.g., psychopathy, lack of control, an attitude that violence is an acceptable behavior, or perhaps that violence is a deliberate way to achieve goals. An optimal needs assessment tool for offenders who are at high risk for *property recidivism* should explore if the offense has arisen from financial reasons, alcohol/drug problems, lack of employable skills, impulsivity, or an attitude that stealing as an acceptable way to achieve goals. Similarly, for high-risk drug offenders, one must examine if they are merely selling for economic reasons, if they are addicted, if they use drugs as an escape due to lack of employable skills, etc.[32] All this to say that significant professional training and insight is needed at this level of youth–juvenile court interaction.

In sum, the main issue with the needs assessment tools is whether the data gained is at all useful in intervention planning. Without research showing that needs-based intervention will reduce recidivism, we cannot reliably say that the needs assessment has any practical value. Research in this area is, however, still in its infancy, and *if* factors derived from the needs assessment *do* turn out to be valid determinants of recidivism amenable to intervention, then it will make sense to address them in intervention programs.

## Common Needs Uncovered in the Needs Assessment

Some of the most commonly identified needs affecting juvenile recidivism are (predictably): problems with parental supervision, school attendance, family relationships, peer relationships, and substance abuse, each having a prevalence of over 30% in adjudicated youth.[24,26] Individual frustration management, poor response to consequences, leisure time influences, and gang involvement are other dynamic needs often uncovered that contribute to recidivism.

[i]Note: Combination Risk/Needs Tools. There are over 20 combination risk/needs assessment tools used across the United States, and all are tailored to state-specific demographics, geographies, and administrator preferences. When assessing the accuracy of the 20 tools to predict needs and recidivism, some are rated higher than others and, generally, those tools using an actuarial approach do better than those using a "structural professional judgment approach." This is different from results gained when a needs assessment is individually administered, in which case an SPJ assessment is currently favored (see previous discussion: SPJ assessments allow the scorer more leeway in assessment and interventions).[55]

### Common Needs Assessment Tools in Use

There are several needs assessment tools in use today, most being extensions of their briefer risk assessment counterparts. The YASI is one of the most widely used combination risk/needs assessment tools. It is now used in over 70 juvenile justice agencies in the United States and has been listed as one of seven promising instruments for predicting youth recidivism (as a *risk* assessment tool).[52] However, YASI's use as a risk assessment tool is quite different from its intent as a *needs* assessment tool. Stratifying youth into low, medium, or high risk of reoffense is quite different from discovering which needs, if addressed in intervention programs, would lead to lower recidivism rates and improved youth lives.

The latest research validates YASI[j] as an effective *risk* assessment tool but concludes that it is ***not*** useful as a needs assessment tool. (The only exception being substance abuse, which *is* assessed in YASI and *is* amenable to treatment in intervention programs.[46]) A serious YASI shortcoming is its inability to discern criminal cognition, attitudinal issues, and antisocial attitudes.[46] This is especially problematic because addressing cognition and attitudinal issues via CBT (see later) is one of the most effective and validated means of intervention affecting recidivism. Thus, unless we have a good means of assessing attitudinal needs and criminal cognition, one of our most effective tools of intervention (CBT) is essentially sidelined. The previous study concludes, "We found little evidence that CA-YASI domain scores labeled as Violence-Aggression, Social-Cognitive Skills, Social Influences, Education/Employment, and Family, specifically translate to treatment-relevant target constructs of anger/hostility, executive function deficits, antisocial peer influence, poor school/work motivation, or problematic parental discipline and monitoring, respectively."

Five other commonly used needs assessment tools deserve mention.

1. The Ohio Youth Assessment Survey (OYAS) is a set of five risk/needs assessments utilized at various stages of contact with the JJS.
2. The Washington State Juvenile Court Assessment (WSJCA) is a combination risk and needs assessment—the risk tool simply being a shortened version of the needs tool. The risk assessment consists of a 27-item "prescreen," while the needs assessment is a full in-depth version of the tool—eight domains/56 primary questions. The WSJCA has been adapted by several states and is claimed to be user friendly.
3. The Positive Achievement Change Tool (PACT), modified from the WSJCA, is a prescreen *risk* assessment tool that has also been validated as a *needs* assessment tool. This 46-item survey has been found useful in assessing the needs of SVC offenders.
4. The Model Youth and Family Assessment of Needs and Strengths stratifies youth into low-, medium-, and high-risk "needs groups" to (theoretically) focus intervention efforts toward the lacking realms.[20]
5. The Child and Adolescent Needs and Strengths (CANS)[k] is another widely used needs assessment tool. It evaluates child behavior and living conditions, assessing the needs and strengths of offending juveniles with queries concerning criminal history, mental health disorders, developmental disabilities, emotional needs, behavioral needs, and family issues.[7] One study found that the top CANS predictors of elevated need were individual frustration management problems and poor response to consequences, family and home issues, school and community factors, and negative peer and leisure time influences. What was surprising was that the study also documented that lack of hope and optimism were significant risk factors for recidivism—a deficit that is, heartbreakingly, all too common among our youth.[7]

## PART III—INTERVENTION PROGRAMS

Although the literature often highlights "collaborative intervention" as the optimal approach to decreasing violent and nonviolent recidivism, no *specific* program has yet been identified as superior.

**In general,** as mentioned, the most effective programs—the ones that made the greatest strides in

[j]Note: It should also be noted in regards to the YASI that administration of the 12-category, 100-item survey takes 2. 5 h and, even in the best circumstances, has been found to be properly administrated and scored by only 60% of trained case workers.[46]

[k]Note: CANS is scored on a 0–3 scale: 0–1 no need for remedial action/watchful waiting; 2 = remedial action is necessary; 3 = immediate/intensive remedial action needed. For rating children's strengths: a score of 0 or 1 = child has a useful strength that can be used as in a strength-based plan; 2 = child has strength but needs strength building efforts; 3 = efforts are needed to identify potential strengths. Each item scored two or three requires intervention.

reducing recidivism—were those that focused on high-risk individuals as stratified in the risk assessment. Second, programs that had a "therapeutic" rather than "disciplinary" philosophy were clearly more effective. (Interestingly, discipline and deterrence programs, such as boot camps and scared straight programs, actually *increased* recidivism.) Third, while some brand name/proprietary programs were effective, they were not necessarily better at reducing recidivism than other generic/nonbrand-name programs. "Indeed some generic programs were more effective than proprietary programs".[20] Thus, when a PCP recommends a "best practices program," they should look at laudable programs of both types.[25] Finally, cognitive behavioral therapy (CBT), especially CBT that includes anger management, conflict resolution, and interpersonal relationship problem solving, has been documented as effective and impacting.[13] Programs incorporating CBT have noted a 25%–50% reduction in recidivism, with no specific CBT program found more effective than another.

Other general recommendations are that intervention programs should target dynamic needs (i.e., factors that are amenable to change), such as peer associations or school performance,[2,1] that intervention be "aimed at different points along the life course," be age-appropriate, and be matched to individual needs.[20]

### Which *Types* of Intervention Programs Are Most Effective and How Effective Are They?

The 2010 Lipsey meta-analysis of intervention programs[28] found an *overall* reduction in recidivism of only 6% when looking at *all* programs across the board—surveillance programs (probation), skill building programs, counseling programs, and mixed/combined programs. However, more significant reductions were found when looking at the individual *types* of programs. Counseling programs, for example, were found to be the most effective type of program with an overall reduction in recidivism of 13%. This was followed by skill building and mixed programs with a 12% reduction, and surveillance programs (probation) with a 6% reduction.[l]

Although the earlier reductions in recidivism may seem fairly insignificant, taking a closer look at program subtypes reveals that more substantial reductions in recidivism are possible. For example, the specific subtypes of counseling interventions found to be most effective were in descending order: (1) group counseling (22% reduction in recidivism); (2) mentoring[m] (21% reduction); (3) mixed programs (16% reduction); and (4) family counseling/therapy (13% reduction). Interestingly, individual counseling was found to reduce recidivism by only 5%—results similar to surveillance alone.

Taking a closer look at skill-building program subtypes, those that emphasized cognitive-behavioral approaches (altering outlook to affect behavior) were most effective with a 26% reduction in recidivism, followed by strictly behavioral programs, with a 22% reduction, social skill building programs (13%), and academic and job skill building programs (5%–10%).

The details of Individual CBT, Group CBT, Family Therapy, Youth Asset Building Intervention based on the 40 Developmental Assets or 5 Promises, Mentoring, and other specific programs are beyond the scope of this chapter. What we have hoped to accomplish in this section is a general overview of intervention, so that after risk factors have been uncovered in screening (and confirmed by a more in-depth interview) the PCP will be better equipped to help in recommending effective intervention.[n]

### Looking Ahead—Monitoring Individuals in Intervention Programs. Moving Beyond the Crude Metric of Recidivism

Individuals who have completed intervention programs might be monitored for the early indicators listed later. Such monitoring may help caseworkers/psychologists to intervene before reoffense can occur and may help

[l]Note: All reductions in recidivism percentages noted in this review are reductions from the national baseline of the 50% seen in "untreated" juveniles. A 20% reduction in recidivism quoted here means a 20% reduction from the baseline, or a recidivism rate of 40% with intervention as opposed to 50% recidivism without intervention.

[m]Note: Generally, mentoring has been found to be of questionable value. A 2011 meta-analysis of 55 studies of community-based mentoring programs[11] found mentoring to have only modest benefits in terms of risky behavior, social competence, and academic and career outcomes. However, despite this relative ineffectiveness of mentoring in the general community, for our purposes (preventing recidivism in *at-risk youth*), there *is* a significant benefit from this type of intervention. As stated earlier, mentoring programs for at-risk youth can reduce recidivism by up to 21%.

[n]Note: When evaluating the effectiveness of intervention programs, follow-up periods ranged from 1 year[27] to 18 months[54] to over 4 years.[18] Obviously, the longer the follow-up, the more validated a program would be.

predict whether or not a youth is beginning along an early positive or negative pathway. Obviously, this has an important health implication for the PCP with adolescent patients in these circumstances. It is important to remember that these "early indicators" are not yet validated by research, but instead are opinion, albeit informed opinion.

- Self-reported factors that might be monitored: self-esteem, purpose, future orientation, time spent with "positive" peers, time with gangs/"negative" peers, time spent with positive adults, family stability (e.g., excessive moving, excess stressors), family adult/adolescent relationships, support outside of the family (e.g., work, school, community), school satisfaction, time spent learning, use of leisure time, amount of parenteral supervision, substance abuse, self-harm, and risk-taking behavior (i.e., Eysenck's Risk-Taking Scale).
- Observed behaviors that might be monitored (by parents, teachers, coaches, guardians, etc.): aggressive episodes, disruptive behaviors, school attendance/performance, amount of parenteral supervision, improved communication, more engaged versus more withdrawn.
- Juvenile–facilitator relationship quality during intervention should be monitored. Our years of experience in the field believe the youth–facilitator relationship is vital to positive youth outcomes. This is not being monitored in any programs that we encountered in our literature review. It might be monitored and perhaps quantified by a simple participant survey.
- Community factors that might be screened: any positive or negative community developments that may have occurred after intervention.

## PART IV—AN OVERVIEW OF *PREVENTION* PROGRAMS

Although the focus of this review is on risk assessment with the intent that PCPs should be aware that such risk factors play a role in not only criminality but also mental and physical health, the PCP should also be aware that general prevention programs exist—programs for all adolescents not just those risk of criminality. General prevention programs focused on violence, substance abuse, and ACE prevention exist and are successful to varying degrees. This is mentioned here only to provide the PCP an open door to investigate such programs should they have an interest in entering into a broader, policy-focused conversation.

## REFERENCES


1. Andrews DA, Bonta J, Wormith JS. The risk-need-responsivity (RNR) model: does adding the good live model contribute to effective crime prevention? *Crim Justice Behav*. 2011;38:735–755.
2. Andrews DA, Bonta J. Rehabilitating criminal justice policy and practice. *Psychol Public Policy Law*. 2010;16:39–55.
3. Andrews DA, Zinger I, Hoge RD, et al. Does correctional treatment work? A clinically relevant and psychologically informed meta-analysis. *Criminology*. 1990;28:369–404.
4. Avviati M, Azzola A, Palix J, et al. Validity and predictive accuracy of the structured assessment of protective factors for violence risk in criminal forensic evaluations: a Swiss cross-validation retrospective study. *Crim Justice Behav*. 2017;44:493–510.
5. Baird C, Healy T, Johnson K, et al. *Comparison of Risk Assessment Instruments in Juvenile Justice. Grant 2010-JR FX-0021 from the Office of Juvenile Justice and Delinquency Prevention, Office of Justice Programs*. US Department of Justice; August 2013.
6. Bernard B. *Fostering Resiliency in Kids: Protective Factors in the Family, School, and Community*. Portland, OR: Northwest Regional Educational Laboratory, Western Regional Center for Drug-Free Schools and Communities, Far West Laboratory; 1991.
7. Cordell KD, Snowden LR, Hosier L. Patterns and priorities of service need identified through the Child and Adolescent Needs and Strengths (CANS) assessment. *Child Youth Serv Rev*. 2016;60:129–135.
8. Cottle C, Lee R, Heilbrun K. The prediction of criminal recidivism in juveniles: a meta-analysis. *Crim Justice Behav*. 2001;28:367–394.
9. Dowden C, Andrews DA. Effective correctional treatment and violent reoffending: a meta-analysis. *Can J Criminol*. 2000;42:449–467.
10. Dowden C, Andrews DA. What works for female offenders: a meta-analytic review. *Crime Del*. 1999;45:438–452.
11. DuBois DL, Holloway BE, Valentine JC, et al. Effectiveness of mentoring programs for youth: a meta-analytic review. *Am J Commun Psychol*. 2002;30:157–197.
12. Emeka TQ, Sorensen JR. Female juvenile risk: is there a need for gendered assessment instruments? *Youth Violence Juv Justice*. 2009;7:313–330.
13. Garrard WM, Lipsey MW. Conflict resolution education and antisocial behavior in U.S. schools: a meta-analysis. *Confl Res Q*. 2007;25:9–38.
14. Garydon KS. *Protective Factors and Recidivism in Latino Juvenile Offenders*. University of California, Santa Barbara: ProQuest Dissertations Publishing; 2007.
15. Gatti U, Tremblay RE, Vitaro F. Iatrogenic effect of juvenile justice. *J Child Psychol Psychiatry*. 2009;50:991–998.
16. Gendreau P, Smith P, French SA. The theory of effective correctional intervention: empirical status and future directions. In: Cullen FT, Wright JP, Blevins KR, eds. *Taking Stock: The Status of Criminological Theory*. Vol. 15. Advances in Criminological Theory. New Brunswick, NJ: Transaction Publishing; 2006:419–446.

17. Gerard J, Beuhler C. Cumulative environmental risk and youth maladjustment: the role of youth attributes. *Child Dev*. 2004;75:1832–1849.
18. Gordon DA, Arbuthnot J, Gustafson KE, et al. Home-based behavioral-systems family therapy with disadvantaged juvenile delinquents. *Am J Fam Ther*. 1998;16:243–255.
19. Green AE, Gesten EL, Greenwald MA, et al. Predicting delinquency in adolescence and young adulthood: a longitudinal analysis of early risk factors. *Youth Violence Juv Justice*. 2008;6:323–342.
20. Howell JC, Lipsey MW, Wilson JJ. *A Handbook for Evidence-Based Juvenile Justice Systems*. NY: Lexington; 2014.
21. Howell JC, Lipsey MW, Wilson JJ. *A Handbook of Evidence-Based Juvenile Justice Systems*. Lanham, MD: Lexington Books; 2004.
22. Huizinga D, Loeber R, Thornberry TP, et al. *Co-occurrence of Delinquency and Other Problem Behaviors, Juvenile Justice Bulletin, Office of Juvenile Justice and Delinquency Prevention*. Washington, DC: U.S. Department of Justice; November 2000.
23. Jones NJ, Brown SL, Robinson D, et al. Validity of the youth assessment and screening instrument: a juvenile justice tool incorporating risks, needs, and strengths. *Law Hum Behav*. 2016;40:182–194.
24. Kelly WR, Macy TS, Mears DP. Juvenile referrals in Texas: an assessment of criminogenic needs and the gap between needs and services. *Prison J*. 2005;85:467–489.
25. Landenberger NA, Lipsey MW. The positive effects of cognitive-behavioral programs for offenders: a meta-analysis of factors associated with effective treatment. *J Exp Criminol*. 2005;1:451–476.
26. Lassiter W, Clarkson S, Howell MQ. *North Carolina Department of Juvenile Justice and Delinquency Prevention Annual Report*. Raleigh, NC: North Carolina Department of Juvenile Justice and Delinquency Prevention; 2008.
27. Lattimore PK, Krebs CP, Graham P, et al. *Evaluation of the Juvenile Breaking the Cycle Program*. Research Triangle Park, North Carolina: RTI International; 2004.
28. Lipsey MW, Howell JC, Kelley MR, et al. *Improving the Effectiveness of Juvenile Justice Programs: A New Perspective on Evidence-Based Practice*. Washington: Center for Juvenile Justice Reform, Georgetown Public Policy Institute, Georgetown University; 2010.
29. Lipsey MW. The primary factors that characterize effective interventions with juvenile offenders: a meta-analytic overview. *Victims Offenders*. 2009;4:124–147.
30. Loeber R, Slot W, Stouthamer-Loeber M. A cumulative developmental model of risk and promotive factors. In: Loeber R, Koot HM, Slot NW, et al., eds. *Tomorrow's Criminals: The Development of Child Delinquency and Effective Interventions*. Hampshire, England: Ashgate Publishing Ltd.; 2008a:133–161.
31. Loeber R, Slot W, Stouthamer-Loeber M. A cumulative developmental model of risk and promotive factors. In: Loeber R, Koot HM, Slott NW, Van der Laan PH, Hoeve M, eds. *Tomorrow's Criminals: The Development of Child Delinquency and Effective Interventions*. Hampshire, England: Ashgate; 2008b:3–17.
32. Miller M. Practitioner compliance with risk/needs assessment tools: a theoretical and empirical assessment. *Crim Justice Behav*. 2013;40:716–736.
33. Moffitt TE. Adolescent-limited and life-course-persistent antisocial behavior: a developmental taxonomy. *Psychol Rev*. 1993;100:674–701.
34. Morrison G, Robertson L, Laurie B, et al. Protective factors related to antisocial behavior trajectories. *J Clin Psychol*. 2002;58:277–290.
35. Mulder E, Brand E, Bullens R, et al. A classification of risk factors in serious juvenile offenders and the relation between patterns of risk factors and recidivism. *Crim Behav Mental Health*. 2010;20:23–38.
36. Mullis RL, Cornille TA, Mullis AK, et al. Female juvenile offending: a review of characteristics and contexts. *J Child Fam Stud*. 2004;13:205–218.
37. National Research Council. Reforming juvenile justice: a developmental approach. In: Bonnie RJ, Johnson RL, Chemers BM, et al., eds. *The Committee on Assessing Juvenile Justice Reform*. Washington, DC: The National Academies Press; 2013.
38. Orbis Partners. *Long-term Validation of the Youth Assessment and Screening Instrument (YASI) in New York State Juvenile Probation*; 2007. Available at: http://www.criminaljustice.ny.gov/opca/pdfs/YASI-Long-Term-Validation-Report.pdf.
39. Orbis Partners. *YASI: Brief Report*. 2007. Unpublished manuscript. Ottawa, Ontario, Canada.
40. Prinzie P, Hoeve M, Stams GJJM. Family processes, parent and child personality characteristics. In: Loeber R, Koot HM, Slot NW, et al., eds. *Tomorrow's Criminals: The Development of Child Delinquency and Effective Interventions*. Hampshire, England: Ashgate Publishing Ltd.; 2008: 91–102.
41. Reingle JM, Jennings WG, Maldonado-Molina MM. Risk and protective factors for trajectories of violent delinquency among a nationally representative sample of early adolescents. *Youth Violence Juv Justice*. 2012;10:261–277.
42. Rice ME, Harris GT. Comparing effect sizes in follow-up studies: ROC Area, Cohen's D, and R. *Law Hum Behav*. 2005;29:615–620.
43. Ryan JP, Williams AB, Courtney ME. Adolescent neglect, juvenile delinquency and the risk of recidivism. *J Youth Adolesc*. 2013;42:454–465.
44. Shepherd SM, Luebbers S, Ogloff JRP. The role of protective factors and the relationship with recidivism for high-risk young people in detention. *Crim Justice Behav*. 2016; 43:863–878.
45. Shook S. Structured decision making in juvenile justice Judges and prbation officers perceptions and use. *Children Youth Serv Rev*. 2007;29:1335–1351.
46. Skeem JL, Kennealy PJ. How well do juvenile risk assessments measure factors to target in treatment? Examining construct validity. *Psychol Assess*. 2017;29: 679–691

47. Soulier M, McBride A. Mental health screening and assessment of detained youth Matthew. *Child Adolesc Psychiatric Clin N Am*. 2016;25:27−39.
48. Stouthamer-Loeber M, Loeber R, Wei E, et al. Risk and promotive effects in the explanation of persistent serious delinquency in boys. *J Consult Clin Psychol*. 2002;70:111−123.
49. van der Put CE, Asscher JJ, Stams GJ, Moonen XM, et al. Differences between juvenile offenders with and without intellectual disabilities in the importance of static and dynamic risk factors for recidivism. *J Intellect Disabil Res*. 2014;58:992−1003.
50. van der Put CE, Stams GJJM, Hoeve M, et al. Changes in the relative importance of dynamic risk factors for recidivism during adolescence. *Int J Offender Ther Comp Criminol*. 2012;56:296−316.
51. van der Put CE. Female adolescent sexual and nonsexual violent offenders: a comparison of the prevalence and impact of risk and protective factors for general recidivism. *BMC Psychiatry*. 2015;15:236.
52. Vincent GM. *Application and Implementation of Risk Assessment in Juvenile Justice for the Courts*. National Courts and Science Institute; 2015. Available at: http://www.macoe.org/sites/macoe.org/files/Vincent_2015.pdf.
53. Vincent GM, Guy LS, Grisso T. *Risk Assessment in Juvenile Justice: A Guidebook for Implementation*. New York, NY: Models for Change; 2012.
54. Washington State Institute for Public Policy. *Outcome Evaluation of Washington State's Research-Based Programs for Juvenile Offenders*. Olympia, Wash: Washington State Institute for Public Policy; 2004.
55. Watcher A. *Statewide Risk Assessment in Juvenile Probation. JJGPS StateScan*. Pittsburgh, PA: National Center for Juvenile Justice; 2014.
56. Wiebush R, ed. *Graduated Sanctions for Juvenile Offenders: A Program Model and Planning Guide*. Reno, NV: Juvenile Sanctions Center, National Council of Juvenile and Family Court Judges; 2002.
57. Gendreau P. The principles of effective intervention with offenders. In: Harland T, ed. *Choosing Correctional Interventions That Work: Defining the Demand and Evaluating the Supply*. Newbury Park, CA: Sage; 1996:117−130.
58. Lipsey MW, Howell JC, Kelley MR, et al. *Improving the Effectiveness of Juvenile Justice Programs: A New Perspective on Evidence-Based Practice*. Washington: Center for Juvenile Justice Reform, Georgetown Public Policy Institute, Georgetown University; 2010.
59. Mihalic SF. *Blueprints for Violence Prevention Report. Office of Justice Programs, Office of Juvenile Justice and Delinquency Prevention*. Washington, DC: U.S. Department of Justice; 2004.

CHAPTER 15

# Screening for Resilience in Adolescents

VINCENT MORELLI, MD

## INTRODUCTION

The harmful physical and psychologic effects of stress are well documented in the medical literature. From chronic low-level stress to posttraumatic stress disorder (PTSD), these burdens are responsible both for direct cardiovascular damage and for the cascading effects on sleep, leading to disordered eating, obesity, and endocrinal and metabolic abnormalities. Stress is a well-recognized slow killer with incalculable societal costs in terms of direct healthcare, absenteeism, occupational injury, risky behaviors, criminal activity, lost productivity, etc. How each of us handle stress is therefore critical to our individual health and longevity and to our society's health and productivity. With this in mind, our goal in this chapter is to help adolescents learn to "deal with" stress—to become resilient—so that they may go on to lead more healthy and productive adult lives and contribute to a healthy and productive society.

Much of the work on resilience comes from studying individuals who have experienced similar or shared traumatic events (e.g., war, rape, domestic violence, displacement, dangerous neighborhoods) and examining differences between the "resilient survivors" who have gone on to lead productive lives and their "traumatized and arrested" counterparts. For example, one study looked at 877 adolescents living in high-risk neighborhoods and examined those who had "adjusted well" i.e., those who had high academic performance, high esteem, high psychologic functioning, and low antisocial behavior. These adolescents were compared with their less-adjusted counterparts to determine what factors had contributed to their success.[1] Researchers believe that studying these "strong survivors" can provide an understanding of resilience. If the individual qualities and characteristics needed to bounce back from adversity can be identified, this knowledge can then be used to help strengthen the more vulnerable.

All of us will face stressful periods and traumatic events in our lifetimes[2]; after which, roughly 25%–50% of us will "naturally" bounce back and thrive, 5%–10% will develop PTSD, and the remainder will suffer lingering, low-grade but manageable effects.[3–10] Owing to the widespread prevalence of trauma and the suboptimal way in which many of us respond, understanding and improving resilience is important if we are to surmount these common events and go on to lead fully productive lives. On a broader scale, resilience is important for a fully engaged and optimized society.

## RESILIENCE FROM WHAT? ADVERSITY AND TRAUMA

When we speak of resilience, we refer to the ability to "quickly" overcome severe adverse conditions or traumatic[a] events—to quickly overcome the intense emotional experiences that ordinarily overwhelm a person's ability to cope. Resilience enables eventual thriving despite single traumatic events (rape, assault) or repetitive ongoing insults (child abuse, neglect, poverty, perceived discrimination).

As the prevalence of trauma is so widespread and the untoward health effects are so impacting (see later discussion and see chapter 7), the importance of resilience cannot be overstated. In the original Adverse Childhood Experiences (ACEs) study,[11] 50% of (mostly) white middle-class participants were found to have experienced at least one traumatic event and 6% had experienced four or more. Other studies have

[a]Adverse childhood experiences (ACEs) consist of five personal traumas, namely, physical abuse, sexual abuse, emotional abuse, physical neglect, and emotional neglect, as well as five household traumas, namely, mother treated violently, household substance abuse, household mental illness, parental separation or divorce, and incarcerated household member. Later studies added death of a parent, witness/victim of neighborhood violence, socioeconomic hardship, and perceived discrimination to the list of impacting ACEs, bringing the current total to 14.[30]

Adolescent Health Screening: An Update in the Age of Big Data. https://doi.org/10.1016/B978-0-323-66130-0.00015-6

noted that 25%–34% of the general US population and 75%–93% of juvenile offenders have experienced at least one ACE.[11–15]

The ubiquity of trauma has spawned a considerable increase in resilience research over the past two decades as funders have begun to appreciate the role of resilience in lifelong health and well-being.[16,17] Studies have highlighted the association of resilience with improved physical and mental health, including lower rates of conduct and behavior issues and lower rates of depression and anxiety. Conversely, lack of resilience has been associated with unsafe sex, poor educational performance, crime, substandard job productivity, and an increased likelihood of poverty.[18–20] Research has also shown that resilience will lead to higher incomes, improved relationships, and more fulfilled lives.[21–27]

Also emphasizing the importance of resilience is the idea that just as the effects of trauma and stress can be passed on to subsequent generations through epigenetic changes and alterations in gene expression, so too (it is believed) can the salutary effects of resilience.[28] These are powerful concepts with incumbent responsibilities on families, communities, and societies. If parents (or societies) can learn to be more resilient, it is possible that they will pass on these epigenetic benefits to their children.

## TRAUMA, ADVERSE CHILDHOOD EXPERIENCES, AND INDIVIDUAL HEALTH

There are several early studies associating childhood trauma with untoward *adult* health outcomes. One of the earliest, the 1964 Isle of Wight study, noted that subjects with low social status, family discord, or stressful early life events had a higher incidence of psychiatric issues (e.g., depression, anxiety).[29] (The term "ACE" had not yet been coined.)

Since then, the links between childhood trauma and untoward adult health effects have been clearly established. The 1998 seminal ACEs study[11] examined 10 traumatic childhood events occurring before age 18 years and monitored the adult health effects up to 50 years later. The study noted that those with 4 or more ACEs had up to a 12 times greater risk of alcoholism, drug abuse, depression, suicide, sexually transmitted diseases, heart disease, liver disease, lung disease, fractures, or cancer. In each of these categories, a graded response was noted with each additional ACE conveying an incrementally greater risk.

Other studies have documented ACEs to be associated with increased risky behaviors, increased substance abuse, higher juvenile offending, lowered socioeconomic achievement, increased obesity, anorexia, increased sleep disturbances, lower self-esteem, and increased psychiatric disorders ranging from depression and anxiety to behavior disorders and PTSD.[11,31,32] An important finding in these studies is that ACEs exhibit a "dose-dependent response," with each additional ACE leading to successively worsening physical and mental health outcomes.[6] For example, each additional ACE in juvenile offenders leads to a harrowing 35% increased risk of recidivism (this will be further discussed later).

## HOW URGENT IS RESILIENCE?

The urgency of addressing childhood adversity lies in looking at the outcomes of ACEs. For example, depression, with causative contributions from ACEs,[33] shaves off an estimated 28.9 years of quality-adjusted life-years (QALYs). This astounding statistic—over twice the QALYs lost through stroke, heart disease, or diabetes[34] highlights the need to manage adversity and enhance resilience.

Other equally distressing examples of the urgent need to address ACEs and promote resilience can be found in studies of juvenile offenders. One such study (mentioned earlier) of 22,575 delinquent youths in Florida[35] found that each additional ACE increased the risk of becoming a violent, chronic offender by an astounding 35%. It is thought that addressing ACEs and enhancing resilience in such youths may improve this devastating downward trajectory.

The urgency to enhance resilience is especially significant in high-risk occupations such as soldiers and rescue workers,[36,37] in whom extreme or ongoing exposure to trauma can lead to PTSD in up to 30% and to markedly higher suicide rates.[38,39]

These are mind-boggling associations with significant economic costs,[40,41] crushing human costs, and pressing "big picture" policy implications. Clearly, addressing trauma and enhancing resilience is an urgent national and worldwide challenge.

With this brief introduction, this chapter will (1) first formally define and discuss the research perspectives on resilience; (2) discuss the factors contributing to *individual* resilience, from genetics and neurobiology to cognitive skills and character traits; (3) discuss the *environmental* factors affecting resilience on a broader scale, i.e., the family and community influences as well as the environment created by national policy; (4) review the screening tools used to assess resilience in individuals; and (5) examine the makeup and effectiveness of resilience enhancement programs that attempt to build resilience in vulnerable individuals. Emphasis is placed on child and adolescent resilience literature because it is here that intervention can set in motion lifelong habits and coping abilities.

## DEFINITIONS AND RESEARCH PERSPECTIVES

### Definition

Resilience is a process rather than a trait. A consensus statement defined resilience as "the process of negotiating, managing, and adapting to significant stress or trauma"—the ability to adapt and thrive despite adversity.[42,43]

Generally, after encountering a stressful event, a person responds in one of the following four ways:

1. the event causes maladaptive, self-destructive behavior;
2. the situation allows for recovery, but with a lingering sense of loss;
3. the event forces a return to baseline, in an effort to "just get past it";
4. the person sees the event as an opportunity for growth.

The more resilient people are, the more likely they are to overcome stress *quickly*, and the more likely they are to view adversity as an occasion for growth—to embrace the situation and take advantage of the opportunities and insights afforded.

### Research Perspectives on Resilience

Researchers have noted that in some, adversity is actually a good thing, encouraging resilience by motivating individuals to seek social support, focus on goal achievement, and inculcate planning behaviors and active coping, which are all important in overcoming future trauma.[9] This is what we will explore in the following sections, i.e., the factors that make 25%50% of us resilient, whereas the rest of us will have difficulty overcoming our experiences and go on to suffer the health, mental health, cognitive, and behavioral consequences. We want to know what makes the resilient, resilient, so that we can attempt to foster the quality in those of us who are more vulnerable.

We will examine resilience from two perspectives. First, from an "individualist" viewpoint and then from a more encompassing environmental or "interactionist" perspective. From the individualist point of view, we will examine the characteristics an individual must possess in order to bounce back from adversity. This view is focused on unearthing and examining the character traits found in resilient individuals in order to foster such characteristics in the less resilient.

From the interactionist point of view, we will take a broader look at resilience—resilience as a dynamic phenomenon evolving with brain development, influenced by character traits and maturing cognitive skills, and dependent on the support of family and that of the wider community. The interactionist viewpoint takes cultural influence, past stress, and life experiences into consideration.[44–47] It also accounts for how resilience may change over time, with periods of acquisition, maintenance, reduction, and loss.[48–50]

From this interactionist viewpoint, we will look at how the overall environment promotes or retards resilience and how family, friends, communities, and societies all contribute. In future works, we will look at why some cultures and countries foster more resilient citizens than others. What aspects of these cultures and countries facilitate this quality? We will look at how the crafting of rules, i.e., policies formed by governments, groups, teams, communities, and corporations, affects the environment to either foster or impede resilience.

## THE INDIVIDUALIST VIEW: INDIVIDUAL TRAITS THAT CONVEY RESILIENCE

At the neurologic level, resilience requires that the cortical areas of the brain be appropriately developed in order to oversee and control a person's "lower limbic, primitive" brain (the area that urges reflexive, automatic, and often disadvantageous response to stress). The cortex exerts its control over the lower brain by developing neural networks that cultivate a set of cognitive skills called executive function (EF). EF skills include planning; decision-making; impulse control; the ability to reframe experiences,[51] focus attention, regulate stress,[52] and exercise restraint[53–55]; and the ability to reason and solve problems. Thus when a person's cortical areas are properly formed and functioning, adequate oversight of lower brain impulses is afforded, proper development of EF will occur, and resilience will be maximized.[52,56–60] Research clearly shows that individuals possessing more developed cortical pathways and stronger EF will have greater resilience.[60–63]

Many factors including sleep, stress, diet, and exercise have been noted to influence cortical networks and EF development. For example, exercise has been proven to enhance brain structure (neurogenesis) and the volume of cortical areas controlling memory processing speed, inhibitory control, and EF, which are all areas critical to resilience.[64–73] One article examining brain plasticity[66] concluded, "the understanding of how exercise promotes long-term cognitive effects is crucial for directing the power of exercise to reduce the burden of neurological and psychiatric disorders." A powerful endorsement of exercise as an underappreciated catholicon. [b]

With this brief overview of the neurologic and cognitive basis for resilience, we must now consider how a person's unique temperament and personality play into creating the characteristics of resilience. Although the terms temperament and personality are sometimes used interchangeably, temperament refers to one's innate, biologically based state (e.g., high-strung, anxious, mellow), whereas personality is formed as an individual's temperament reacts with his or her environment. Temperament, then, is more of a fixed foundation for the more malleable and evolving personality.[74] All this to say that both a person's innate temperament and evolving personality will account for some of the observed individual differences in resilience.

Now, on to the characteristics found in resilient individuals. As stated, much of data on the characteristics of resilience comes from studies of individuals exposed to adverse conditions such as war, poverty, neglect, abuse, etc. Studies of combat veterans, for example, have shown that altruism and the ability to bond socially, reframe experiences (reconsolidate memories),[75–77] and act effectively in the face of fear are all qualities possessed by resilient soldiers.[78] Findings from other studies have illuminated several other characteristics/traits that promote resilience and mental health in youths and adults. These factors include physical health[79,80]; social competence (i.e., one's ability to possess and maintain good relationships with peers, love interests, family members) and social support[81]; optimism, positivity,[c] and the ability to elicit positive responses from others[10]; adaptability, self-esteem, self-confidence, self-efficacy (belief that one can accomplish goals)[82]; future orientation[83]; school/work/community connectedness[84]; engagement in activities outside the home[6]; spiritual beliefs and practices[85,86]; a sense of purpose and the ability to forgive[87]; creativity[88]; achievement motivation, insight and skills that lead to an efficient use of abilities, and the belief that one controls the events in one's life[89]; college education[9]; humor and the ability to learn from adverse events[78,90,91]; determination, flexibility, active coping styles, problem-solving skills[92–95]; hardiness; and other grouped characteristics.[d] Other characteristics of resiliency noted from different cultural perspectives include having a sense of "Atman" (true self); a sense of "kokoro" (heart), also known as the indomitable fighting spirit; having a totem (an animal spirit that lives inside), and being able to cultivate Chi or internal energy.[94,96–98]

Two studies[99–101] have documented the association of these resilience characteristics with mental health outcomes in traumatized individuals in the real world. Both studies noted that despite significant trauma (e.g., sexual/physical abuse, low education, low employment, low salary), individuals with more resilience characteristics/traits experienced fewer depressive episodes or other mental health issues. It must be remembered, however, that this association is *not* the same as documenting that training programs built around cultivating these characteristics will be effective. (We will discuss this further in the later sections.)

This simple grouping of attributes is useful because hardiness encompasses characteristics possessed by the individual, while resilience can entail a broader concept incorporating environmental protective factors such as family and community support. Other groupings of characteristics can be seen in some of the resiliency screening tools. For example, the Resiliency Scale for Children and Adolescents (RSCA) groups characteristics into (1) sense of mastery (belief in one's abilities, optimism, and adaptability), (2) sense of relatedness (trust,

[b]Perhaps even more interesting is that exercise has been shown to produce epigenetic changes (e.g., DNA methylation, histone modification, micro-RNAs). Such changes can alter gene expression and may be passed down to future generations. It is amazing to think that a parent's exercise habits might affect a child's mental abilities, executive function capacity, and resilience.

[c]Positivity refers to the way one views life—the lens through which one views reality.[101,102] It makes one to see events as predictable and generally occurring in one's best interest. It is felt to be the key factor in adjusting to life stressors.[103] This "positive outlook trait" has been proven to be associated with health, quality of friendships, and, important from our point of view, ego-resiliency—the flexible and resourceful adaptation to changing environmental and internal dysphonic states.[102,104]

[d]An additional note that might help the reader who wishes to study resilience further. While each of the abovementioned individual characteristics and skills are associated with and, important for, enhancing resilience, some researchers have found that grouping these traits also leads to helpful insights. One such grouping of traits is referred to as "hardiness," and it is composed of three components: (1) a belief that one can *control* or influence the events of their experience, (2) a *commitment* to the activities of their lives (achievement motivation mentioned earlier), and (3) an ability to see *change* as an exciting challenge.[105]

perceived social support, comfort, and tolerance), and (3) emotional reactivity (a person's vulnerability—his or her sensitivity, recovery potential, and impairment). Those scoring highly in self-mastery and relatedness have proven to exhibit greater resilience in the face of stressful events.

Thus athough receiving limited study to date, it may be that such groupings/combinations of factors will add to the understanding of resilience. A final grouping example, a study by Lenzi et al.[106] found that having four protective factors (e.g., social support, optimism, self-efficacy, emotional regulation) allowed one to reach a "protective tipping point" and avoid school victimization. More research into combinations and groupings of resilience factors is needed.

## INTERACTIONALIST VIEW: ENVIRONMENTAL INFLUENCES ON RESILIENCE

The majority of research to date has focused on the *individual* characteristics associated with resilience—characteristics woven into our American, "pull yourself up by your bootstraps," mentality. However, this view fails to adequately consider the family, community, and governmental factors at play. This tendency to approach systems-level problems with individual-only solutions is shortsighted. To tell a person that the only impediment to their overcoming adversity is their own limited commitment sets them up for additional failure. A further injurious practice is holding up an "ideal individual" as an example of resilience, intimating that, "they too could overcome adversity if only they work harder." These two scenarios discount the family, community, and societal factors that can be significantly influential.[107]

A review favoring the interactionalist slant on resilience stated, " … resilience results from a complex interplay between genetics, temperament, knowledge, skills, past experiences, social supports, and cultural and societal resources,[108] where individuals are seen as nested within communities, within cities, within countries."[50]

### The Family's Role in Resilience

Stressful family situations (e.g., divorce, poverty, family members with addiction)[109–111] can adversely affect the entire family, with trickle-down effects on individual family members. Such stress can erode mental bandwidth and impede an individual's resilience. Conversely, well-functioning families can positively influence child outcomes in the face of adversity by providing support and belonging and helping alleviate usual life stressors.[112]

Research has found that families supporting resilience have remarkably similar processes in place. Several studies[6,7,112,113] have organized these salutary family processes into four domains.

1. Family beliefs and expectations: These include encouraging children to learn from failures, commit to family life, develop a realistic but optimistic/hopeful outlook, maintain a sense of purpose and meaningful activities, develop self-efficacy (i.e., "can do" spirit and confidence in one's abilities), and see adversity as normal and as an opportunity to learn.
2. Emotional connectedness: This includes mutual support and respect, pleasurable/humor-filled interactions, consistent communication, shared fair decision-making, and effective conflict resolution.
3. Organizational aspects: These include consistent family routines (i.e., stability where EF is allowed to develop), clear roles and responsibilities, clear child behavior guidelines and expectations, monitoring of children's activities, extended kin and social support, and activities connecting with the wider community.
4. Family learning opportunities: These include following routines that support learning activities, supporting academic and social skills acquisition, and affording explicit feedback.

Researchers have noted that these four "family processes" act in synergy, meaning that contributions from each of the four domains are necessary for a child's academic success and resilience. Researchers have also noted that these family processes are more impacting than factors such as divorce or a single parent home. A corroborating study[114] highlighting the importance of "family processes" in academic resilience (performing well in school despite adverse conditions) found that only 25% of the variance in student reading achievement was explained by social class or "intact versus divorced family," whereas 60% of the variance was explained by family interactions and family processes.

Family involvement in resilience training, therefore, is critical. Understanding families in terms of the stressful worlds they inhabit and understanding culturally distinct parenting styles is vital. Family education programs focused on creating a set of shared beliefs and expectations when facing stressful situations can help eliminate feelings of helplessness and can help build mutual support among family members. Family emotional connectedness can be enhanced by sharing stories of adversity and by framing stressful situations as "natural life events. Coaching parents on how best to approach difficult conversations such as sexual activity, drug and alcohol use, etc. can further enhance emotional connection. Such discussions give parents a chance to both share and express their own hopes and desires for their children. Communication and sharing can reduce blame, shame, and guilt and encourage active coping. Family organizational processes can be improved by reviewing family habits and resource utilization. Creating family learning opportunities, although time consuming, is a place where facilitators can help provide information about learning resources that are available and what parents can do at home to foster their child's exposure to opportunities and learning environments. It is important to show parents that improving these "family processes" has been shown to have positive effects in all families, regardless of their economic and social resources.

Schools and communities can be instrumental in initiating such programs. A counselor's main goal should be to develop an atmosphere and relationships that will foster a school–family partnership in the critical process of educating their children. This, of course, is not an easy task, especially when parents are socioeconomically disadvantaged, have limited time, or live in school districts where a significant distrust exists between parents and the school system.

### Community Influences on Resilience

Community factors such as high crime rates, poverty, institutionalized racism, sexism—all influenced by societal values and government policies—can also contribute to stress and tax resilience on a persistent basis. This ongoing stress consumes mental bandwidth,[115] alters brain development, contributes to suboptimal esteem and social position (placement on the lower rungs of established systems of school, work, etc.), and will erode resilience.

If we are to enhance individual resilience, reducing and overcoming adverse community conditions (e.g., poverty, crime, social exclusion) is vital. Programs bent on strengthening individual resilience cannot be expected to fully overcome larger community and societal issues. Indeed, researchers looking at individual resilience–building programs have documented the limited efficacy of such programs. Thus despite the most well-intentioned and well-implemented efforts, if adverse social conditions are allowed to exist, lower rates of resilience will be evident.[116]

When discussing individual versus community resilience, the literature often uses the phrases *beating the odds* versus *changing the odds. Beating the odds* refers to individual resilience, and *changing the odds* refers to the community and policy efforts needed foster resilience on a larger scale.[117] Policies that strengthen the notions of fairness of opportunity, social justice, social inclusion, access to resources, involvement, and mutual respect will help foster mental health[e] and individual resilience.[107,118–120]

In conclusion, designers of resilience programs should consider the following:

1. Individual factors such as neurobiological condition, cognitive skills, EF, temperament, personality, character traits, age, stage of development, race/ethnicity, education, diet, exercise, sleep, income, social support, state of health/disease, and recent and past life stressors.[122] Designers should be aware that those experiencing chronic stress, ongoing trauma, etc. can have slowed brain maturation resulting in poor EF, suboptimal trait and characteristic development, and poor resilience. It may take time to heal the involved neurobiological condition, allow EF to mature, and to promote the salutary traits and characteristics needed for resilience.
2. Community norms and values and the effects that government policies have on an individual. Thus programs designed to enhance resilience should focus on both strengthening individual attributes and on championing larger-scale policy efforts.

## RESILIENCE SCREENING

Remembering that 25%–50% of those experiencing adversity will be "naturally resilient," and do not require any help in overcoming adversity, screening should help separate these individuals from the more vulnerable. Screening should also help illuminate which specific aspects of EF, character traits, and environmental factors might be lacking, thus helping to tailor future resilience enhancement interventions.

In the literature, there are multiple resiliency tools used to screen for and assess resiliency, with no established gold standard. A cataloging of 38 such scales was conducted by Darlene Kordich Hall of the Child & Family Partnership in Toronto. Nineteen of these scales underwent a 2011 systematic review to assess validity, consistency, and interpretability.[123] Of the five most commonly used scales, the Ego Resiliency Scale,[124] Psychological Hardiness Scale,[125] Resilience

[e]By mental health, here, we mean more than just the absence of mental illness. We mean the healthy mental state required for human flourishing—a mindset dependent on relationships with families, schools, jobs, available resources, opportunities, etc.[121]

Scale for Adults (RSA),[126] Connor-Davidson Resilience Scale (CD-RISC),[127] and the Brief Resilience Scale (BRS),[128] the three most highly rated were CD-RISC, RSA, and BRS.[123] Although these three scales were the most highly rated in comparison to the other tools evaluated, they were still only of moderate overall quality. All three scales were developed for adults but were deemed useful in both adolescents and adult populations.

A review[45] looked at 17 resilience measures and noted the four highest scoring measures to be the Psychological Capital Questionnaire (PCQ), RSA, BRS, and CD-RISC. Again, however, the authors noted various shortcomings, commenting that most of the scales placed an undue emphasis on individual resiliency traits and did not adequately consider family, community, or other dynamic or broader environmental factors—a shortcoming that is surprising in light of the importance that families and communities play in resilience. Other studies have corroborated these shortcomings.[129]

In adolescents, CD-RISC (http://www.connordavidson-resiliencescale.com/.) and the Resiliency Scales for Children and Adolescents (RSCA) are perhaps the most widely used. They are discussed briefly in the following to give the reader a general appreciation of resilience screening tools.

### The Connor-Davidson Resilience Scale

Originally developed in 2003, the CD-RISC screens several main categories associated with resilience: (1) personal competence, (2) high standards, (3) trust in one's own instincts, (4) tenacity, (5) tolerance of negative outcomes (e.g., with humor, patience), (6) strengthening effects of stress, (7) acceptance of change, (8) secure relationships, (9) sense of control, and (10) spiritual influences. The tool consists of 25 questions based on these categories and can be completed in 5–10 min.[130] Each question is scored 0 to 4, resulting in a maximum score of 100, with higher scores indicating enhanced resilience. The scale has been validated in adolescents,[131] older adults, and across cultures and countries.[42,132] It has also been validated when assessing resiliency in athletes[133,134] and in the US military, where it has successfully predicted depression, overall psychologic functioning, and which soldiers would likely experience PTSD if stressed under wartime conditions.[135,136]

Despite the generally accepted validity of the CD-RISC, the scale has been criticized for its failure to adequately take into account the environmental, interactive, and dynamic characteristics of resilience.[137]

Statistical validation is corroborated by the scale's "Cronbach's alpha." Cronbach's alpha estimates the reliability of psychometric tests on tools such as the CD-RISC, where a screening tool is compared to a gold standard." Alpha values range from 0 to 1, with higher values indicating a more reliable test. Usually, researchers require an alpha of 0.70 or higher before they will use an instrument in research, although this is an arbitrary cutoff. CD-RISC has a Cronbach's alpha of 0.89, which is an excellent indicator of its reliability. However, as no true gold standard exists for resilience, one cannot calculate a *true* Cronbach's alpha for CD-RISC.

### The Resiliency Scales for Children and Adolescents

The RSCA, created in 2005, is a 64-item survey designed for 9- to 18-year-old individuals with at least third-grade reading skills. This tool groups questions into three main categories: sense of mastery, sense of relatedness, and emotional reactivity. The tool's construction provides a resource index, which identifies perceived strengths (mastery and relatedness), and a vulnerability index, which notes the discrepancy between strengths and emotional reactivity. Its use has been validated[138,139] and endorsed[85,138,140] by several researchers.

Several studies have administered RSCA to normal youths, youths with mental health issues, and incarcerated juveniles.[141–145] The tool was validated across all studies, with high levels of self-mastery (ability, optimism, adaptability) and relatedness (social support and connection) promoting resilience and high levels of emotional reactivity indicating vulnerability. The structure of the tool implies that those with shortcomings in emotional reactivity might overcome these deficits with a high sense of self-mastery and relatedness. This approach might be taken into consideration when formulating treatment plans; an individual's self-mastery and relatedness might be enhanced in order to compensate for any vulnerability in emotional reactivity.

## RESILIENCE ENHANCEMENT PROGRAMS

Resilience enhancement exists in two distinct formats: resilience *promotion*, which is important for *all* youths, and resilience *intervention*, which is focused on the 25%–50% of youths who have been screened and deemed lacking in individual or environmental factors ordinarily associated with resilience. This said, however, there is considerable confusion in the literature between promotion and intervention. Often times the terms are used interchangeably and often a single program may be used in both instances. Please note, however, that this is quite different from the *treatment* of ACEs and psychologic trauma.

Consensus guidelines generally recommend pretrauma resilience enhancement, *promotion or intervention*, programs to prepare for future traumatic events[146,147] as well as posttraumatic *treatment* programs to help surmount trauma and build future resilience. Despite the fact that evidence supporting the efficacy of resilience enhancement programs is thin, guidelines generally recommend a multimodal approach focusing on individual, family, and community factors. In addition, broad-based policy interventions are recommended to support an environment that provides safety, stability, and fair access to opportunities and generally an environment that supports healthy individuals, families, and communities.[148,149]

Some general concepts useful in designing resilience enhancement programs are listed in the following:

1. Programs are best served by first assessing vulnerability using screening tools such as the RSCA or CD-RISC. Intervention can then be focused on the 50%−75% of those lacking in "natural resilience." Effective programs such as group cognitive behavior therapy (CBT), life skills programs, and youth mentoring have been documented as effective in enhancing resilience (and also in reducing juvenile recidivism).
2. If mentoring is the chosen intervention, it should not only address vulnerabilities but also highlight and strengthen a child's unique strengths and skills, which are important aspects of esteem and efficacy building. Mentoring programs should include the most effective ways to solidify a mentor–mentee relationship, alleviate strain, and enhance resilience in at-risk youths. Such methods include modeling and teaching emotional regulation, imparting conflict resolution skills, instilling future orientation, and modeling active listening.[149,150] Active listening was perceived as the most useful approach to deal with mentee stress and was seen as the foundation for solidifying the mentoring relationship.[151] Similar insights can be gained from the literature if group CBT or life skills programs are chosen for resilience intervention.
3. Programs that target individual attributes and skill building should aid in developing EF, active coping, promote exercise, sleep, and self-care.[152–154] Identifying individual strengths and interests is also important, as this can help channel energy into engaging extracurricular activities and help foster a sense of accomplishment and confidence. Building self-efficacy, which can aid in building strong peer and "other adult" relationships, is important in promoting resilience.
4. Programs should address family and parenting factors. They should emphasize stable and consistent routines.[155] Families with at least one "very caring" parent have been found to foster significantly more resilience than those lacking concerned parents (62% of those with caring parents have been documented to be resilient versus 20% of those without a caring parent).[4] Programs should convey to mothers that they are doing a good job, as maternal feelings are also important in developing resilience in their offspring. They should also make every attempt to mitigate for high levels of psychosocial stress, which makes optimal parenting difficult.[156]
5. In both individual and family intervention programs, education about stress and trauma is important. Children who have experienced chronic stress or trauma rarely spontaneously speak of their experiences, as they are often not aware that their situation is abnormal or that it can be mitigated. They tend to have little insight about the relationship between their experiences and how they feel and act. Parents and mentors need to be aware of this. Several studies have shown the positive impact of trauma education on children's mental health outcomes.[157–159] Well-designed programs should incorporate such education into their curriculum (see the chapter 7 for a discussion of Trauma Informed Care).
6. Specially focused intervention programs designed for at-risk youths should take into consideration the fact that stress from disadvantaged conditions (e.g., chaotic family life, violence, abuse, poverty, lack of academic or social support)[160] can make resilience and transitioning into adulthood difficult.[161,162] Instead of growing, learning, exploring identities, setting goals, and choosing career paths, such youths are in "financial, social, and emotional survival mode," forced to focus on lower Maslow needs rather than on self-discovery and self-actualization.[163,164] Programs bent on enhancing resilience in this population should take all this into consideration, allowing adequate time for the prerequisite neurobiological, cognitive, EF, and behavior changes to take hold.

## Specific Resilience Promotion/Intervention Programs

Several programs fashioned to enhance resilience exist.[f] Some of those programs are Empower, Spark, Psychological Capital Model, Spiritual Based, Psychoeducational Based, Problem Solving Emphasis, Cognitive Behavioral Coaching, Stress Inoculation Training (SIT), Attention and Interpretation Therapy (Living in a World With Higher Principles), Child-Caregiver-Advocacy Resilience Intervention (Childcare), Resilience and Coping Intervention (RCI), Promoting Resilience in Stress Management (Prism), Psychological First Aid (PFA) Guided Preparedness Planning (GPP), the Penn Resiliency Program, Positive Psychology Techniques, CBT, Transformational Coping, Acceptance and Commitment Therapy, Mindfulness, Interpersonal Therapy, Attention and Interpretation Therapy, Relaxation and Diaphragmatic Breathing, and the US Army Comprehensive Soldier Fitness Program (CSF).

## Resilience Intervention Programs

Once screening had identified vulnerable individuals, resilience intervention can be implemented.

Ideally, intervention entails enhancing both "microlevel" individual characteristics and the "macrolevel" environment. It is likely that a properly functional macroenvironment is needed before individual resilience can be optimized.[165]

Two reviews have been conducted on the effectiveness of resilience-focused interventions.[37,166] The first review included studies of resilience intent on steeling individuals against future traumatic events. Of the 2333 articles examined in this review, only seven adult trials (randomized controlled trials) were of sufficient quality to be included in the analysis. These seven studies measured resilience characteristics (via one of the abovementioned screening tools), implemented a resilience training program, and then measured how much a subject's resilience survey answers changed after the training. Six of the seven studies showed a modest improvement in the resilience characteristics surveyed at the completion of the program. These results indicate an acquisition of *knowledge of resilience*, rather than an acquisition of the characteristics, skills, or abilities necessary to overcome adverse experiences in real life. Not a ringing endorsement of resilience enhancement programs and not the same as proving efficacy under real-world adverse conditions. In addition to these glaring limitations, other shortcomings of these studies included poor methodology, poor reporting, and limited length of follow-up (longest follow-up period was 10 weeks), all resulting in the authors' low level of confidence in their conclusion that resilience promotion programs were efficacious.

The second review of randomized controlled trials by Leppin et al.[166] found 25 studies that met the inclusion criteria. Again, the overall results noted a modest but consistent benefit of resiliency training programs on measured outcomes—in this case, mental health outcomes of improved stress, anxiety, and depression. As before, however, this review noted that studies were limited by poor methodology and only considered patient-reported measures as a measure of success (i.e., before and after survey results). Several similar studies have been conducted but had the same limitations: short-term results and unknown real-world impact.[167–169] In conclusion, although all these studies had encouraging results, they all had quality limitations and did not measure the real-world effectiveness of resiliency training. Still, the efforts are a well-intentioned foundation on which future research can be built.

## Resilience Promotion

One exception to the abovementioned "lack of ability to demonstrate real-world effectiveness" was seen in the SIT program[g] instituted in certain schools in Israel. The SIT program was added to the curriculum for all students in schools located in high-risk-for-armed-conflict areas. After an ensuing 3-week "traumatic exposure" (constant mortar shelling), children in the SIT schools were found to have significantly less PTSD, depression, anxiety, or other symptoms of distress

[f]As an example, the SPARK (*S*ituation, *P*erception, *A*utopilot, *R*eaction, and *K*nowledge) program teaches children how, in everyday *S*ituations, their *P*erceptions can trigger *A*utomatic emotional *R*eactions. Reflections on the scenarios used in the program help children gain *K*nowledge, help them challenge their cognitive distortions, and help them identify and modify their automatic reactions. It helps them to refrain from blaming, judging, and seeing themselves as losers or "giver-uppers" and also helps them refrain from catastrophizing or minimization. Children are also taught assertiveness, problem-solving skills, and to enhance their strengths and social support in an effort to build their "resilience muscles." The program is administered in 12 1-h sessions over 3–4 months by teachers who have been trained in a 2-day workshop.

[g]Stress Inoculation Training (SIT) involves three phases: (1) cognitive preparation, (2) skills acquisition and rehearsal, and (3) application and practice of coping techniques. SIT has also been shown to be effective in reducing stress in public speaking, sports, police work, military, and in preparation for hospital admission for children.[170,171]

when compared with children in schools that did *not* receive such training.[147]

## WHAT WE *DON'T* KNOW ABOUT RESILIENCE

Although much is known about resilience, much work remains. Areas of future research include the following:

1. Determining if the factors and resources needed to bounce back from acute stressors (e.g., job loss, death of a loved one) are different from those needed to overcome chronic stressors (e.g., poverty, ongoing abuse).[85]
2. Determining if specific trauma treatments in the face of specific traumas could be used proactively in resilience promotion and intervention.
3. Designing and evaluating resilience programs focused on individual, dynamic, developmental, family, and community factors, with the intent of finding an optimal resilience enhancement program because, as of yet, no gold standard program exists.
4. Documenting the effectiveness of resilience programs in the real world. Despite the presence of multiple resilience enhancement programs, most studies are only substantiated as effective by pre- and postsurvey analyses.
5. Standardizing outcome measurements in resilience research so that conclusions across studies can be clearly understood and compared. For example, some studies say a person is resilient if he or she has endured adverse conditions and has emerged without any overt mental health issues, whereas other studies define resilience as the return to "normal functioning" after adversity. Still others determine resilient outcomes only in terms of posttraumatic growth (i.e., strength and steeling in the face of trauma).[45]
6. Continuing to explore and clarify areas of debate in the resilience literature. For example, the debate over whether trauma is inoculating or sensitizing. Does one traumatic event steel you against further events (inoculating) or make you more susceptible (sensitized) to future events? In which types of individuals which types of events would inoculate, which would sensitize, and which would immobilize[172]?
7. Exploring the macroenvironment. We know comparatively little about the role that government policies, community norms, or corporate culture play in setting the stage for resilience, either fostering or impeding individual resilience. Several other areas of inquiry will come to light as research in the area continues.

## CONCLUSIONS

Government policies, corporate codes, and cultural values must minimize environmental stressors and help promote stable families and communities. Such an environment can then provide the foundation for resiliency in individuals who have yet to be exposed to trauma. Although much work has been done in this area, much work remains if we are to illuminate truth, foster actualized individuals, and develop actualized societies.

## END NOTE: *GRIT* BY ANGELA DUCKWORTH

Duckworth's book is focused on helping people succeed by first helping them discover their true career interests (e.g., not just money, fame, or parental expectations) and then by providing insights to help them overcome setbacks along the path to success. Duckworth says that once this foundation of "true interest" has been prepared, deliberate, effortful, and ongoing practice; a desire for continual improvement; a purpose greater than one's self; and active coping can push one past obstacles and move him or her toward success. (She calls active coping "hope" but what she really means is active coping and a belief in self-efficacy.)

As grit, in her view, relies first on finding one's interest (this is what will sustain one over the long run), she devotes significant time on how such interest is acquired. She indicates the following:

1. Interest takes time—you won't have interest right away, and you certainly won't have passion right away. It starts with play and exploration, followed by a little interest, then slowly more involvement and more interest. Most people don't find their interests quickly.
2. Interest is not discovered by introspection but rather by interaction with the outside world (i.e., some *experience* sparks your interest). This usually occurs unconsciously (i.e., when you are bored, you are always aware that you are bored, but when you are "interested" you are often so engaged in what you are doing that you are unaware that you are "interested."
3. Interest is spurred on by success and encouragement from others. In a sense, interest becomes a part of one's "chosen" identity—that part of identity that is not fixed by race, sex, ethnicity, etc.

Following the acquisition of interest, deliberate practice, working with a purpose intent on serving others, belief in one's abilities, and active coping when problems arise are all contributing attributes in achieving mastery, overcoming obstacles, and achieving grit.

A critique of Duckworth's book[173] challenged her claims on the value of grit. The authors stated that she exaggerated the impact that grit has upon success—a critique that Duckworth, in a written response, actually agreed with. The authors of the critique also note that grit is nearly identical to conscientiousness, i.e., organization, self-control, thoughtfulness, and goal-directed behavior, a group of traits that have been studied by psychologists for decades, thus making grit a case of "old wine in new bottles." The critical review goes on to say that Duckworth suggests that grit is a skill that can be taught and learned, whereas conscientiousness is more of a trait (part genetics and part environment) that *may* change with time as one ages but is not something that can be taught with direct instructions. The critique concludes, "Our results suggest that interventions designed to enhance grit may only have weak effects on performance and success, that the construct validity of grit is in question," and that the limited effect that grit may have on success is due to the effort/perseverance facet of grit.

Despite this criticism of Duckworth's work,[173] her writing still deserves merit, as it helps solidify the distinctions between grit and resilience and highlights a useful discussion of perseverance and overcoming obstacles.

## REFERENCES

1. Tiet QQ, Huizinga D, Byrnes FH. Predictors of resilience among inner city youths. *J Child Fam Stud.* 2010;19: 360−378.
2. Norris FH. Epidemiology of trauma: frequency and impact of different potentially traumatic events on different demographic groups. *J Consult Clin Psychol.* 1992;60(3):409−418.
3. Bonanno GA, Westphal M, Mancini AD. Resilience to loss and potential trauma. *Annu Rev Clin Psychol.* 2011;7: 511−535.
4. Collishaw S, Pickles A, Messer J, et al. Resilience to adult psychopathology following childhood maltreatment: evidence from a community sample. *Child Abuse Negl.* 2007;31(3):211−229.
5. Dubowitz H, Thompson R, Proctor L, et al. Adversity, maltreatment, and resilience in young children. *Acad Pediatr.* 2016;16(3):233−239.
6. Kwong TY, Hayes DK. Adverse family experiences and flourishing amongst children ages 6-17 years: 2011/12 National Survey of Children's Health. *Child Abuse Negl.* 2017;70:240−246.
7. McGloin JM, Widom CS. Resilience among abused and neglected children grown up. *Dev Psychopathol.* 2001 Fall;13(4):1021−1038.
8. Stevenson J. The treatment of the long-term sequelae of child abuse. *J Child Psychol Psychiatry.* 1999;40(1): 89−111.
9. Thomson P, Jaque SV. Adverse childhood experiences (ACE) and adult attachment interview (AAI) in a non-clinical population. *Child Abuse Negl.* 2017;70:255−263.
10. Werner EE. The children of Kauai: resiliency and recovery in adolescence and adulthood. *J Adolesc Health.* 1992; 13(4):262−268.
11. Felitti VJ, Anda RF, Nordenberg D, et al. Relationship of childhood abuse and household dysfunction to many of the leading causes of death in adults. The Adverse Childhood Experiences (ACE) Study. *Am J Prev Med.* 1998;14(4):245−258.
12. Finkelhor D, Turner HA, Shattuck A, et al. Violence, crime, and abuse exposure in a national sample of children and youth: an update. *JAMA Pediatr.* 2013;167(7): 614−621.
13. Dierkhising CB, Ko SJ, Woods-Jaeger B, et al. Trauma histories among justice-involved youth: findings from the national child traumatic stress network. *Eur J Psychotraumatol.* 2013 Jul 16;4.
14. Evans-Chase M. Addressing trauma and psychosocial development in juvenile justice-involved youth: a synthesis of the developmental neuroscience, juvenile justice and trauma literature. *Laws.* 2014;3(4):744−758.
15. Rutter M. Isle of Wight revisited: twenty-five years of child psychiatric epidemiology l. *J Am Acad Child Adoles Psychiatry.* 1989;28:633−653.
16. Friedli L. *Mental Health, Resilience and Inequalities.* Denmark: World Health Organisation; 2009. Available at: http://www.euro.who.int/document/e92227.pdf. Accessed 08.15.17.
17. The Scottish Government. *Equally Well: Report of the Ministerial Task Force on Health Inequalities.* Edinburgh: The Scottish Government. Available at: http://www.scotland.gov.uk/Publications/2008/06/09160103/0. Accessed 08.15.17.
18. Keyes CL. The nexus of cardiovascular disease and depression revisited: the complete mental health perspective and the moderating role of age and gender. *Aging and Mental Health.* 2004;8:266−274.
19. Pressman SD, Cohen S. Does positive affect influence health? *Psychol Bullet.* 2005;131:925−971.
20. Sylva K, Melhuish E, Sammons P, et al. *Effective Pre-school and Primary Education 3-11 Project a Longitudinal Study Funded by the DFES.* London: Institute of Education; 2007.
21. Csikszentmihalyi M. *Flow: e Psychology of Optimal Experience.* New York: HarperCollins; 1991.
22. Csikszentmihalyi M. *Finding Flow: The Psychology of Engagement with Everyday Life.* New York: HarperCollins; 1997.
23. Jackson SA, Eklund RC. Assessing flow in physical activity: the flow state scale-2 and the dispositional flow scale-2. *J Sport Exerc Psychol.* 2002;24:133−150.
24. Swann C, Keegan RJ, Piggot D, et al. A systematic review of experience, occurrence and controllability of flow states in elite sport. *Psychol Sport Exerc.* 2012;13: 807−819.
25. Golby J, Sheard M. Mental toughness and hardiness at different levels of rugby league. *Personality Individ Differ.* 2004;37:933−942.

26. Sheard M, Golby J. Personality hardiness differentiates elite-level performers. *Int J Sport Exercise Psychol.* 2010;8: 160–169.
27. Vealey RS, Perritt NC. Hardiness and optimism as predictors of the frequency of flow in collegiate athletes. *J Sport Behav.* 2015;38:321–338.
28. Masten AS, Cicchetti D. Developmental cascades. *Dev Psychopathol.* 2010;22(3):491–495.
29. Costello EJ, Costello AJ, Edelbrock C, et al. Psychiatric disorders in pediatric primary care. Prevalence and risk factors. *Arch Gen Psychiatry.* 1988;45:1107–1116.
30. Shonkoff JP, Garner AS, Committee on Psychosocial Aspects of Child and Family Health; Committee on Early Childhood, Adoption, and Dependent Care; Section on Developmental and Behavioral Pediatrics. The lifelong effects of early childhood adversity and toxic stress. *Pediatrics.* 2012;129(1):e232–e246.
31. Merrick MT, Ports KA, Ford DC, et al. Unpacking the impact of adverse childhood experiences on adult mental health. *Child Abuse Negl.* 2017;69:10–19.
32. Metzler M, Merrick MT, Klevens J, et al. Adverse childhood experiences and life opportunities: shifting the narrative. *Child Youth Serv Rev.* 2017;72:141–149.
33. Center for Behavioral Health Statistics and Quality. *Behavioral Health Trends in the United States: Results from the 2014 National Survey on Drug Use and Health;* 2015 (HHS Publication No. SMA 15-4927, NSDUH Series H-50). Available at: https://www.samhsa.gov/data/sites/default/files/NSDUH-FRR1-2014/NSDUH-FRR1-2014.pdf. Accessed 08.15.17.
34. Jia H, Zack MM, Thompson WW, et al. Impact of depression on quality-adjusted life expectancy (QALE) directly as well as indirectly through suicide. *Soc Psychiatry Psychiatr Epidemiol.* 2015;50(6):939–949.
35. Fox BH, Perez N, Cass E, et al. Trauma changes everything: examining the relationship between adverse childhood experiences and serious, violent and chronic juvenile offenders. *Child Abuse Negl.* 2015;46:163–173.
36. Casey GW Jr. Comprehensive soldier fitness: a vision for psychological resilience in the U.S. Army. *Am Psychol.* 2011;66(1):1-3.
37. Macedo T, Wilheim L, Gonçalves R, et al. Building resilience for future adversity: a systematic review of interventions in non-clinical samples of adults. *BMC Psychiatry.* 2014;14:227.
38. Marmar CR. Mental health impact of Afghanistan and Iraq deployment: meeting the challenge of a new generation of veterans. *Depress Anxiety.* 2009;26:493–497.
39. Hoge CW, Castro CA, Messer SC, et al. Combat duty in Iraq and Afghanistan, mental health problems, and barriers to care. *N Engl J Med.* 2004;351:13–22.
40. Cohen MA. The monetary value of saving a high-risk youth. *J Quant Criminol.* 1998;14:5–33.
41. Cohen MA, Piquero AR. New evidence on the monetary value of saving a high risk youth. *J Quant Criminol.* 2009;25:25–49.
42. Windle G. What is resilience? A systematic review and concept analysis. *Rev Clin Gerontol.* 2010;21:1–18.
43. Langeland K, Manheim D, McLeod G, et al. *How Civil Institutions Build Resilience: Organizational Practices Derived from Academic Literature and Case Studies.* Santa Monica, CA: RAND Corporation; 2016. https://www.rand.org/pubs/research_reports/RR1246.html. Accessed 08.13.17.
44. Cameron CA, Ungar M, Liebenberg L. Cultural understandings of resilience: roots for wings in the development of affective resources for resilience. *Child Adolesc Psychiatr Clin N Am.* 2007;16:285–301, vii–viii.
45. Pangallo A, Zibarras L, Lewis R, et al. Resilience through the lens of interactionism: a systematic review. *Psychol Assess.* 2015;27:1–20.
46. Gillespie BM, Chaboyer W, Wallis M. Development of a theoretically derived model of resilience through concept analysis. *Contemp Nurse.* 2007;25:124–135.
47. Lepore S, Revenson T. Resilience and posttraumatic growth: recovery, resistance, and reconfiguration. In: Calhoun L, Tedesch R, eds. *Handbook of Posttraumatic Growth: Research and Practice.* Mahwah, NJ: Lawrence Erlbaum Associates; 2006:24–46.
48. Ungar M. A constructionist discourse on resilience: multiple contexts, multiple realities among at risk children and youth. *Youth Soc.* 2004;35:341–365.
49. Ungar M. Resilience across cultures. *Br J Soc Work.* 2008; 38:218–235.
50. Khanlou N, Wray R. A whole community approach toward child and youth resilience promotion: a review of resilience literature. *Int J Ment Health Addiction.* 2014; 12:64–79.
51. Insel K, Morrow D, Brewer B, et al. Executive function, working memory, and medication adherence among older adults. *J Gerontol B Psychol Sci Soc Sci.* 2006;61: P102–P107.
52. Shields GS, Moons WG, Slavich GM. Better executive function under stress mitigates the effects of recent life stress exposure on health in young adults. *Stress.* 2017; 20(1):75–85.
53. Lowe CJ, Hall PA, Staines WR. The effects of continuous theta burst stimulation to the left dorsolateral prefrontal cortex on executive function, food cravings, and snack food consumption. *Psychosom Med.* 2014;76:503–511.
54. Hall PA. Executive-control processes in high-calorie food consumption. *Curr Dir Psychol Sci.* 2016;25:91–98.
55. Hall PA, Marteau TM. Executive function in the context of chronic disease prevention: theory, research and practice. *Prev Med.* 2014;68:44–50.
56. Casey BJ, Trainor RJ, Orendi JL, et al. A developmental functional MRI study of prefrontal activation during performance of a go-No-go task. *J Cogn Neurosci* 1997;9: 835–847.
57. Rothbart MK, Bates JE. Temperament. In: Damon WW, Eisenberg N, eds. *Handbook of Child Psychology. Vol. 3.* Social, emotional and personality development, 5th ed. NewYork: Wiley; 1998:105–176.
58. Gyurak A, Goodkind MS, Kramer JH, et al. Executive functions and the down-regulation and up-regulation of emotion. *Cogn Emot.* 2012;26:103–118.

59. Ochsner KN, Silvers JA, Buhle JT. Functional imaging studies of emotion regulation: a synthetic review and evolving model of the cognitive control of emotion. *Ann N Y Acad Sci*. 2012;1251:E1–E24.
60. Schmeichel BJ, Tang D. Individual differences in executive functioning and their relationship to emotional processes and responses. *Curr Dir Psychol Sci*. 2015;24:93–98.
61. Eisenberg N, Spinrad TL, Fabes RA, et al. The relations of effortful control and impulsivity to children's resiliency and adjustment. *Child Dev*. 2004;75(1):25–46.
62. Eisenberg N, Valiente C, Fabes RA, et al. The relations of effortful control and ego control to children's resiliency and social functioning. *Dev Psychol*. 2003;39(4):761–776.
63. Buckner JC, Mezzacappa E, Beardslee WR. Characteristics of resilient youths living in poverty: the role of self-regulatory processes. *Dev Psychopathol*. 2003;15:139–162.
64. Colcombe SJ, Erickson KI, Scalf PE, et al. Aerobic exercise training increases brain volume in aging humans. *J Gerontol A Biol Sci Med Sci*. 2006;61:1166–1170.
65. Hsu CL, Best JR, Davis JC, et al. Aerobic exercise promotes executive functions and impacts functional neural activity among older adults with vascular cognitive impairment. *Br J Sports Med*. 2018;52:184–191.
66. Kramer AF, Erickson KI. Capitalizing on cortical plasticity: influence of physical activity on cognition and brain function. *Trends Cogn Sci*. 2007;11:342–348.
67. Erickson KI, Hillman CH, Kramer AF. Physical activity, brain, and cognition. *Curr Opin Behav Sci*. 2015;4:27–32.
68. Hillman CH, Erickson KI, Kramer AF. Be smart, exercise your heart: exercise effects on brain and cognition. *Nat Rev Neurosci*. 2008;9:58–65.
69. Smith PJ, Blumenthal JA, Hoffman BM, et al. Aerobic exercise and neurocognitive performance: a meta-analytic review of randomized controlled trials. *Psychosom Med*. 2010;72:239–252.
70. Chang YK, Labban JD, Gapin JI, et al. The effects of acute exercise on cognitive performance: a meta-analysis. *Brain Res*. 2012;1453:87–101.
71. Zang J, Liu Y, Li W, et al. Voluntary exercise increases adult hippocampal neurogenesis by increasing GSK-3β activity in mice. *Neuroscience*. 2017;354:122–135.
72. Jonasson LS, Nyberg L, Kramer AF, et al. Aerobic exercise intervention, cognitive performance, and brain structure: results from the physical influences on brain in aging (PHIBRA) study. *Front Aging Neurosci*. 2017;18(8):336.
73. Lowe CJ, Staines WR, Hall PA. Effects of moderate exercise on cortical resilience: a transcranial magnetic stimulation study targeting the dorsolateral prefrontal cortex. *Psychosom Med*. 2017;79:143–152.
74. Rothbart MK, Ahadi SA, Evans DE. Temperament and personality: origins and outcomes. *J Pers Soc Psychol*. 2000;78:122–135.
75. Debiec J, LeDoux JE, Nader K. Cellular and systems reconsolidation in the hippocampus. *Neuron*. 2002;36:527–538.
76. Milekic MH, Alberini CM. Temporally graded requirement for protein synthesis following memory reactivation. *Neuron*. 2002;36:521–525.
77. Myers KM, Davis M. Systems-level reconsolidation: reengagement of the hippocampus with memory reactivation. *Neuron*. 2002;36:340–343.
78. Charney DS. Psychobiological mechanisms of resilience and vulnerability: implications for successful adaptation to extreme stress. *Am J Psychiatry*. 2004;161:195–216.
79. Bell CC, Gamm S, Vallas P, et al. Strategies for the prevention of youth violence in Chicago public schools. In: Shafii M, Shafii S, eds. *School Violence: Contributing Factors, Management, and Prevention*. Washington, DC: American Psychiatric Press; 2001:251–272.
80. Mattis JS, Bell CC, Jagers RJ, et al. Towards a critical approach to stress-related disorders in African-Americans. *J Natl Med Assoc*. 1999;91:80–85.
81. Taylor SE, Brown JD. Illusion and well-being: a social psychological perspective on mental health. *Psychol Bull*. 1988;103:193–210.
82. Taylor SE, Kemeny ME, Reed GM, et al. Psychological resources, positive illusions, and health. *Am Psychol*. 2000;55:99–109.
83. Kerpelman JL, Mosher LS. Rural African American adolescents' future orientation: the importance of self-efficacy, control and responsibility, and identity development. *Identity*. 2004;4:187–208.
84. Sinclair VG, Wallston KA. The development and psychometric evaluation of the brief resilient coping scale. *Assessment*. 2004;11(1):94–101.
85. Masten AS. Ordinary magic. Resilience processes in development. *Am Psychol*. 2001;56:227–238.
86. Brewer-Smyth K, Koenig HG. Could spirituality and religion promote stress resilience in survivors of childhood trauma? *Issues Ment Health Nurs*. 2014;35:251–256.
87. Banyarda V, Hambyb S. Health effects of adverse childhood events: identifying promising protective factors at the intersection of mental and physical well-being. *Child Abuse Negl*. 2017;65:88–98.
88. Dornbusch SM, Erickson KG, Laird J, et al. The relation of family and school attachment to adolescent deviance in diverse groups and communities. *J Adoles Res*. 2001;16:396–422.
89. Frijda NH. The laws of emotion. *Am Psychol*. 1988;43(5):349.
90. Joseph S, Linley PA. Growth following adversity: theoretical perspectives and implications for clinical practice. *Clin Psychol Rev*. 2006;26:1041–1053.
91. Southwick SM, Vythilingam M, Charney DS. The psychobiology of depression and resilience to stress: implications for prevention and treatment. *Annu Rev Clin Psychol*. 2005;1:255–291.
92. Aspinwall LG, Taylor SE. A stitch in time: self-regulation and proactive coping. *Psychol Bull*. 1997;121:417–436.
93. Richardson GE. The metatheory of resilience and resiliency. *J Clin Psychol*. 2002;58:307–321.

94. Masten AS, Coatsworth JD. The development of competence in favorable and unfavorable environments. Lessons from research on successful children. *Am Psychol.* 1998;53:205–220.
95. Bell CC. Cultivating resiliency in youth. *J Adolesc Health.* 2001;29:375–381.
96. Apfel RJ, Simon B, eds. *Minefields in Their Hearts: The Mental Health of Children of War and Communal Violence.* New Haven: Yale University Press; 1996:9–11.
97. Wolin S, Wolin SJ. The challenge model: working with strengths in children of substance-abusing parents. *Child Adol Psych Cl.* 1996;5:243–256.
98. Bell CC, Suggs H. Using sports to strengthen resiliency in children. Training heart. *Child Adolesc Psychiatr Clin N Am.* 1998;7(4):859–865.
99. Wingo AP, Wrenn G, Pelletier T, et al. Moderating effects of resilience on depression in individuals with a history of childhood abuse or trauma exposure. *J Affect Disord.* 2010;126(3):411–414.
100. Beutel ME, Tibubos AN, Klein EM, et al. Childhood adversities and distress - the role of resilience in a representative sample. *PLoS One.* 2017;12(3):e0173826.
101. Caprara GV, Eisenberg N, Alessandri G. Positivity. The dispositional basis of happiness. *J Happiness Stud.* 2016: 1–19.
102. Alessandri G, Caprara GV, Tisak J. The unique contribution of positive orientation to optimal functioning: further exploration. *Europ Psychol.* 2012a;17:44–45.
103. Hobfoll SE. Conservation of resources. A new attempt at conceptualizing stress. *Am Psychol.* 1989;44(3): 513–524.
104. Milioni M, Alessandri G, Eisenberg N, et al. The role of positivity as predictor of ego-resiliency from adolescence to young adulthood. *Personal Individ Differ.* 2016;101: 306–311.
105. Maddi SR. Personal views survey II. In: Zalaquett CP, Wood RJ, eds. *Evaluating Stress: A Book of Resources.* Lanham, MD: Scarecrow Press, Inc.; 1997:293–309.
106. Lenzi M, Furlong MJ, Dowdy E, et al. The quantity and variety across domains of psychological and social assets associated with school victimization. *Psychol Viol.* 2015; 5:411–421.
107. Shaw J, McLean K, Taylor B, et al. Beyond resilience: why we need to look at systems too. *Psychol Viol.* 2016;6: 34–41.
108. Traub F, Boynton-Jarrett R. Modifiable resilience factors to childhood adversity for clinical pediatric practice. *Pediatrics.* 2017;139:e20162569.
109. Rolland JS, Walsh F. Systemic training for healthcare professionals: the chicago center for family health approach. *Family Process.* 2005;44:283–301.
110. Kelly JB, Emery RE. Children's adjustment following divorce: risk and resilience perspectives. *Family Relations.* 2003;52:352–362.
111. Landau J, Garret J. Invitational intervention: the ARISE model for engaging reluctant alcohol and other drug abusers in treatment. *Alcohol Treatment Q.* 2008;26: 147–168.
112. Amatea ES, Smith-Adcock S, Villares E. From family deficit to family strength: viewing families' contributions to children's learning from a family resilience perspective. *Prof School Couns.* 2006;9:177–189.
113. Walsh F. Family resilience: a framework for clinical practice. *Family Process.* 2003;42:1–18.
114. Walberg HJ. Families as partners in educational productivity. *Phi Delta Kappan.* 1984;65:397–400.
115. Mullainathan S, Shafir E. *Scarcity. Why Having So Little Means So Much.* New York: Henry Holt & Company; 2013.
116. Vanderbilt-Adriance E, Shaw DS. Conceptualizing and re-evaluating resilience across levels of risk, time and domains of competence. *Clin Family Psychol Rev.* 2008;11:30–58.
117. Seccombe K. "Beating the odds" versus "changing the odds": poverty, resilience and family policy. *J Marriage Family.* 2002;64:384–394.
118. Barankin T, Khanlou N. *Growing up Resilient: Ways to Build Resilience in Children and Youth.* Toronto: CAMH (Centre for Addiction and Mental Health); 2007.
119. Miller GE, Lachman ME, Chen E, et al. Pathways to resilience: maternal nurturance as a buffer against the effects of childhood poverty on metabolic syndrome at midlife. *Psychol Sci.* 2011;22:1591–1599.
120. Teti M, Martin AE, Ranade R, et al. "I'm a keep rising. I'm a keep going forward, regardless": exploring Black men's resilience amid sociostructural challenges and stressors. *Qual Health Res.* 2012;22:524–533.
121. Lahtinen E, Lehtinen V, Riikonen E, eds. *Framework for Promoting Mental Health in Europe.* Hamina: Ministry of Social Affairs and Health, STAKES, National Research and Development Centre for Welfare and Health; 1999.
122. Bonanno GA, Galea S, Bucciarelli A, et al. What predicts psychological resilience after disaster? The role of demographics, resources, and life stress. *J Consult Clin Psychol.* 2007;75(5):671–682.
123. Windle G, Bennett KM, Noyes J. A methodological review of resilience measurement scales. *Health Qual Life Outcomes.* 2011;9:8.
124. Block J, Kremen AM. IQ and ego-resiliency: conceptual and empirical connections and separateness. *J Pers Soc Psychol.* 1996;70(2):349–361.
125. Bartone PT, Ursano RJ, Wright KM, Ingraham LH. The impact of a military air disaster on the health of assistance workers. A prospective study. *J Nerv Ment Dis.* 1989;177(6):317–328.
126. Wagnild GM, Young HM. Development and psychometric evaluation of the resilience scale. *J Nurs Meas.* 1993 Winter;1(2):165–178.
127. Connor KM, Davidson JR. Development of a new resilience scale: the connor-davidson resilience scale (CD-RISC). *Depress Anxiety.* 2003;18(2):76–82.
128. Smith BW, Dalen J, Wiggins K, Tooley E, Christopher P, Bernard J. The brief resilience scale: assessing the ability to bounce back. *Int J Behav Med.* 2008;15(3):194–200.
129. Folkman S, Lazarus RS, Dunkel-Schetter C, et al. Dynamics of a stressful encounter: cognitive appraisal, coping, and encounter outcomes. *J Pers Soc Psychol.* 1986;50(5):992–1003.

130. Campbell-Sills L, Stein MB. Psychometric analysis and refinement of the connor-davidson resilience scale (CD-RISC): validation of a 10-item measure of resilience. *J Trauma Stress*. 2007;20(6):1019–1028.
131. Duong C, Hurst CP. Reliability and validity of the Khmer version of the 10-item connor-davidson resilience scale (Kh-CD-RISC10) in Cambodian adolescents. *BMC Res Notes*. 2016;9:297.
132. Wang L, Shi Z, Zhang Y, et al. Psychometric properties of the 10-item connor-davidson resilience scale in Chinese earthquake victims. *Psychiatry Clin Neurosci*. 2010;64(5): 499–504.
133. Gucciardi DF, Jackson B, Coulter TJ, et al. The Connor-Davidson Resilience Scale (CD-RISC): dimensionality and age-related measurement invariance with Australian cricketers. *Psychol Sport Exercise*. 2011;12:423–433.
134. Gonzalez SP, Moore EWG, Newton M, et al. Validity and reliability of the connor-davidson resilience scale (CD-RISC) in competitive sport. *Psychol Sport Exercise*. 2016; 23:31–39.
135. Bezdjian S, Schneider KG, Burchett D, et al. Resilience in the United States air force: psychometric properties of the connor-davidson resilience scale (CD-RISC). *Psychol Assess*. 2017;29(5):479–485.
136. Green KT, Calhoun PS, Dennis MF, Mid-Atlantic Mental Illness Research, Education and Clinical Center Work-group, Beckham JC. Exploration of the resilience construct in posttraumatic stress disorder severity and functional correlates in military combat veterans who have served since September 11, 2001. *J Clin Psychiatry*. 2010;71(7):823–830.
137. Galli N, Gonzalez SP. Psychological resilience in sport: a review of the literature and implications for research and practice. *Int J Sport Exercise Psychol*. 2015;13:243–257.
138. Prince-Embury S, Courville T. Comparison of one, two and three factor models of personal resiliency using the Resiliency Scales for Children and Adolescents. *Canad J School Psychol*. 2008;23:11–25.
139. Prince-Embury S, Courville T. Measurement invariance of the resiliency scales for children and adolescents with respect to sex and age cohorts. *Canad J School Psychol*. 2008;23:26–40.
140. Masten AS. Regulatory processes, risk and resilience in adolescent development. *Ann N Y Acad Sci*. 2004;1021: 310–319.
141. Mowder M, Cummings JA, McKinney R. Resiliency scales for children and adolescents: profiles of juvenile offenders. *J Psychoeducat Assess*. 2010;28(4):326–337.
142. Prince-Embury S. The resiliency scales for children and adolescents: psychological symptoms and clinical status in adolescents. *Canad J School Psychol*. 2008;23: 41–56.
143. Prince-Embury S. The Resiliency Scales for Children and Adolescents as related to parent education level and race/ethnicity in children. *Canad J School Psychol*. 2009; 24:167–182.
144. Prince-Embury S. Profiles of personal resiliency for normative and clinical samples of youth assessed by the resiliency scales for children and adolescents TM. *J Psychoeducat Assess*. 2010;28(4):303–314.
145. Deblinger E, Runyon MK. Profiles of personal resiliency in youth who have experienced physical or sexual abuse. *J Psychoeduc Assess*. 2014;32(6):558–566.
146. Masten AS, Obradovic J. Disaster preparation and recovery: lessons from research on resilience in human development. *Ecol Society*. 2008;13(1):9–24.
147. Wolmer L, Hamiel D, Laor N. Preventing children's post-traumatic stress after disaster with teacher-based intervention: a controlled study. *J Am Acad Child Adolesc Psychiatry*. 2011;50(4):340–348, 348, e1–e2.
148. Oral R, Ramirez M, Coohey C, et al. Adverse childhood experiences and trauma informed care: the future of healthcare. *Pediatr Res*. 2016;79(1–2):227–233.
149. Izard CE, King KA, Trentacosta CJ, et al. Accelerating the development of emotion competence in Head Start children: effects on adaptive and maladaptive behavior. *Dev Psychopathol*. 2008 Winter;20(1):369–397.
150. Oyserman D, Terry K, Bybee D. A possible selves intervention to enhance school involvement. *J Adolesc*. 2002; 25(3):313–326.
151. Wesely JK. Mentoring at-risk youth: an examination of strain and mentor response strategies. *Am J Crim Justice*. 2017;42:198–217.
152. Diamond A, Lee K. Interventions shown to aid executive function development in children 4 to 12 years old. *Science*. 2011;333(6045):959–964.
153. Nurius PS, Green S, Logan-Greene P, et al. Life course pathways of adverse childhood experiences toward adult psychological well-being: a stress process analysis. *Child Abuse Negl*. 2015;45:143–153.
154. Evans GW, Gonnella C, Marcynyszyn LA, et al. The role of chaos in poverty and children's socioemotional adjustment. *Psychol Sci*. 2005;16(7):560–565.
155. Blair C, Raver CC. Poverty, stress, and brain development: new directions for prevention and intervention. *Acad Pediatr*. 2016;16(suppl 3):S30–S36.
156. Savage-McGlynn E, Redshaw M, Heron J, et al. Mechanisms of resilience in children of mothers who self-report with depressive symptoms in the first postnatal year. *PLoS One*. 2015;10(11):e0142898.
157. Ghosh IC, Harris WW, Van Horn P, et al. Traumatic and stressful events in early childhood: can treatment help those at highest risk? *Child Abuse Negl*. 2011;35: 504–513.
158. Cohen JA, Deblinger E, Mannarino AP, Steer RA. A multisite, randomized controlled trial for children with sexual abuse-related PTSD symptoms. *J Am Acad Child Adolesc Psychiatry*. 2004;43(4):393–402.
159. Dorsey S, Conover KL, Revillion Cox J. Improving foster parent engagement: using qualitative methods to guide tailoring of evidence-based engagement strategies. *J Clin Child Adolesc Psychol*. 2014;43(6):877–889.
160. Agnew R. Foundation for a general strain theory of crime and delinquency. *Criminology*. 1992;30(1):47–88.
161. Goodkind S, Schelbe LA, Shook JJ. Why youth leave care: understandings of adulthood and transition successes

and challenges among youth aging out of child welfare. *Child Youth Serv Rev.* 2011;33:1039–1048.

162. Sulimani-Aidan Y. Barriers and resources in transition to adulthood among at-risk young adults. *Child Youth Serv Rev.* 2017;77:147–152.
163. Arnett JJ. Emerging adulthood. A theory of development from the late teens through the twenties. *Am Psychol.* 2000;55(5):469–480.
164. Hendry LB, Kloep M. How universal is emerging adulthood? An empirical update. *J Youth Stud.* 2010;13(2): 169–179.
165. Greenberg MT. Promoting resilience in children and youth: preventive interventions and their interface with neuroscience. *Ann N Y Acad Sci.* 2006;1094:139–150.
166. Leppin AL, Bora PR, Tilburt JC, et al. The efficacy of resiliency training programs: a systematic review and meta-analysis of randomized trials. *PLoS One.* 2014;9(10): e111420.
167. Pluess M, Boniwell I, Hefferon K, et al. Preliminary evaluation of a school-based resilience-promoting intervention in a high-risk population: application of an exploratory two-cohort treatment/control design. *PLoS One.* 2017;12(5):e0177191.
168. Li X, Harrison SE, Fairchild AJ, et al. A randomized controlled trial of a resilience-based intervention on psychosocial well-being of children affected by HIV/AIDS: effects at 6- and 12-month follow-up. *Soc Sci Med.* 2017;190:256–264. pii: S0277-9536(17)30087-4.
169. Houston JB, First J, Spialek ML, et al. Randomized controlled trial of the Resilience and Coping Intervention (RCI) with undergraduate university students. *J Am Coll Health.* 2017;65(1):1–9.
170. Mace R, Carroll D. Stress inoculation training to control anxiety in sport: two case studies in squash. *Br J Sports Med.* 1986;20(3):115–117.
171. Jaremko ME. The use of stress inoculation training in the reduction of public speaking anxiety. *J Clin Psychol.* 1980; 36(3):735–742.
172. Bonanno GA, Brewin CR, Kaniasty K, et al. Weighing the costs of disaster: consequences, risks, and resilience in individuals, families, and communities. *Psychol Sci Public Interest.* 2010;11(1):1–49.
173. Credé M, Tynan MC, Harms PD. Much ado about grit: a meta-analytic synthesis of the grit literature. *J Pers Social Psychol.* 2017;113:492–511.

## FURTHER READING

1. Bell CC. *Eight Pieces of Brocade.* Chicago: Community Mental Health Council, Inc.; 2000.
2. Cohen KS. *The Way of Qigong: The Art and Science of Chinese Energy Healing.* New York: Ballantine Books; 1997.
3. Betancourt TS, Borisova II, Williams TP, et al. Sierra Leone's former child soldiers: a follow-up study of psychosocial adjustment and community reintegration. *Child Dev.* 2010;81(4):1077–1095.
4. Bradley R, Greene J, Russ E, et al. A multidimensional meta-analysis of psychotherapy for PTSD. *Am J Psychiatry.* 2005;162:214–227.
5. Duckworth AL, Peterson C, Matthews MD, et al. Grit: perseverance and passion for long term goals. *J Pers Soc Psychol.* 2007;92:1087–1101.
6. Ehring T, Welboren R, Morina N, et al. Meta-analysis of psychological treatments for posttraumatic stress disorder in adult survivors of childhood abuse. *Clin Psychol Rev.* 2014;34:645–657.
7. Gilbert LK, Breiding MJ, Merrick MT, et al. Childhood adversity and adult chronic disease: an update from ten states and the District of Columbia, 2010. *Am J Prev Med.* 2015;48(3):345–349.
8. Giller E. *What Is Psychological Trauma?* Sidran Institute; 1999. Available at: http://www.sidran.org/resources/for-survivors-and-loved-ones/what-is-psychological-trauma/.
9. Heckman J, Krueger A, eds. *Inequality in America: What Role for Human Capital Policy?* MIT Press; 2003. Available at: https://www.irp.wisc.edu/publications/focus/pdfs/foc233a.pdf. Accessed 08.17.17.
10. Lee S, Aos S, Drake E, et al. *Return on Investment: Evidence-Based Options to Improve Statewide Outcomes.* April 2012 update. Olympia, WA: Washington State Institute for Public Policy; 2012. Available at: http://www.wsipp.wa.gov/ReportFile/1102/Wsipp_Return-on-Investment-Evidence-Based-Options-to-Improve-Statewide-Outcomes-April-2012-Update_Full-Report.pdf. Accessed 08.17.17.
11. Shipherd JC, Street AE, Resick PA. Cognitive therapy for posttraumatic stress disorder. In: Follette VM, Rosef JI, eds. *Cognitive-behavioral Therapies for Trauma.* 2nd ed. New York: Guilford Press; 2006:96–106.
12. Twohig MP. Acceptance and commitment therapy for treatment-resistant posttraumatic stress disorder: a case study, Utah State University. *Cogn Behav Prac.* 2009;16: 243–252.

CHAPTER 16

# Spiritual Screening in Adolescents

DALJEET RAI, MD • ALI STUHL, MTS, BA • VINCENT MORELLI, MD •
NAVDEEP RAI, MD

## INTRODUCTION

In literature, the terms religiosity and spirituality are often used interchangeably, although there is a difference between the two. Religiosity is associated with institutions, scriptures, rituals, and organizational membership,[1] while spirituality refers to a more subjective search for peace, harmony, meaning, and connection with the sacred.[2] For the purposes of this chapter, when possible, we will use spirituality or religiosity/spirituality (R/S), as the broader more encompassing terms.

Whether spirituality is an innate part of human nature or is engraved upon us by culture and environment has long been debated. The adherents of the "nature" argument see the commonalities of spirituality across cultures and historical periods as undeniable evidence that R/S is hardwired. The "nurture" proponents, on the other hand, see culture/socialization as inculcating our spiritual values. Most scholars today, however, instead of an either–or proposition, view nature and nurture as additives, with nature providing the biological foundation and nurture contributing to the cultural aspects of our spirituality.[3]

Regardless of where one stands in the debate, the value of human spirituality cannot be denied. There is a consensus that R/S serves the purposes of helping to establish identity, enhance health, and form a connection to community and the divine. In adolescents, the importance of spirituality is evidenced in overarching documents such as the United Nations Convention on the Rights of the Child, which mandates a child's right "to develop physically, mentally, morally, spiritually, and socially in a healthy, normal manner in conditions of freedom and dignity."[4]

Yet despite the common acceptance that spirituality is integral to develop youths, there is a relative paucity of literature addressing the topic in this age group and even less on the focus of this chapter—adolescent spiritual *screening*. In addition, the studies that do exist on adolescent screening often use tools that fail to take into account an adolescent's developmental stage. For example, a 13-year-old adolescent's emotional insight, abstract thinking, and spirituality differ significantly from that of one who is 18 years old. In addition, most tools fail to consider the effect of family and peers on spirituality, are not well validated, or are simply too general to offer meaningful insight.[5] These are all glaring shortcomings because adolescents are in a state of ever-changing development where family and peers still play a significant role in identity formation, habits, beliefs, and adapted spiritual values.

Keeping these shortcomings in mind, there is still much to be gained from reviewing the adolescent literature on the health impacts of spiritualty and spiritual screening, and much to be gleaned from the adult literature as well. In this chapter, we will first review the proposed mechanisms through which R/S is thought to impact health. Then we will examine the literature connecting spirituality to *adult* health, providing a context from which to examine the less-studied health associations of adolescent spirituality. With this background, we will next examine the extant work on adolescent spirituality and health, highlighting the importance of establishing healthy adolescent spiritual habits that are likely to go on to affect adult health. Much like heart disease and diabetes can largely be prevented by establishing healthful habits early, spirituality in adolescence may serve as a "habit" which can be expected to convey health benefits into adulthood.[6–8] Finally, in this chapter, we will discuss three of the most common methods at our disposal to screen for adolescent spirituality. All this is an attempt to help our adolescent patients, parents,

Adolescent Health Screening: An Update in the Age of Big Data. https://doi.org/10.1016/B978-0-323-66130-0.00016-8

and primary care providers (PCPs) become more aware of the health impacts of spirituality; to choose appropriate methods of screening; to know the limitations of our current state of knowledge; and, hopefully, to help instill lifelong healthful habits in our youths.

### Mechanisms by Which Spirituality Conveys Health Benefits

Spirituality imparts its beneficial health effects through at least four mechanisms:

1. Behavior mechanisms: Certain spiritual practices advocate healthy diets and advise against smoking, alcohol, drugs, and other risky behaviors.
2. Social mechanisms: R/S groups can provide supportive communities that can, like family and other social groups, convey healthful equanimity through a sense of belonging.
3. Psychologic and emotional mechanisms: These provide support, especially in the face of stress or chronic illness.
4. Physical mechanisms: These include neurohormonal responses brought on by a spiritual mindset in the face of stressors. These physiologic changes are measurable (e.g., heart rate, blood pressure, cortisol levels) and have been termed the "relax response" of spirituality.[9]

Given that spirituality is believed to bestow such health benefits, we can easily appreciate how it could play a significant role in our current epidemic of noncommunicable diseases (NCDs). NCDs such as heart disease, smoking-induced respiratory disease, diabetes, etc. have become a major source of mortality and premature deaths,[10] killing over 41 million people per year (71% of all deaths globally),[11] and although such NCDs are obviously caused by a combination of genetic, environmental, and behavioral factors, individual behaviors, influenced by spirituality, are certainly significant contributors.[12]

## ADULT SPIRITUALITY

Because up to 90% of patients believe spirituality to be important in health[13] and coping with illness,[14] and because research has been increasingly illuminating spirituality's association with health outcomes, the Joint Commission on Accreditation of Healthcare Organizations (JCAHO) now requires that a spiritual assessment be done on all patients admitted to the hospital.[15] Although they do not specify how exactly spirituality should be assessed, there are several spiritual history tools available and judged as "superior" for use in adults.[a]

A 2013 review of 25 spiritual history instruments noted 5 as "superior" and useful in the clinical setting.[18] The five tools were FICA (2000), SPIRITual History (1996), FAITH (2009), HOPE (2001), and The Royal College of Psychiatrists' Assessment. Although only one of these has been validated in any way, all five were deemed superior because they met several of the 16 criteria the authors *felt* were important. Criteria such as "easy to remember in the clinical setting" and "not too time consuming," as well as 14 others, were decided to be important.

Overall, there is a need for spiritual history tools to become academically validated and a need for academic spiritual screening tools to become more useful in the clinical setting. That being said, the academically validated spiritual assessment tools provide a more accurate way of approaching spirituality, that is, spirituality as a multidimensional concept best assessed by examining the individual components of spirituality. These individual components can then be evaluated and discussed more easily in terms of health outcomes. We will discuss this multidimensional approach to spiritualty later in our in-depth look into adolescent spirituality screening tools.

### Assessing Spirituality in Adults

There are over 120 adult spiritual assessment or spiritual history tools documented in the literature,[19] and because of the multitude and heterogeneity of the tools, it can be difficult to draw precise conclusions regarding the impact of spirituality on health. There are essentially two ways to approach the issue. First, one may consider spirituality as a "single construct." This approach regards each of the many spiritual history/assessment tools as equal and adequate, and they simply examine the health outcomes associated with each. In doing this, one assumes that each tool measures spirituality

[a]Taking a *spiritual history* in the clinical setting is quite different from using psychometrically validated *spiritual screening tools* as we will see later. The spiritual history is simply a "set of questions designed to invite patients to share their spiritual beliefs and help identify spiritual issues." In other words, the history is a just method of getting patients to talk about their spirituality, whereas the spiritual screening tools used in research are designed to tease out the components of spirituality. They are more psychometrically validated and more useful in assessing health outcomes. Thus the "superior" spiritual history tools mentioned earlier will extract some useful information from patients but will leave us with little insight into which aspects of spirituality might be lacking or how such deficits might lead to untoward health effects.[16,17]

equally and adequately and then can be associated with health outcomes. The second way to approach the subject is much more analytic. It involves breaking down spirituality into its elemental components then examining each component's association to health. For example, we might tease out forgiveness or meaning as essential components of spirituality and then examine each separately with regard to their respective health impact. In the following sections, we will first provide an overview of the health outcomes associated with "single-construct spirituality" in adults. Later, when we discuss adolescent spirituality, we will review the literature in both regards: first examining the health association of single-construct spirituality and then breaking down spirituality into its elemental components and looking at each component individually as it relates to health. (Spirituality as a "multidimensional" construct.)

### Single-Construct Spirituality in Adult Physical Health

When one looks at spirituality as a single construct, its impact on adult physical health can be assessed in the literature. A comprehensive review[20] found that a slight majority of high-quality studies document a beneficial effect of R/S on cardiovascular disease, cognitive function, self-reported health, and overall mortality. Cardiovascular disease seems particularly strongly associated with spiritual influences, with one study noting a 20% decrease in 5-year mortality from congestive heart failure in spiritual patients.[21] Another of the clearest benefits of spirituality can be seen in overall mortality, where over 75% of well-performed studies have documented R/S as being associated with improved longevity. One particularly well-performed meta-analysis of over 126,000 study participants[22] noted that after accounting for all confounding variables, religion still conferred a small but clear mortality benefit. The slight increased longevity was seen most robustly in those who were "publicly religious" that is, those who frequently attended services or were involved in religious groups. Authors believed this robustness was confirmed by the inherent psychosocial benefits of group involvement.

### Single-Construct Spirituality in Adult Mental and Behavioral Health

The majority of published studies have also documented a beneficial association between single-construct spirituality and adult mental health. Those with a strong sense of R/S have been shown to

- be less likely to develop anxiety and depression,
- be less likely to suffer from eating disorders,
- have higher esteem and psychologic competence,
- have an enhanced ability to deal with adversity,
- experience less posttraumatic stress disorder (PTSD),
- be less likely to abuse alcohol or engage in other risky behaviors,
- have less suicidal ideation.[20,22–27]

Spirituality also conveys a protective effect on personality and behavior disorders; those with greater spirituality are being less likely to develop borderline personality disorder,[28] antisocial behavior disorder (lack of regard for the rights of others), impulse control disorder, and criminality.[29] An adult's sense of spiritual well-being (SWB) is also associated with greater overall "psychologic well-being" (social, emotional, mental, and functional health involving self-acceptance, autonomy, mastery, purpose, growth, and relations to others),[30–32] higher levels of optimism and hope, higher levels of social support, and greater life satisfaction and happiness.[33,34]

Overall then, "single-construct" adult spirituality has been associated with better physical, mental, and behavioral health and better overall psychologic well-being. However, the reader should consider three caveats before lauding these above benefits. First, not all studies show a salutary effect of R/S on health. A minority of studies have documented an *increase* in anxiety, depression, cardiovascular disease, hypertension, cognitive functioning, physical functioning, and cancer in those considered to have greater R/S. Authors explain these untoward effects by the guilt, stress, or anxiety felt by some adherents when they fail to live up to religious standards.[20] The second caveat to consider is that the effect that R/S has on each of the health domains (i.e., physical, mental, behavioral health) is small, and thus should not be overweighted.[35] The final caveat is that research has documented only an *association* of spirituality with health outcomes. It has not documented causation. Saying that a lack of spirituality is associated with depression is quite different from saying that spiritual deficits *cause* depression, or that enhancing spirituality can help *treat* the affliction.

### Multidimensional Spirituality in Adults

We will not discuss the multidimensional aspects of spirituality in adults, that is, spirituality broken down into its component parts. As discussed, the rationale for presenting the previous section on the health impacts of single-construct adult spirituality is to illuminate what may happen if subpar adolescent spiritual habits are allowed to continue into adulthood. From the perspective of this chapter, the multidimensional aspects of spirituality are better looked at in terms *adolescent* spirituality, as we will discuss in the following.

## ADOLESCENT SPIRITUALITY

As mentioned in our introductory chapter, adolescence is a time of transition, identity formation, and the establishment of habits[36,37] that will carry over into adulthood. It is also a time when teens often begin their search for identity, meaning,[b] and spirituality.

Naturally, there are many other factors at play in identity formation and making meaning, such as family, peers, extracurricular activities, technology, etc. The fact remains, however, that spirituality can be a significant contributor.

This is especially true in the United States where the vast majority of teens, 84%, identify themselves as being religious and roughly half report that religion is very important to them. Although researchers have noted a decrease in religious interest and a small increase in more personalized spirituality, religion still remains an important aspect in the lives and identities of many of America's youths.[42–45]

With this in mind, questions naturally arise: "Do the 50% of the youth who regard religion as very important have better physical, emotional, behavioral, cognitive, or mental health outcomes than their less-religious counterparts? Are those without the guidance of spirituality more susceptible to poor habits, risky behaviors, delinquency, depression, and other physical and emotional maladies? Will those who are more spiritual in adolescence go on to have better health as adults?" To answer these questions, we will first have to review how one assesses spirituality in this age group.

## SPIRITUAL SCREENING IN ADOLESCENCE

As noted earlier, there is a relative lack of research discussing adolescent R/S. There are fewer spiritual assessment tools available, they are less validated, and there is less data examining health outcomes. Those adolescent screening tools that do exist are complicated by several factors including the following:

1. The difficulty in crafting "one tool" to account for the differences in developmental levels between "young" and "old" adolescents. (In a review, only 15 of 100 articles examining adolescent screening took developmental issues into account.[46])
2. Varying parental and peer influences a youth experiences are infrequently explored.
3. The influences of community, ethnic, and cultural norms are similarly not often incorporated into screening.
4. The multidimensional aspects of spirituality are not easily or adequately screened for in adolescents, especially in "short-form" assessment tools. This is important because some dimensions of spirituality (e.g., prayer, attending services, feelings of equanimity) may prove more health affecting than others.
5. The fact that over 66% of studies examining adolescent screening tools make no mention of psychometric validity and over 80% of such studies report on tools that have not been previously tested in adolescents.[46]

These difficulties are only part of the problem. There are also the obvious practical problems of addressing adolescent spirituality in short clinical encounters and the fact that most PCPs (60%) feel a lack of experience in approaching the subject.[47,48] Such considerations, as well as the "only modest" impact that spirituality has on health, leaves many questioning the utility of adolescent spiritual screening with the tools now available.

With this said, there are over 35 adolescent R/S screening tools in use and,[49] although there is no gold standard,[50] the most frequently used tools are the Multidimensional Measure of Religiousness/Spirituality (MMRS); its truncated version, the Brief MMRS (BMMRS)[9]; the Spiritual Well-Being Scale (SWBS)[51]; adolescent versions of the Religious Coping (RCOPE) scale[52]; the Religious Orientation Scale (ROS)[53]; and the Systems of Belief Inventory.[54] We will discuss three of the most commonly used tools, the MMRS, BMMRS, and SWBS, in our analysis to give the reader a general overview and to offer a practical, evidenced-based approach to screening and associated health outcomes. An in-depth discussion and comparison of *each* of the abovementioned tools is beyond the scope of this chapter.

As in our section on Adult Spirituality, we will first look at spirituality as a "single construct" in adolescence followed by a closer analysis of spirituality as a multidimensional construct, reviewing the health impacts associated with each.

## ADOLESCENT SPIRITUALITY AS A SINGLE CONSTRUCT

### Ties to Mental, Behavioral, and Physical Health and Positive Youth Development

#### *Mental and behavioral health*

The literature has demonstrated that, generally, R/S teens exhibit less risky health behaviors, have fewer mental health issues, have fewer behavior problems,

[b]Although R/S has been shown to help establish identity and meaning, it is not *necessary* to accomplish either.[38–41]

have less suicidal ideation, and better utilize spiritual coping to manage stress and physical illness.[50,55–59] Spirituality has been noted to be particularly strongly associated with teens coping well with chronic illness[60,61] and avoiding alcohol, substance use, smoking, and risky sexual behavior. Indeed, roughly 90% of well-performed studies document an associated beneficial effect of R/S in these categories.[20] R/S teens are also less likely to develop delinquent and antisocial behaviors (e.g., violence, stealing, trouble with police),[62–64] less prone to substandard academic achievement,[20] and more likely to have higher self-esteem, holding more positive attitudes about life than their nonspiritual peers.[35]

Systemic reviews and meta-analyses have also found spirituality to render youths slightly less susceptible to anxiety and depression,[35,65] an important consideration in adolescents, of whom 65% will experience significant depressive symptoms and almost 20% will experience a full-blown depressive episode.[66,67] Depression, of course, has been proven to lead to academic problems, difficulties in relationships, and increased psychopathologic conditions as adults.[68] These mental health associations are important, as spirituality's potential impact in this area could be highly significant in a world where over 430 million people are affected by mental health disorders.[83]

#### *Physical health*

Physical health and "single-construct spirituality" is a bit more difficult to examine, as adolescents are generally healthy and many somatic health effects tied to R/S will only become evident over the long term. In this regard, it is helpful to look at the impact of R/S on *adult* physical health, as we have done earlier, and then extrapolate back to adolescence; our point being that encouraging spirituality and other healthful habits in youths will confer salutary benefits later in adulthood.

### Spirituality and Positive Youth Development

A new concept in adolescent growth is that of positive youth development (PYD). Slowly gaining a foothold since the 1990s, PYD programs are designed to help youths progress toward a healthy adulthood. The construct is defined by adolescent attainment of the five *C*'s, namely, competence, confidence, character, connection, and caring/compassion, along with a sixth *C*, contribution, becoming integral as an adolescent begins to "thrive."[69] Spirituality is often considered an essential component of these programs, supporting character, connection, and compassion.[70,71] The association between PYD and spirituality has been explored in the literature and has been positively correlated with PYD.[71] The association seems particularly strong in younger (and presumably more impressionable) adolescents and when a teen's spirituality is coherently organized and can be clearly articulated.[70]

### Adolescent Single-Construct Spirituality: The Caveats

As with adult caveats, we must again note the potentially negative influence that R/S can have on adolescent health. A minority of studies have documented an *increase* in anxiety, depression, sedentary lifestyle, and obesity.[20,57] Also, remember that the overall effect that R/S has on adolescent health (mental and behavioral health) is small,[35] and we are only documenting an *association* between spirituality and health, not causation.

In summary, despite the fact that the beneficial effects of "single-construct spirituality" on adolescent mental, emotional, and behavioral health are small and that a minority of adolescents will experience untoward health effects because of R/S, overall, spirituality can still be considered a positive attribute in adolescents. Too little or too much R/S may be detrimental, but a moderate amount may be "just right."

## ADOLESCENT SPIRITUALITY AS A MULTIDIMENSIONAL CONSTRUCT

### The Commonly Used Scale: The Multidimensional Measure of Religiousness/Spirituality/Brief Multidimensional Measure of Religiousness/Spirituality

In 1999, in response to the lack of uniformity in spiritual assessment tools and the realization that "spirituality" represented more than just a single construct, the Fetzer Institute convened a group of experts and tasked them with breaking down spirituality into its essential components. The collaboration resulted in the creation of a scale that is now one of the most commonly used and most widely vetted methods of evaluating spirituality for use in research, namely, the MMRS. The scale divides spirituality into 12 subdomains, each contributing to one's "overall spirituality." The 12 subdomains agreed upon were daily spiritual experiences, meaning, values, beliefs, forgiveness, private religious practices (PRP), religious/spiritual coping, religious support (RS), religious/spiritual history, commitment, organizational religiousness, and religious preference. This was a conscientious effort to tease out the basic building blocks of spirituality so that researchers could then examine each subdomain's impact on health.

Although researchers are just beginning to examine the individual subdomains of the MMRS, the current literature does allow us to look critically at the health impacts of a few of them. Some of the better studied and more validated subdomains in relation to health outcomes are meaning/purpose, daily spirituality experiences (confusingly called "spirituality" in some studies), religious practices/organized religiousness (OR), religious coping, and forgiveness.[52,72–74] In the following sections, we will take a closer look at these five subdomains in an effort to present some of the strongest evidence tying adolescent spirituality to health outcomes.

## Meaning

The literature examining meaning/purpose and health can be confusing for at least two reasons. First, when speaking of meaning, the difference between one who has found meaning (an *outcome*) and one who is searching for meaning (a *process*) is often not differentiated in the literature. This distinction is important, as each may be associated with different health outcomes and thus *should* be examined separately.[75] Second, the terms "meaning" and "purpose" are often used interchangeably or combined as a single metric in assessment tools. This is despite the fact that meaning and purpose are better thought of as distinct concepts: "meaning" defined as a sense of understanding the significance of life and "purpose" being more of a goal orientation or direction in life.[76] Although the two concepts should be viewed as distinct entities, too often they are not.

Although many of the multidimensional spiritual assessment tools in use today make this error, they can still be useful as "combined measures" (i.e., measuring outcome and process, meaning and purpose) and are thus mentioned here. The most common combined meaning/purpose assessment tools the reader is likely to encounter in the literature are the Purpose in Life (PIL) scale, the Seeking of Noetic Goals (SONG) scale, Ryff's PIL subscale, the Life Regard Index (LRI), the Sense of Coherence (SOC) Scale, and perhaps the most validated of these, the MMRS's meaning subdomain.

Since the 1999 and 2003 Fetzer Institute[9] reports espousing the importance of tying meaning to health outcomes, there have been a few studies associating meaning with adolescent health. Extracting conclusions from the studies do exist; however, we can say that, overall in adolescents, a sense of meaning and purpose is beneficial. Meaning combined with purpose has been associated with lower rates of substance abuse, less risky sexual behaviors,[77] better dietary habits, increased physical activity,[77] greater self-esteem,[78] greater optimism and happiness,[79,80] greater psychologic well-being,[81] and greater life satisfaction.[82]

Meaning, specifically teased out from purpose, has only been associated with greater resilience and posttraumatic growth,[76] but it has not been specifically studied with regard to other health outcomes. Purpose, teased out from meaning, has been associated with fewer intrusive thoughts and less anxiety, but, as with meaning, it is less studied with regard to other health outcomes (Table 16.1).[76]

## Daily Spiritual Experiences

The Daily Spiritual Experience Scale (DSES) is a 16-item scale (see Table 16.2) that checks for daily experiences of connection with the divine. It includes measures of awe, gratitude, and mercy; feelings of connection; compassionate love; and a sense of inner peace. It was designed both for the religious and the "spiritual but not religious" and has been psychometrically validated across cultures, countries, and languages, as well as in adolescents.

DSES has been validated in ethnically diverse adolescents[83] and is highly predictive of lower psychologic stress,[84] greater positive affect and life satisfaction, less depressive symptoms,[85] more compliant health behaviors,[86] and lower levels of substance abuse.

Since habits begun in adolescence often carry over into adulthood, we will briefly mention the associations of DSES with *adult* health. Again, our intent is to illuminate the potential long-term fallout associated with spiritual habits formed during adolescence. In terms of adult physical, mental, and behavioral health, fewer DSES have been associated with worse self-reported psychologic and physical health[87,88]; deficient healthful behaviors such as dietary indiscretions and physical inactivity[89]; worse mental outlooks in chronic pain patients[90,91]; more depression, anxiety, loneliness,[92] and work burnout[93,94]; more substance abuse[73,95]; lower self-reported marital happiness in both men and women[96]; more days of long-term care in nursing homes or rehab centers for older adults[97]; and lower levels of happiness, self-esteem, optimism, and life satisfaction.[98]

## Private Religious Practices, Religious Support, and Organized Religiousness

This category combines the MMRS subdomains of PRP, RS, and OR. It queries items such as attendance at

**TABLE 16.1**
**Meaning/Purpose Subscale Based on the Multidimensional Measure of Religiousness/Spirituality**

**Meaning-Long Form (No Short Form)**

1. My spiritual beliefs give meaning to my life's joys and sorrows.
   a. Strongly disagree
   b. Disagree
   c. Neutral
   d. Agree
   e. Strongly agree
2. The goals of my life grow out of my understanding of God.
   a. Strongly disagree
   b. Disagree
   c. Neutral
   d. Agree
   e. Strongly agree
3. Without a sense of spirituality, my daily life would be meaningless.
   a. Strongly disagree
   b. Disagree
   c. Neutral
   d. Agree
   e. Strongly agree
4. The meaning in my life comes from feeling connected to other living things.
   a. Strongly disagree
   b. Disagree
   c. Neutral
   d. Agree
   e. Strongly agree
5. My religious beliefs help me find a purpose in even with painful and confusing events.
   a. Strongly disagree
   b. Disagree
   c. Neutral
   d. Agree
   e. Strongly agree
6. When I lose touch with God, I have a harder time feeling there is purpose and meaning in life.
   a. Strongly disagree
   b. Disagree
   c. Neutral
   d. Agree
   e. Strongly agree
7. My spiritual beliefs give my life a sense of significance and purpose.
   a. Strongly disagree
   b. Disagree
   c. Neutral
   d. Agree
   e. Strongly agree

**TABLE 16.1**
**Meaning/Purpose Subscale Based on the Multidimensional Measure of Religiousness/Spirituality—cont'd**

**Meaning-Long Form (No Short Form)**

8. My mission in life is guided/shaped by my faith in God.
   a. Strongly disagree
   b. Disagree
   c. Neutral
   d. Agree
   e. Strongly agree
9. When I am disconnected from the spiritual dimension of my life, I lose my sense of purpose.
   a. Strongly disagree
   b. Disagree
   c. Neutral
   d. Agree
   e. Strongly agree
10. My relationship with God helps me find meaning in the ups and downs of life.
    a. Strongly disagree
    b. Disagree
    c. Neutral
    d. Agree
    e. Strongly agree
11. My life is significant because I am part of God's plan.
    a. Strongly disagree
    b. Disagree
    c. Neutral
    d. Agree
    e. Strongly agree
12. What I try to do in my day-to-day life is important to me from a spiritual point of view.
    a. Strongly disagree
    b. Disagree
    c. Neutral
    d. Agree
    e. Strongly agree
13. I am trying to fulfill my God-given purpose in life.
    a. Strongly disagree
    b. Disagree
    c. Neutral
    d. Agree
    e. Strongly agree
14. Knowing that I am a part of something greater than myself gives meaning to my life.
    a. Strongly disagree
    b. Disagree
    c. Neutral
    d. Agree
    e. Strongly agree

*Continued*

**TABLE 16.1**
**Meaning/Purpose Subscale Based on the Multidimensional Measure of Religiousness/Spirituality—cont'd**

| Meaning-Long Form (No Short Form) |
|---|
| 15. Looking at the most troubling/confusing events from a spiritual perspective adds meaning.<br>a. Strongly disagree<br>b. Disagree<br>c. Neutral<br>d. Agree<br>e. Strongly agree |
| 16. My purpose in life reflects what I believe God wants for me.<br>a. Strongly disagree<br>b. Disagree<br>c. Neutral<br>d. Agree<br>e. Strongly agree |
| 17 Without my religious foundation, my life would be meaningless.<br>a. Strongly disagree<br>b. Disagree<br>c. Neutral<br>d. Agree<br>e. Strongly agree |
| 18. My feelings of spirituality add meaning to the events in my life.<br>a. Strongly disagree<br>b. Disagree<br>c. Neutral<br>d. Agree<br>e. Strongly agree |
| 19. God plays a role in how I choose my path in life.<br>a. Strongly disagree<br>b. Disagree<br>c. Neutral<br>d. Agree<br>e. Strongly agree |
| 20. My spirituality helps define the goals I set for myself.<br>a. Strongly disagree<br>b. Disagree<br>c. Neutral<br>d. Agree<br>e. Strongly agree |

From Fetzer Institute/National Institute on Aging Working Group. *Multidimensional measurement of religiousness/spirituality for use in health research: A report of the Fetzer Institute/National Institute on aging working group*. Kalamazoo: John E. Fetzer Institute; 1999, Accessed November 2018. http://fetzer.org/sites/default/files/images/resources/attachment/%5Bcurrent-date%3Atiny%5D/Multidimensional_Measurement_of_Religousness_Spirituality.pdf.

religious services or participation in choir or youth groups (OR), how supportive one's spiritual group is (RS), and PRP such as prayer, saying grace, and watching religious videos, which are activities that individuals may exercise outside the confines of institutional religion (Table 16.3).

In adolescents, PRP, RS, and OR have been associated with lower rates of depression, suicidal ideation,[99] substance abuse,[100] and initiation of smoking.[101]

In adults, PRP, RS, and OR, though not optimally validated, have been significantly associated with greater physical/psychologic health and well-being,[102] as well as overall improved health. They have been associated with lower rates of substance abuse, smoking, mood disorders, and[103] suicide.[104] Again, we mention these adult effects so that the reader will realize that the effects of spiritual habits—in this case, PRP, RS, and OR—begun in adolescence will carry over to adulthood and perhaps have long-term implications on adult health.

## Religious/Spiritual Coping

One of the early scales designed for measuring religious/spiritual coping was called the RCOPE scale.[105] The scale was internally consistent, reliable, and valid and allowed for three styles of spiritual coping to be considered (a deferring style, a self-directing style, and a collaborative style). However, the lengthy, time-consuming RCOPE scale did not achieve widespread use. In response, researchers developed the Brief RCOPE scale,[106] a shortened 14-item measure that was proven internally consistent, reliable, and valid (concurrent validity, predictive validity, and incremental validity) (see Table 16.4).

It is currently the most commonly used measure of religious coping and has been validated across cultures[74,107–109] and in adolescents.[110,111]

The Brief RCOPE scale surveys both positive coping (i.e., the use of faith for comfort during crisis) and negative coping (i.e., the struggles or doubts experienced because of spiritual outlooks during times of stress). The way in which one copes with life's trying situations can have either a calming or a deleterious effect on health. Positive coping has been found to be associated with lower distress and a greater sense of well-being in people with several chronic conditions such as asthma, cystic fibrosis,[60] diabetes, cancer, and epilepsy.[61] Negative religious coping, on the other hand, has emerged as a robust predictor of negative health outcomes during stress.[9] Increased depression,[112] eating disorders,[113]

TABLE 16.2
The Daily Spiritual Experience Scale (With Item Numbers Added)

| | | Many Times a Day | Every Day | Most Days | Some Days | Once in a While | Never or Almost Never |
|---|---|---|---|---|---|---|---|
| 1[a] | I feel God's presence. | | | | | | |
| 2 | I experience a connection to all of life. | | | | | | |
| 3 | During worship, or at other times when connecting with God, I feel joy which lifts me out of my daily concerns. | | | | | | |
| 4[a] | I find strength in my religion or spirituality. | | | | | | |
| 5[a] | I find comfort in my religion or spirituality. | | | | | | |
| 6[a] | I feel deep inner peace or harmony. | | | | | | |
| 7 | I ask for God's help in the midst of daily activities. | | | | | | |
| 8 | I feel guided by God in the midst of daily activities. | | | | | | |
| 9[a] | I feel God's love for me directly. | | | | | | |
| 10[a] | I feel God's love for me through others. | | | | | | |
| 11[a] | I am spiritually touched by the beauty of creation. | | | | | | |
| 12 | I feel thankful for my blessings. | | | | | | |
| 13 | I feel a selfless caring for others. | | | | | | |
| 14 | I accept others even when they do things I think are wrong. | | | | | | |
| 15[a] | I desire to be closer to God or in union with the divine | | | | | | |
| | | **Not close** | **Somewhat close** | **Very close** | **As close as possible** | | |
| 16 | In general, how close do you feel to God? | | | | | | |

Introduction: The list that follows includes items you may or may not experience. Please consider how often you directly have this experience and try to disregard whether you feel you should or should not have these experiences. A number of items use the word "God." If this word is not a comfortable one for you, please substitute another word that calls to mind the divine or holy for you.

[a] Items that were used to form part of the Brief Multidimensional Measure of Religiousness/Spirituality six-item scale, Daily Spiritual Experience domain. Items 4 and 5 were combined: "I find strength and comfort in my religion." Items 9 and 10 were also combined: "I feel God's love for me directly or through others." These form part of the six-item Daily Spiritual Experience Scale referred to in the text.

and substance abuse[114] have all been associated with the Brief RCOPE scale's negative coping scale.

## Forgiveness

Forgiveness has been theorized to link spirituality to physical and psychologic health.[115] However, it was not known how significant a factor "forgiveness alone" was in this regard. It was not known if forgiveness could convey health benefits to those with the ability to forgive regardless of their "overall spirituality."

A 2018 article[116] examined just that—the association of forgiveness (forgiveness of self, of others, and of divine forgiveness) with psychosocial, mental, behavioral, and physical health outcomes. Although the authors found no association between forgiveness and physical or behavioral health in the 6-year study,

**TABLE 16.3**
**Private Religious Practices, Religious Support, and Organized Religiousness Scales**

**Private Religious Practices Long Form (No Short Form)**

1. How often do you pray privately in places other than at church or synagogue?
   a. Several times a day
   b. Once a day
   c. A few times a week
   d. Once a week
   e. A few times a month
   f. Once a month
   g. Less than once a month
   h. Never
2. How often do you watch or listen to religious programs on TV or radio?
   a. Several times a day
   b. Once a day
   c. A few times a week
   d. Once a week
   e. A few times a month
   f. Once a month
   g. Less than once a month
   h. Never
3. How often do you read the Bible or other religious literature?
   a. Several times a day
   b. Once a day
   c. A few times a week
   d. Once a week
   e. A few times a month
   f. Once a month
   g. Less than once a month
   h. Never
4. How often are prayers or grace said before or after meals in your home?
   a. At all meals
   b. Once a day
   c. At least once a week
   d. Only on special occasions
   e. Never

Scoring: Lower scores represent higher levels of private religious experiences.

**Religious Support: Short Form From BMMRS**
The following questions deal with relationships you have with the people in your congregation.

**EMOTIONAL SUPPORT RECEIVED FROM OTHERS**

1. How often do the people in your congregation make you feel loved and cared for?
   a. Very often
   b. Fairly often
   c. Once in a while
   d. Never

**TABLE 16.3**
**Private Religious Practices, Religious Support, and Organized Religiousness Scales—cont'd**

**Private Religious Practices Long Form (No Short Form)**

2. How often do the people in your congregation listen/talk about your problems and concerns?
   a. Very often
   b. Fairly often
   c. Once in a while
   d. Never

**EMOTIONAL SUPPORT PROVIDED TO OTHERS**

3. How often do you make the people in your congregation feel loved and cared for?
   a. Very often
   b. Fairly often
   c. Once in a while
   d. Never
4. How often do you listen to the people in your congregation talk about problems and concerns?
   a. Very often
   b. Fairly often
   c. Once in a while
   d. Never

**NEGATIVE INTERACTION: CONTACT WITH OTHERS IN YOUR CONGREGATION IS NOT ALWAYS PLEASANT**

5. How often do the people in your congregation make too many demands on you?
   a. Very often
   b. Fairly often
   c. Once in a while
   d. Never
6. How often are the people in your congregation critical of you/things you do?
   a. Very often
   b. Fairly often
   c. Once in a while
   d. Never

**ANTICIPATED SUPPORT**

7. If you were ill, how much would the people in your congregation be willing to help out?
   a. A great deal
   b. Some
   c. A little
   d. None
8. If you had a problem or were faced with a difficult situation, how much comfort would the people in your congregation be willing to give you?
   a. A great deal
   b. Some
   c. A little
   d. None

TABLE 16.3
Private Religious Practices, Religious Support, and Organized Religiousness Scales—cont'd

**Private Religious Practices Long Form (No Short Form)**

Scoring: Score these responses in the following manner (points in parentheses): Very often (4), fairly often (3), once in a while (2), and never (1). Higher scores represent more of a feeling of religious support.

**Organizational Religiousness: Short Form From BMMRS**
**ATTENDANCE (GENERAL SOCIAL SURVEY)**

1. How often do you attend religious services?
   a. Never
   b. Less than once a year
   c. About once or twice a year
   d. Several times a year
   e. About once a month
   f. Two to three times a month
   g. Nearly every week
   h. Every week
   i. Several times a week
2. Besides religious services, how often do you take part in other activities at a place of worship?
   a. Never
   b. Less than once a year
   c. About once or twice a year
   d. Several times a year
   e. About once a month
   f. Two to three times a month
   g. Nearly every week
   h. Every week
   i. Several times a week

*BMMRS*, Brief Multidimensional Measure of Religiousness/Spirituality.
Fetzer Institute/National Institute on Aging Working Group. *Multidimensional measurement of religiousness/spirituality for use in health research: A report of the Fetzer Institute/National Institute on aging working group*. Kalamazoo: John E. Fetzer Institute; 1999. http://fetzer.org/sites/default/files/images/resources/attachment/%5Bcurrent-date%3Atiny%5D/Multidimensional_Measurement_of_Religousness_Spirituality.pdf.

TABLE 16.4

**BRIEF RCOPE SCALE ITEMS**

- Positive spiritual coping reflects the use of faith for comfort.
- Negative spiritual coping reflects struggle, doubt, or doubt with God/faith during crisis.

**BRIEF RCOPE SCALE**

The Brief RCOPE scale is divided into two subscales, each consisting of seven items, which identify clusters of positive and negative religious coping methods. The 14 items (7 positive and 7 negative) are rated on a 4- point scale ("not at all" [0] to "a great deal"). Scores are added and averaged, with higher scores indicating higher levels of positive and negative spiritual coping, respectively. When in a crisis, I …

**Positive Religious Coping Subscale Items**

1. Looked for a stronger connection with God.
2. Sought God's love and care.
3. Sought help from God in letting go of my anger.
4. Tried to put my plans into action together with God.
5. Tried to see how God might be trying to strengthen me in this situation.
6. Asked forgiveness for my sins.
7. Focused on religion to stop worrying about my problems.

**Negative Religious Coping Subscale Items**

8. Wondered whether God had abandoned me.
9. Felt punished by God for my lack of devotion.
10. Wondered what I did for God to punish me.
11. Questioned God's love for me.
12. Wondered whether my church had abandoned me.
13. Decided the devil made this happen.
14. Questioned the power of God.

*RCOPE*, Religious Coping.
Fetzer Institute/National Institute on Aging Working Group. *Multidimensional measurement of religiousness/spirituality for use in health research: A report of the Fetzer Institute/National Institute on aging working group*. Kalamazoo: John E. Fetzer Institute; 1999. http://fetzer.org/sites/default/files/images/resources/attachment/%5Bcurrent-date%3Atiny%5D/Multidimensional_Measurement_of_Religousness_Spirituality.pdf.

they did find that those with a greater capacity to forgive had enhanced psychologic well-being and those with a lesser capacity for forgiveness were at an increased risk of anxiety and depression. Other researchers have noted similar results.[117,118] Interestingly, these and other studies[119] have noted self-forgiveness to be more health-impacting than forgiveness of others or divine forgiveness, possibly because self-forgiveness may involve different emotional and cognitive processes such as the resolution of guilt, shame, and anxiety,[120] whereas forgiveness of others is more related to the resolution of anger.[121] The authors also theorized that divine forgiveness may be a pathway through which self-forgiveness is attained.

**TABLE 16.5**
**Forgiveness Short Form**

| Forgiveness Short Form |
|---|
| 1. I have forgiven myself for things that I have done wrong.<br>a. Always or almost always<br>b. Often<br>c. Seldom<br>d. Never |
| 2. I have forgiven those who hurt me.<br>a. Always or almost always<br>b. Often<br>c. Seldom<br>d. Never |
| 3. I know that God forgives me.<br>a. Always or almost always<br>b. Often<br>c. Seldom<br>d. Never |

Fetzer Institute/National Institute on Aging Working Group. *Multidimensional measurement of religiousness/spirituality for use in health research: A report of the Fetzer Institute/National Institute on aging working group*. Kalamazoo: John E. Fetzer Institute; 1999. http://fetzer.org/sites/default/files/images/resources/attachment/%5Bcurrent-date%3Atiny%5D/Multidimensional_Measurement_of_Religousness_Spirituality.pdf.

The MMRS Forgiveness Scale is shown in Table 16.5.

## Multidimensional Measure of Religiousness/Spirituality and Brief Multidimensional Measure of Religiousness/Spirituality Scoring

The scoring of the MMRS and BMMRS is not meant to be interpreted in an actuarial fashion (i.e., a score of X indicates a lack of spirituality and thus represents a Y% chance of unhealthy consequences). Instead, the tool is meant to be used by researchers when designing studies to assess possible health effects of specific domains of spiritual deficiency. When the clinical provider examines the survey results and scoring, the intent is that each deficient area could be discussed with patients in a general manner—a general discussion to improve a youth's mental, behavioral, and emotional well-being, as well as his or her future adult physical health—without an intent to "treat" the individual. The data is not yet there to support any specific type of intervention.

## The Second Commonly Used Scale: The Spiritual Well-Being Scale

Another of the most studied and most commonly used spiritual screening tools is the SWBS.[2,122] Its origins can be traced to the 1960 and 1970s when the movement to develop "quality-of-life" metrics virtually ignored spirituality as a significant factor in life quality. In response to this oversight, two researchers developed the SWBS,[123,124] with the idea that spirituality was also an important aspect of a balanced, fulfilled life.

SWB refers to one's subjective sense of spiritual contentment. SWBS measures this in two domains: (1) religious well-being (RWB), emphasizing one's relationship to God, and (2) existential well-being (EWB), focusing on one's sense of meaning, purpose, and life satisfaction. The tool and contains 10 religion-oriented questions and 10 existential (spiritual but necessarily not religious) items. The proprietary set of 20 questions is available for $2.25 at https://lifeadvance.com/spiritual-well-being-scale.html and is attached here in Table 16.6. About half of the items in the survey are "reverse worded" (and therefore reverse scored) as a guard against bias, with each item scored from 1 to 6, thus rendering total scores ranging from 20 to 120, with higher scores representing greater SWB. The tool allows three subscale scores to be evaluated by researchers: (1) a total score for overall SWB, (2) an RWB subscale score, and (3) an EWB subscale score. The EWB subscale also yielded two small subfactors: one connoting life satisfaction and one connoting life purpose.

The SWBS has been translated and psychometrically validated (it is reliable with consistent performance across time, individuals, and situations and it is valid, measuring what it sets out to measure) in Greek adults,[125] Jordanian Arab Christian adults,[126] Iranian Muslim adults,[127] Korean Christians and unaffiliated Korean adults,[128] Jordanian and Malaysian Muslim college students,[129] Thai adults,[130] Chinese adults,[131] and Czech and American adolescents. A short form of the SWBS was also found valid and reliable in these studies of both religious and secular adolesents.[132,133]

Although SWBS has been statistically and psychometrically validated and it allows researchers to measure both religious and existential spirituality, the tool does not break down R/S into it's more essential building blocks (forgiveness, meaning, daily religious practice, etc.) as the MMRS does. These factors, perhaps, make SWBS less optimal in the research setting.

In addition to these shortcomings, a relatively few studies on SWBS and health outcomes have been performed. Those studies that have been done in this regard reveal that higher *total* SWBS scores are associated with greater adolescent psychologic well-being,[134] less risky behaviors (if combined with religious attendance),[135] greater adolescent posttraumatic growth and adaptation,[136] and greater overall quality of life.[137]

**TABLE 16.6**
**The Spiritual Well-Being Scale**

| | | | | | | |
|---|---|---|---|---|---|---|
| 1. I don't find much satisfaction in private prayer with God. | SA | MA | A | D | MD | SD |
| 2. I don't know who I am, where I came from, or where I'm going. | SA | MA | A | D | MD | SD |
| 3. I believe that God loves me and cares about me. | SA | MA | A | D | MD | SD |
| 4. I feel that life is a positive experience. | SA | MA | A | D | MD | SD |
| 5. I believe that God is impersonal and not interested in my daily situations. | SA | MA | A | D | MD | SD |
| 6. I feel unsettled about my future. | SA | MA | A | D | MD | SD |
| 7. I have a personally meaningful relationship with God. | SA | MA | A | D | MD | SD |
| 8. I feel very fulfilled and satisfied with life. | SA | MA | A | D | MD | SD |
| 9. I don't get much personal strength and support from my God. | SA | MA | A | D | MD | SD |
| 10. I feel a sense of well-being about the direction my life is headed in. | SA | MA | A | D | MD | SD |
| 11. I believe that God is concerned about my problems. | SA | MA | A | D | MD | SD |
| 12. I don't enjoy much about life. | SA | MA | A | D | MD | SD |
| 13. I don't have a personally satisfying relationship with God. | SA | MA | A | D | MD | SD |
| 14. I feel good about my future. | SA | MA | A | D | MD | SD |
| 15. My relationship with God helps me not to feel lonely. | SA | MA | A | D | MD | SD |
| 16. I feel that life is full of conflict and unhappiness. | SA | MA | A | D | MD | SD |
| 17. I feel most fulfilled when I'm in close communion with God. | SA | MA | A | D | MD | SD |
| 18. Life doesn't have much meaning. | SA | MA | A | D | MD | SD |
| 19. My relation with God contributes to my sense of well-being. | SA | MA | A | D | MD | SD |
| 20. I believe there is some real purpose for my life. | SA | MA | A | D | MD | SD |

For each of the following statements circle the choice that best indicates the extent of your agreement or disagreement, as it describes your personal experience.
*SA*, Strongly agree; *D* = Disagree; *MA* = Moderately agree; *MD* = Moderately disagree; *A* = Agree; *SD* = Strongly disagree.
Craig W. Ellison and Raymond F. Paloutzian. See www.lifeadvance.com.

EWB but not RWB has been associated with less depressive symptoms in adolescents[59,138] and less anxiety in young adults.[139] Cotton et al.[140] have found EWB but not RWB to be significantly associated with predicting risky health behaviors and depression in adolescents, with higher scores in EWB associated with less risky behaviors and less depression. The authors go on to state EWB (and thus a wider sense of spirituality beyond RWB) is important in adolescent mental and physical health. They also note EWB (but not necessarily RWB) is important in developing resilience in adolescents, with the important aspects of resilience being hope, optimism, future orientation, purpose, and meaning, all factors related to EWB (see chapter 15).

In adults, higher SWBS scores have been associated with less depressive symptoms and higher resilience. (Again, we present the adult data here so that PCPs might project what future problems might arise if adolescent spirituality is not addressed.) This is important, as resilience can play such a significant role in combating, and aiding remission of, depression and other psychiatric conditions.[141–143] Higher SWBS scores have also been found to be associated with less substance abuse[144]; better quality of life; improved coping with chronic illness[146]; lower chronic pain scores[147]; less loneliness[148]; a greater sense of hope[149] (important because hope is a critical factor in resilience; see chapter 15); better sleep; better mental and physical health self-assessments in patients with chronic diseases such as AIDS,[150] diabetes,[151] and end-stage renal disease[152]; and improved overall quality of life.[145,148]

When separated out from SWBS, EWB in adults has been found to be associated with lower suicidal rates in patients with PTSD,[153] lower rates of depression and stress,[154] greater resilience, more pro-social behavior, and a greater sense of purpose and satisfaction in life.[155]

In conclusion, although SWBS is commonly used, it fails to break down spirituality into its more basic building blocks and thus appears less useful as a research tool for measuring health outcomes. The health outcome studies that exist seem to favor EWB over RWB in terms of beneficial associations.

## TREATMENT: DELIVERING SPIRITUAL CARE

Although the focus of our chapter is adolescent spiritual *screening*, a brief overview of spiritual *treatment* is provided in order to help the reader understand where we are in terms of evidence-based spiritual therapies[c]—the idea being that, in future, once spiritual deficits are illuminated by a spiritual assessment, spiritual intervention may be considered.

As mentioned, good data on spiritual treatments for mental or physical health issues is lacking. The studies that do exist are usually small, often have methodological flaws, and, overall, have mixed results, with some documenting small benefits with spiritual treatment and others failing to do so. Spiritual intervention in these small, flawed studies has been found to be beneficial in cancer patients[157] and in those with other chronic physical illnesses, offering improved mental health and psychologic well-being. Spiritual therapy has also been shown to improve depressive symptoms,[158,159] help with eating disorders (e.g., anorexia, bulimia) in women (even more so than cognitive behavior therapy [CBT] or emotional support in one study),[158,159] increase compliance with other mental health therapies when integrated into treatment plans,[160] and beneficially impact overall quality of life (QAL).[161]

Other studies, however, have found spiritual practices *not* to be beneficial. A 2016 randomized trial of depressed patients found spirituality (religious CBT) to be no better than conventional intervention (conventional CBT).[162] Similarly, spiritual intervention in alcohol abuse and eating disorders has, surprisingly, been shown to *not* to offer any added benefit over standard treatment.[163,164]

Treating a diagnosed malady with spiritual intervention is quite different from what we are trying to do—break down spirituality into essential components, associate these individual components with health outcomes, then preventatively screen adolescents for "component deficits," and finally initiate some as-yet-undefined treatment to prevent associated untoward health effects. There is much work to be done, for in this realm the literature is essentially nonexistent.

Despite this, the association of spiritual deficiencies with untoward health effects has led the WHO to advocate a holistic approach to mental health treatment, an approach that includes spirituality in most communities. Indeed, the WHO includes spiritual care as the fourth dimension of the care of the whole person, the other three being physical, emotional, and social care.[12,165] It should be noted that, in 2013, the *Diagnostic and Statistical Manual of Mental Disorders* (Fourth Edition) (*DSM-IV*) acknowledged a new diagnostic category called "religious or spiritual problems." It stipulated that spiritual deficits might cause "nonpathologic" problems. Conventional psychiatry finally, formally recognized the role of spirituality in mental and behavioral health.

## CONCLUSIONS

Researchers will continue to tease out the impact of spirituality's subdomains on health outcomes, and they will continue to improve upon the screening tools used in both adolescents and adults. In this regard, an ideal tool should include measures that (1) have demonstrated validity across all developmental stages of adolescence, (2) can separately assess the multiple domains of R/S so that the most health-impacting attributes may be illuminated, and (3) are brief enough to be used clinically yet thorough enough to yield meaningful results.[83]

From this discussion, we can reasonably conclude that, generally, R/S can help convey a sense of psychologic well-being to adolescents, meaning a sense of social, emotional, mental, and functional health

[c]Several different methods of spiritual counseling exist, including pastoral care, pastoral counseling, spiritual direction, spiritually oriented psychotherapy, and spiritual care. Each of these modes of counseling has its own training, certification, and methods of approaching spiritual and mental health issues. Concise definitions of each approach is set out nicely in a review by Sperry.[156]

involving self-acceptance, autonomy, mastery, purpose, growth, and good relations to others. More specifically, the individual components of spirituality, as discussed earlier, can be associated with beneficial health effects in adolescents. Self-forgiveness has been associated with less depressive symptoms and a greater sense of overall well-being. DSES, PRP/RS/OR, and meaning/purpose are also protective against depression, anxiety, suicidal ideation, and substance abuse. Meaning/purpose has also been associated with resilience and posttraumatic growth.

Although these associations hold true, it is still too early to know definitively if any spiritual counseling/treatment will be beneficial to adolescents screened and found to have spiritual deficits. There is conflicting evidence on spiritual counseling's impact on depression, substance abuse, eating disorders, and overall quality of life.

As research moves toward evidenced-based spiritual screenings and interventions, PCPs must be mindful of these issues with adolescents. Developmental stage, life experiences, familial influences, and social and cultural contexts must be considered when screening in this critical age group.[166] As our knowledge continues to grow, it is likely that better screening methods and spiritual interventions will slowly emerge, both of which will improve our ability to give youths a more positive adolescence and, eventually, a healthier, more satisfying adulthood.

## REFERENCES


1. Zinnbauer BJ, Pargament KI, Cole B, et al. Religion and spirituality: unfuzzying the fuzzy. *J Sci Stud Relig*. 1997; 36:549–564.
2. Koenig HG. Concerns about measuring 'spirituality' in research. *J Nerv Ment Dis*. 2008;196:349–355.
3. Granqvist P, Nkara F. Nature meets nurture in religious and spiritual development. *Br J Dev Psychol*. 2017;35: 142–155.
4. UN High Commissioner for Refugees. UN Convention on the Rights of the Child. http://www.unhcr.org/uk/4d9474b49.pdf.
5. Cotton S, McGrady ME, Rosen SL. Measurement of religiosity/spirituality in adolescent health outcomes research: trends and recommendations. *J Relig Health*. 2010;49: 414–444.
6. Tripodi A, Severi S, Midili S, et al. Community projects" in Modena (Italy): promote regular physical activity and healthy nutrition habits since childhood. *Int J Pediatr Obes*. 2011;6(suppl 2):54–56.
7. te Velde SJ, Twisk JW, Brug J. Tracking of fruit and vegetable consumption from adolescence into adulthood and its longitudinal association with overweight. *Br J Nutr*. 2007;98:431–438.
8. Cleland V, Dwyer T, Venn A. Which domains of childhood physical activity predict physical activity in adulthood? A 20-year prospective tracking study. *Br J Sports Med*. 2012;46(8):595–602.
9. Fetzer Institute/National Institute on Aging Working Group. *Multidimensional Measurement of Religiousness/spirituality for Use in Health Research: A Report of the Fetzer Institute/National Institute on Aging Working Group*. Kalamazoo: John E. Fetzer Institute; 1999.
10. Luskin F. Review of the effect of spiritual and religious factors on mortality and morbidity with a focus on cardiovascular and pulmonary disease. *J Cardiopulm Rehabil*. 2000;20(1):8–15.
11. World Health Organization. Noncommunicable diseases. http://www.who.int/news-room/fact-sheets/detail/noncommunicable-diseases, June 2018.
12. Dhar N, Chaturvedi SK, Nandan D. Spiritual health, the fourth dimension: a public health perspective. *WHO South-East Asia J Public Health*. 2013;2(1):3–5.
13. King DE, Bushwick B. Beliefs and attitudes of hospital inpatients about faith healing and prayer. *J Fam Pract*. 1994; 39(4):349–352.
14. Koenig HG. Religious attitudes and practices of hospitalized medically ill older adults. *Int J Geriatr Psychiatry*. 1998;13(4):213–224.
15. *The Joint Commission. Advancing Effective Communication, Cultural Competence, and Patient- and Family-Centered Care: A Roadmap for Hospitals*. Oakbrook Terrace, Ill: The Joint Commission; 2010.
16. Hill PC, Hood Jr RW, eds. *Measures of Religiosity*. Birmingham, AL: Religious Education Press; 1999.
17. Monod S, Brennan M, Rochat E, et al. Instruments measuring spirituality in clinical research: a systematic review. *J Gen Intern Med*. 2011;26(11):1345–1357.
18. Lucchetti G. Taking spiritual history in clinical practice: a systematic review of instruments. *Explore*. 2013;9(3): 159–170.
19. Hill PC, Hood Jr RW, eds. *Measures of Religiosity*. Birmingham, AL: Religious Education Press; 1999. Birmingham.
20. Koenig HG. Religion, spirituality, and health: the research and clinical implications. ISRN Psychiatry; Volume 2012, Article ID 278730:33.
21. Park CL, Aldwin CL, Choun S, et al. Spiritual peace predicts 5-year mortality in congestive heart failure patients. *Health Psychol*. 2016;35(3):203–210.
22. McCullough ME, Hoyt WT, Larson DB, et al. Religious involvement and mortality: a meta-analytic review. *Health Psychol*. 2000;19(3):211–222.
23. Sharmaa V, Marina DB. Religion, spirituality, and mental health of U.S. military veterans: results from the national health and resilience in veterans study. *J Affect Disord*. 2017;217:197–204.
24. Boisvert JA, Harrell WA. The impact of spirituality on eating disorder symptomatology in ethnically diverse Canadian women. *Int J Soc Psychiatry*. 2013;59(8): 729–738.
25. Bennett K, Shepherd J, Janca A. Personality disorders and spirituality. *Curr Opin Psychiatry*. 2013;26(1):79–83.

26. Toussaint LL, Marschall JC, Williams DR. Prospective associations between religiousness/spirituality and depression and mediating effects of forgiveness in a nationally representative sample of United States adults. *Depress Res Treat.* 2012;2012:10. Article ID 267820.
27. O'Laoire S. An experimental study of the effects of distant, intercessory prayer on self-esteem, anxiety, and depression. *Altern Ther Health Med.* 1997;3(6):38–53.
28. Forbis SK. Religion/spirituality status and borderline personality symptomatology among outpatients in an internal medicine clinic. *Int J Psychiatry Clin Pract.* 2012; 16:48–52.
29. Laird RD, Marks LD, Marrero MD. Religiosity, self-control and antisocial behavior. *J Appl Dev Psychol.* 2011;32, 78-75.
30. Whitford HS, Olver IN, Peterson M. Spirituality as a core domain in the assessment of quality of life in oncology. *Psychooncology.* 2008;17:1121–1128.
31. Whitford HS, Olver IN. The multidimensionality of spiritual wellbeing: peace, meaning, and faith and their association with quality of life and coping in oncology. *Psychooncology.* 2012;21:602–610.
32. Lazenby M, Khatib J, Al-Khair F, et al. Psychometric properties of the functional assessment of chronic illness therapy—spiritual well-being (FAICT-Sp) in an Arabic speaking, predominantly Muslim population. *Psychooncology.* 2013;22:220–227.
33. Moreira-Almeida A, Koenig HG. Clinical Implications of Spirituality to mental health - review of evidence and practical guidelines. *Braz J Psychiat.* 2014;36:176–182.
34. Bonelli R, Dew RE, Koenig HG, et al. Religious and spiritual factors in depression: review and integration of the research. *Depress Res Treat.* 2012;2012:1–8.
35. Yonker JE, Schnabelrauch CA, DeHaan LG. The relationship between spirituality and religiosity on psychological outcomes in adolescents and emerging adults: a meta-analytic review. *J Adolesc.* 2012;35:299–314.
36. Erikson EH. *Identity: Youth and Crisis.* New York: Norton; 1968.
37. Arnett JJ. Emerging adulthood. a theory of development from the late teens through the twenties. *Am Psychol.* 2000;55(5):469–480.
38. Hunsberger B, Pratt M, Pancer SM. Adolescent identity formation: religious exploration and commitment. *Identity.* 2001;1(4):365–386.
39. Marksttrom-Adams C, Smith M. Identity formation and religious orientation among high school students from the United States and Canada. *J Adolesc.* 1996;19: 247–261.
40. Dimitrova R, van de Vijver FJR, Taušová J. Ethnic, familial, and religious identity of Roma adolescents in Bulgaria, Czech Republic, Kosovo, and Romania in relation to their level of well-being. *Child Dev.* 2017;88(3): 693–709.
41. Ebstyne King P. Religion and identity: the role of ideological, social, and spiritual contexts. *Appl Dev Sci.* 2003; 7(3):197–204.
42. University of Notre Dame. National Study of Youth and Religion. https://youthandreligion.nd.edu/research-findings/reports.
43. Smith C, Denton ML, Faris R, Regnerus M. Mapping American adolescent religious participation. *J Sci Stud Relig.* 2002;41(4):597–612.
44. Gallup GJ, Bezilla R. *The Religious Life of Young Americans.* Princeton, NJ: The George H. Gallup International Institute; 1992.
45. Smith CL, Denton ML. *Soul Searching: The Religious and Spiritual Lives of American Teenagers.* New York, NY: Oxford University Press; 2005.
46. Cotton S, McGrady ME, Rosenthal SL. Measurement of religiosity/spirituality in adolescent health outcomes research: trends and recommendations. *J Relig Health.* 2010;49(4):414–444.
47. Lucchetti G, Bassi RM, Lucchetti ALG. Taking spiritual history in clinical practice: a systematic review of instruments. *Explore.* 2013;9(3):159–170.
48. Ellis MR, Vinson DC, Ewigman B. Addressing spiritual concerns of patients: family physicians' attitudes and practices. *J Fam Pract.* 1999;48(2):105–109.
49. Monod S, Brennan M. Instruments measuring spirituality in clinical research: a systematic review. *J Gen Intern Med.* 2011;26(11):1345–1357.
50. Cotton S, Zebracki K. Religion/spirituality and adolescent health outcomes: a review. *J Adolesc Health.* 2006;38: 472–480.
51. Ellison CW. Spiritual well-being: conceptualization and measurement. *J Psychol Theol.* 1983;11(4):330–340.
52. Pargament KI, Koenig HG, Perez LM. The many methods of religious coping: development and initial validation of the RCOPE. *J Clin Psychol.* 2000;56(4):519–543.
53. Allport G, Ross J. Personal religious orientation and prejudice. *J Pers Soc Psychol.* 1967;5(4):432.
54. Holland JC, Kash KM, Passik S, et al. A brief spiritual beliefs inventory for use in quality of life research in life-threatening illness. *Psychooncology.* 1998;7(6): 460–469.
55. Miller L, Gur M. Religiousness and sexual responsibility in adolescent girls. *J Adolesc Health.* 2002;31(5):401–406.
56. Cochran JK. The effects of religiosity on adolescent self-reported frequency of drug and alcohol use. *J Drug Issues.* 1992;22(1):91–104.
57. Pearce MJ, Little TD, Perez JE. Religiousness and depressive symptoms among adolescents. *J Clin Child Adolesc Psychol.* 2003;32(2):267–276.
58. Pendleton SM, Cavalli KS, Pargament KI, Nasr SZ. Religious/spiritual coping in childhood cystic fibrosis: a qualitative study. *Pediatrics.* 2002;109(1):E8.
59. Cotton S, Larkin E. The impact of adolescent spirituality on depressive symptoms and health risk behaviors. *J Adolesc Health.* 2005;36, 529.e7–529.e14.
60. Shelton S, Linfield K, Carter B, Morton R. Spirituality and coping with chronic life-threatening pediatric illness: cystic fibrosis and severe asthma. *Proc Am Thorac Soc.* 2005;2:520.

61. Zehnder D, Prchal A, Vollrath M, Landolt MA. Prospective study of the effectiveness of coping in pediatric patients. *Child Psychiatry Hum Dev*. 2006;36:351. e68.
62. Pearce LD, Haynie DL. Intergenerational religious dynamics and adolescent delinquency. *Social Forces*. 2004;82(4):1553–1572.
63. Regnerus MD. Moral communities and adolescent delinquency: religious contexts and community social control. *Sociol Q*. 2003;44(4):523–554.
64. Nonnemaker JM, McNeely CA, Blum RW. Public and private domains of religiosity and adolescent health risk behaviors: evidence from the National Longitudinal Study of Adolescent Health. *Soc Sci Med*. 2003;57(11): 2049–2054.
65. Smith TB, McCullough ME, Poll J. Religiousness and depression: evidence for a main effect and the moderating influence of stressful life events. *Psychol Bull*. 2003; 129(4):614–636.
66. Hankin B, Abramson L, Moffitt T, et al. Development of depression from preadolescence to young adulthood: emerging gender differences in a 10-year longitudinal study. *J Abnorm Psychol*. 1998;107:128–140.
67. Hammen C, Compas B. Unmasking unmasked depression in children and adolescents: the problem of comorbidity. *Clin Psychol Rev*. 1994;14(6):585–603.
68. Rutter M, Kim-Cohe J, Maughan B. Continuities and discontinuities in psychopathology between childhood and adult life. *J Child Psychol Psychiatry*. 2006;47(3–4): 276–295.
69. Lerner RM, Lerner JV, Almerigi J, et al. Positive youth development, participation in community youth development programs, and community contributions of fifth grade adolescents: findings from the first wave of the 4-H study of positive youth development. *J Early Adolesc*. 2005;25:17–e71.
70. James AG, Fine MA. Relations between youths' conceptions of spirituality and their developmental outcomes. *J Adolesc*. 2015;43:171–e180.
71. James A, Fine MA, Turner J. An empirical examination of youths' self-perceived spirituality as an internal developmental asset during adolescence. *Appl Dev Sci*. 2012;16: 181–e194.
72. Stewart C, Koeske GF. A preliminary construct validation of the multidimensional measurement of religiousness/ spirituality instrument: a study of Southern USA samples. *Int J Psychol Relig*. 2006;16(3):181–196.
73. Underwood LG, Teresi JA. The daily spiritual experience scale: development, theoretical description, reliability, exploratory factor analysis, and preliminary construct validity using health-related data. *Ann Behav Med*. 2002;24: 22–33.
74. Pargament K, Feuille M, Burdzy D. The brief RCOPE: current psychometric status of a short measure of religious coping. *Religions*. 2011;2(1):51–76.
75. Dufton BD, Perlman D. The association between religiosity and the Purpose-in- Life test: does it reflect purpose or satisfaction. *J Psychol Theol*. 1986;14:42–48.
76. George LS, Park CL. Are meaning and purpose distinct? An examination of correlates and predictors. *J Posit Psychol*. 2013;8(5):365–375.
77. Brassai L, Piko BF, Steger MF. Meaning in life: is it a protective factor for adolescents' psychological health? *Int J Behav Med*. 2011;18:44–51.
78. Halama P, Medova M. Meaning in life and hope as predictors of positive mental health: do they explain residual variance not predicted by personality trait? *Stud Psychol*. 2007;49:191–200.
79. Siahpush M, Spittal M, Singh GK. Happiness and life satisfaction prospectively predict self-rated health, physical health, and the presence of limiting, long-term health conditions. *Am J Health Prom*. 2008;23:18–26.
80. Steger MF, Frazier P, Oishi S, Kaler M. The meaning in life questionnaire: assessing the presence of and search for meaning in life. *J Couns Psychol*. 2006;53:80–93.
81. Rathi N, Rastogi R. Meaning in life and psychological well-being in pre-adolescents and adolescents. *J Ind Acad Appl Psychol*. 2007;33:31–38.
82. Steger M, Kashdan T. Stability and specificity of meaning in life and life satisfaction over one year. *J Happiness Stud*. 2007;8:161–179.
83. Harris SK, Sherritt LR, Holdeer DW, et al. Reliability and validity of the brief multidimensional measure of religiousness/spirituality among adolescents. *J Relig Health*. 2008;47:438–457.
84. Van Dyke CJ, Glenwick D, Cecero J, et al. The relationship of religious coping and spirituality to adjustment and psychological distress in urban early adolescents. *Ment Health Relig Cult*. 2009;12:369–383.
85. Desrosiers A, Miller L. Relational spirituality and depression in adolescent girls. *J Clin Psychol*. 2007;63: 1021–1037.
86. Park CL, Edmondson D, Hale-Smith A, et al. Religiousness/spirituality and health behaviors in younger adult cancer survivors: does faith promote a healthier lifestyle? *J Behav Med*. 2009;32:582–591.
87. Koenig HG, George LK, Titus P. Religion, spirituality and health in medically ill hospitalized older patients. *J Am Geriatr Soc*. 2004;52:554–562.
88. Skarupski K, Fitchett G, Evans D, et al. Daily spiritual experiences in a biracial community-based population of older adults. *Aging Men Health*. 2010;14:779–789.
89. Boswell GH, Kahana E, Dilworth-Anderson P. Spirituality and healthy lifestyle behaviors: stress counter-balancing effects on the well-being of older adults. *J Relig Health*. 2006;45:587–602.
90. Keefe FJ, Affleck G, Lefebvre J, et al. Living with rheumatoid arthritis: the role of daily spirituality and daily religious and spiritual coping. *J Pain*. 2001;2:101–110.
91. Rippentrop AE, Altmaier EM, Chen JJ. The relationship between religion/spirituality and physical health, mental health, and pain in a chronic pain population. *Pain*. 2005;116:311–321.
92. Kalkstein S, Tower RB. The Daily Spiritual Experience Scale and well-being: demographic comparisons and

scale validation with older Jewish adults and a diverse internet sample. *J Relig Health*. 2009;48:401–417.
93. Ng SM, Ted CT, Fong E, et al. Validation of the Chinese version of underwood's daily spiritual experience scale—transcending cultural boundaries? *Int J Behav Med*. 2009;16:91–97.
94. Holland JM, Neimeyer RA. Reducing the risk of burnout in end-of-life care settings: the role of daily spiritual experiences and training. *Palliat Support Care*. 2005;3: 173–181.
95. Shorkey C, Uebel M, Windsor LC. Measuring dimensions of spirituality in chemical dependence treatment and recovery: research and practice. *Int J Ment Health Addict*. 2008;6:286–305.
96. Bell Jr DE. *The Relationship Between Distal Religious and Proximal Spiritual Variables and Self Reported Marital Happiness*. Florida State University College of Medicine; 2009. Ph.D dissertation.
97. Koenig HG, George LK, Titus P, et al. Religion, spirituality, and acute care hospitalization and long-term care by older patients. *Arch Intern Med*. 2004;164: 1579–1585.
98. Underwood LG. The daily spiritual experience scale: overview and results. *Religions*. 2011;2:29–50.
99. Cole-Lewis YC, Gipson PY, Opperman KJ, et al. Protective role of religious involvement against depression and suicidal ideation among youth with interpersonal problems. *J Relig Health*. 2016;55(4):1172–1188.
100. Tavares BF, Beria JU, Lima MA. Factors associated with drug use among adolescent students in Southern Brazil. *Rev Saude Publica*. 2004;38(6):787–796.
101. Nonnemaker J, McNeely CA, Blum RW. Public and private domains of religiosity and adolescent smoking transitions. *Soc Sci Med*. 2006;62(12):3084–3095.
102. Levin JS, Chatters LM, Taylor RJ. Religious effects on health status and life satisfaction among Black Americans. *J Gerontol B Psychol Sci Soc Sci*. 1995;50B: S154–S163.
103. Koenig LB, Vaillant GE. A prospective study of church attendance and health over the lifespan. *Health Psychol*. 2009;28(1):117–124.
104. Rasic DT, Robinson JA, Bolton J, et al. Longitudinal relationships of religious worship attendance and spirituality with major depression, anxiety disorders, and suicidal ideation and attempts: findings from the Baltimore epidemiologic catchment area study. *J Psychiatr Res*. 2011;45:848–854.
105. Pargament KI, Koenig HG. *A Comprehensive Measure of Religious Coping. Development and Initial Validation of the RCOPE. Report presented at: Retirement Research Foundation*. 1997. Chicago, Ill.
106. Pargament KI, Smith BW, Koenig HG, Perez L. Patterns of positive and negative religious coping with major life stressors. *J Sci Stud Relig*. 1998;37:711–725.
107. *The Psychometric Study of the Attachment to God Inventory and the Brief Religious Coping Scale in a Taiwanese Christian Sample*. Liberty University, ProQuest Dissertations Publishing; 2011.
108. Gonzalez-Morkos B. *Preliminary Reliability Analysis of a Spanish Translation of the Brief RCOPE*. Pepperdine University, ProQuest Dissertations Publishing; 2005.
109. Tang KNS, Chan CS, Ng J, et al. Action type-based factorial structure of brief COPE among Hong Kong Chinese. *J Psychopathol Behav Assess*. 2016;38(4):631–644.
110. Cotton S, Grossoehme D, Rosenthal SL, et al. Religious/spiritual coping in adolescents with sickle cell disease: a pilot study. *J Pediatr Hematol Oncol*. 2009;31(5): 313–318.
111. Reynolds N, Mrug S, Guion K. Spiritual coping and psychosocial adjustment of adolescents with chronic illness: the role of cognitive attributions, age, and disease group. *Adolesc Health*. 2013;52(5):559–565.
112. Carpenter TP, Laney T, Mezulis A. Religious coping, stress, and depressive symptoms among adolescents: a prospective study. *Psychol Relig Spiritual*. 2012;4(1): 19–30.
113. Latzer Y, Weinberger-Litman SL, Gerson B, et al. Negative religious coping predicts disordered eating pathology among Orthodox Jewish adolescent girls. *J Relig Health*. 2015;54(5):1760–1771.
114. Parenteau SC. Religious coping and substance use: the moderating role of sex. *J Relig Health*. 2017;56(2): 380–387.
115. Worthington Jr EL, Sandage SJ. *Forgiveness and Spirituality in Psychotherapy: A Relational Approach*. Washington, DC: American Psychological Association; 2016.
116. Chen Y, Harris SK, Worthington Jr EL, et al. Religiously or spiritually-motivated forgiveness and subsequent health and well-being among young adults: an outcome-wide analysis. *J Posit Psychol*; 2018. https://doi.org/10.1080/17439760.2018.1519591. https://arxiv.org/abs/1810.10164.
117. Worthington Jr EL, Griffin BJ, Provencher C. Forgiveness. In: Maddux JE, ed. *Social Psychological Foundations of Well-Being and Life Satisfaction*. New York, NY: Routledge; 2018:148–167.
118. Toussaint LL, Worthington EL, Williams DR. *Forgiveness and Health: Scientific Evidence and Theories Relating Forgiveness to Better Health*. New York, NY: Springer; 2015.
119. Macaskill A. Differentiating dispositional self-forgiveness from other-forgiveness: associations with mental health and life satisfaction. *J Soc Clin Psychol*. 2012;31:28–50.
120. Griffin BJ, Moloney JM, Green JD. Perpetrators' reactions to perceived interpersonal wrongdoing: the associations of guilt and shame with forgiving, punishing, and excusing oneself. *Self Identity*. 2016;15:650–661.
121. Enright RD, Fitzgibbons RP. *Forgiveness Therapy: An Empirical Guide for Resolving Anger and Restoring Hope*. 2nd ed. Washington, DC: American Psychological Association; 2015.
122. Ellison CW, Smith J. Toward an integrative measure of health and well-being. *J Psychol Theol*. 1991;19(1):35–48.
123. Paloutzian RF, Ellison CW. Loneliness, spiritual well-being and quality of life. In: Peplau LA, Perlman D, eds. *Loneliness: A Sourcebook of Current Theory, Research and Therapy*. New York: Wiley Inter- science; 1982.

124. Elllison CW. Spiritual Well-Being: conceptualization and measurement. *J Psychol Theol.* 1983;11(4): 330–340.
125. Darvyri P, Galanakis M, Avgoustidis A, et al. The spiritual well-being scale (SWBS) in Greek population of attica. *Psychol.* 2014;5(13):1575–1582.
126. Musa AS, Pevalin DJ. Psychometric evaluation of the Arabic version of the spiritual well-being scale on a sample of Jordanian Arab Christians. *J Psychol Theol.* 2014; 42(3):293–301.
127. Biglari AM, Fisher JW, Kheiltash A. Validation of the Persian version of spiritual well-being questionnaires. *Iran J Med Sci.* 2018;43(3):276–285.
128. You S, Yoo JE. Evaluation of the spiritual well-being scale in a sample of Korean adults. *J Relig Health.* 2016;55(4): 1289–1299.
129. Musa AS. Factor structure of the spiritual well-being scale: cross-cultural comparisons between Jordanian Arab and Malaysian Muslim university students in Jordan. *J Transcult Nurs.* 2016;27(2):117–125.
130. Chaiviboontham S, Phinitkhajorndech N, Hanucharurnkul S, et al. Psychometric properties of the Thai spiritual well-being scale. *Palliat Support Care.* 2016;14(2):109–117.
131. Tang WR, Kao CY. Psychometric testing of the Spiritual Well-Being Scale-Mandarin version in Taiwanese cancer patients. *Palliat Support Care.* 2017;15(3):336–347.
132. Cotton S, Larkin E, Hoopes A, et al. The impact of adolescent spirituality on depressive symptoms and health risk behaviors. *J Adolesc Health.* 2005;36: 529.e527–529.e514.
133. Malinakova K, Kopcakova J, Kolarcik P. The spiritual well-being scale: psychometric evaluation of the shortened version in Czech adolescents. *J Relig Health.* 2017; 56(2):697–705.
134. Mohan J, Sehgal M, Tripathi A. Psychological well-being, spiritual well-being and personality. *J Psychosoc Res.* 2008; 3(1):81–97.
135. Malinakova K, Kopcakova J, Madarasova G, et al. I am spiritual, but not religious": does one without the other protect against adolescent health-risk behaviour? *Int J Public Health.* 2018. https://doi.org/10.1007/s00038-018-1116-4.
136. Sehgal M, Sethi K, Vaneet K. Psychosocial factors contributing to post traumatic growth. *J Psychosoc Res.* 2016; 11(2):437–445.
137. Sawatzky R, Gadermann A, Pesut B. An investigation of the relationships between spirituality, health status and quality of life in adolescents. *Appl Res Qual Life.* 2009; 4(1):5–22.
138. Wenger S. Religiosity in relation to depression and well-being among adolescents: a comparison of findings among the Anglo-Saxon population and findings among Austrian high school students. *Ment Health Relig Cult.* 2011;14(6):515–529.
139. Fabbris JL, Mesquita AC, Caldeira S. Anxiety and spiritual well-being in nursing students: a cross-sectional study. *J Holist Nurs.* 2017;35(3):261–270.
140. Cotton S, Larkin E, Hoopes A, et al. The impact of adolescent spirituality on depressive symptoms and health risk behaviors. *J Adolesc Health.* 2005;36(6):529.
141. Steinhardt M, Dolbier C. Evaluation of a resilience intervention to enhance coping strategies and protective factors and decrease symptomatology. *J Am Coll Health.* 2008;56:445–453.
142. Mela MA, Marcoux E, Baetz M, et al. The effect of religiosity and spirituality on psychological well-being among forensic psychiatric patients in Canada. *Ment Health Relig Cult.* 2008;11(5):517–532.
143. Ozawaa C, Suzukia T, Mizunoa Y. Resilience and spirituality in patients with depression and their family members: a cross-sectional study. *Compr Psychiatry.* 2017;77: 53–59.
144. Jalali A, Shabrandi B, Jalali R, et al. Methamphetamine abusers' personality traits and its relational with spiritual well-being and perceived social support. *Curr Drug Abuse Rev.* 2018;11. https://doi.org/10.2174/1874473711666181017121256.
145. Anye ET, Gallien TL, Bian H, et al. The relationship between spiritual well-being and health-related quality of life in college students. *J Am Coll Health.* 2013;61(7): 414–421.
146. Aktürk S, Aktürk Ü. Determining the spiritual well-being of patients with spinal cord injury. *J Spinal Cord Med.* June 29, 2018:1–8.
147. Bai J, Brubaker A, Meghani SH. Spirituality and quality of life in black patients with cancer pain. *J Pain Symptom Manage.* 2018;56(3):390–398.
148. Paloutzian RF, Bufford RK, Wildman AJ. Spiritual well-being scale: mental and physical health relationships. In: Puchalski C, Rumbold B, eds. *Oxford Textbook of Spirituality in Healthcare.* New York, NY: Oxford University Press; 2012:353–358; Vol. XVI.
149. Yaghoobzadeh A, Soleimani MA. Relationship between spiritual well-being and hope in patients with cardiovascular disease. *J Relig Health.* 2018;57:938–950.
150. Coleman CL, Holzemer. Spirituality, psychological well-being, and HIV symptoms for African-Americans living with HIV disease. *J Assoc Nurses AIDS Care.* 1999;10(1): 42–50.
151. Landis BJ. Uncertainty, spiritual well-being, and psychosocial adjustment to chronic illness. *Issues Ment Health Nurs.* 1996;17(3):217–231.
152. Tanyi RA, Werner JS. Spirituality in African American and Caucasian women with end-stage renal disease on hemodialysis treatment. *Health Care Women Int.* 2007;28(2): 141–154.
153. Nad S, Marcinko D, Vuksan-Æusa B, et al. Spiritual wellbeing, intrinsic religiosity, and suicidal behavior in predominantly Catholic Croatian war veterans with chronic posttraumatic stress disorder: a case control study. *J Nerv Ment Dis.* 2008;196(1):79–83.
154. Lee Y. The relationship of spiritual well-being and involvement with depression and perceived stress in Korean nursing students. *Glob J Health Sci.* 2014;6: 169–176.

155. Wilkins TA, Piedmont RL, Magyar-Russell GM. Spirituality or religiousness: which serves as the better predictor of elements of mental health? *Res Social Scientific Study Relig.* 2012;23:53–73.
156. Sperry L. Varieties of religious and spiritual treatment: spirituality oriented psychotherapy and beyond. *Spiritual Clin Pract.* 2016;3(1):1–4.
157. Kaplar ME, Wachholtz AB, O'Brien WH. The effect of religious and spiritual interventions on the biological, psychological, and spiritual outcomes of oncology patients: a meta-analytic review. *J Psychosoc Oncol.* 2004; 22(1):39–49.
158. McCullough ME. Research on religion-accommodative counseling: review and meta-analysis. *J Couns Psychol.* 1999;46:92–98.
159. Richards PS, Berrett ME, Hardman RK, et al. Comparative efficacy of spirituality, cognitive, and emotional support groups for treating eating disorder inpatients. *Eating Disord.* 2006;14(5):401–415.
160. Touchet B, Youman K, Pierce A, et al. The impact of spirituality on psychiatric treatment adherence. *J Spiritual Ment Health.* 2012;14(4):259–267.
161. Sajadi M, Niazi N, Khosravi S, et al. Effect of spiritual counseling on spiritual well-being in Iranian women with cancer: a randomized clinical trial. *Complement Ther Clin Pract.* 2018;30:79–84.
162. Pearce MJ, Koenig HG. Spiritual struggles and religious cognitive behavioral therapy: a randomized clinical trial in those with depression and chronic medical illness. *J Psychol Theol.* 2016;44(1):3–15.
163. Miller WR, Forcehimes A, O'Leary MJ, et al. Spiritual direction in addiction treatment: two clinical trials. *J Subst Abuse Treat.* 2008;35(4):434–442.
164. Tonkin KM. Obesity, bulimia, and binge-eating disorder: the use of a cognitive behavioral and spiritual intervention. *Diss Abstr Int.* 2005;67:563. ProQuest Information & Learning, 2006. AAI3201378.
165. World Health Organization. Mental Disorders. http://www.who.int/mediacentre/factsheets/fs396/en/.
166. Johnson KS, Elbert-Avila KI, Tulsky JA. The influence of spiritual beliefs and practices on the treatment preferences of African Americans: a review of the literature. *J Am Geriatr Soc.* 2005;53(4):711–719.

CHAPTER 17

# Screening for Strengths and Assets in Adolescents

GINA FRIEDEN, PHD

## INTRODUCTION

Including strengths as part of a thorough clinical assessment has gained more prominence among mental health practitioners in recent years. Yet many clinicians remain focused on using pathological labels and limit assessment and treatment to what is going wrong rather than what is going right when working with clients. The study of strengths has its roots in the humanistic psychology tradition.[1] In the past decade, the emphasis on research into the study of well-being and mindfulness and the contributions of the positive psychology movement[2,3] has added increasing credibility to adopting a strengths perspective. Positive psychologists have suggested that by adopting a strength perspective, certain disorders may never reach the point of becoming problematic.[3] This approach moves away from a wholesale endorsement of the medical model by focusing on well-being and individual strengths as important dimensions to consider in clinical assessment and treatment.

Different definitions of strengths are used in the research literature. If viewed as individual traits, strengths could be defined as the talents, assets, and capabilities that are naturally occurring and stable.[4] Strengths have also been described as psychological competencies that develop over time[5] and may vary by context. Additionally, resources in families and communities that contribute to the adolescent's well-being are sometimes included under the heading of strengths.[6]

It should also be noted that resilience and strengths are sometimes used interchangeably. However, they represent different constructs, with resilience typically discussed as a process that happens following an adverse experience, while strengths are considered natural assets that grow out of an individual's capabilities and interests.[7,8] Although strengths can be used to describe individuals who have gone through challenging situations, experiencing hardship is not a requisite for possessing them. Strengths will be used here to mean an individual's capabilities, assets, and competencies that develop over time and contribute to a sense of mastery and well-being.

With this definition in place, the benefits of a strength-based assessment will be explored. Besides the added benefits of building a positive therapeutic alliance and developing a comprehensive treatment plan, a strength-based assessment conveys a broader context for discussion of the client's needs. Referral to other professionals for medication review or case management can be viewed in the context of holistic healthcare offering a more accurate picture of overall well-being and better guidance about how to collaborate as part of a treatment team.[9–11] Other disciplines are beginning to address strengths in their practice as well. Strength-based approaches are being used in schools, community psychology, social work, and prevention.[12–15]

## ADOLESCENCE AND STRENGTHS

Nowhere has a focus on strengths been more important than in the field of adolescent health and well-being. In the mental health field, counseling, psychology, and social work are disciplines that are united in acknowledging the importance of strengths in working with children and teens (Laursen 2003; Seligman, 2002).[16,16a,17,17a] The strength perspective assumes that even if emotional and behavioral disorders are identified, all youth have the ability to access and act on strengths.[18–20] Strengths-based perspectives developed as a way to empower children and adolescents to be experts in their own lives and find solutions to the challenges they face.[20a] A strength-based approach recognizes that all youth have strengths, but may not have had the opportunities to identify personal assets or develop the competencies needed to feel empowered.[21] Strengths-based practice is built on the premise that

Adolescent Health Screening: An Update in the Age of Big Data. https://doi.org/10.1016/B978-0-323-66130-0.00017-X

people can use their assets and inner resources to overcome even the most intractable of problems.[22] In essence, a strengths-based approach draws on the youth's capabilities to achieve goals.

In spite of renewed interest in the field, researchers have spent more time developing and validating measures that focus on mental disorders such as depression, anxiety, or substance abuse.[23,24] Research is often oriented to the study of psychopathology and a focus on vulnerabilities rather than assets. Masten, Burt, and Coatsworth,[25] however, have advocated for a more integrated and balanced approach in studying risk and protective factors. For example, children who experience adversity are likely to experience both negative and positive outcomes but those who have a variety of strengths will likely experience more positive outcomes.[5] The development of strengths has been associated with resilience[26] and life satisfaction.[27]

Identifying strengths as part of an overall health assessment can provide a more balanced picture of how the teen is doing in multiple contexts of their lives. Additionally, integrating strengths into screening and assessment protocols can lead to a more collaborative relationship between the adolescent and mental health professional and more investment in meeting goals.[8] Treatment planning that incorporates strengths and resiliencies leads to outcomes associated with increased motivation and greater empowerment for making decisions and solving problems.[28]

## DEVELOPMENTAL COMPETENCIES AND TASKS IN ADOLESCENCE

Using strength-based approaches in adolescent assessment and treatment creates the opportunity to support positive, proactive, and developmentally appropriate behaviors even in the face of challenging experiences. Professionals who work with adolescents can benefit from using this approach.[29] However, without a developmental perspective, problematic behaviors that are the source of referral become the focus of attention while strengths, which are closely tied to developmental competencies may be overlooked. Because adolescence is marked by changes in cognitive complexity, emotional development, and social relationships, it is up to the practitioner to differentiate between normal behavior of typically developing teens and symptoms that may require further assessment and diagnosis.

For example, typically developing teens will go through mood fluctuations, be concerned about relationships with peers, and test limits and boundaries.[30] Understanding that these behaviors can represent normal developmental markers in adolescence can prevent conflict and frustration from creating more tension at home. Before discussing the role of strengths in development, it is important to note how strengths relate to developmental competencies and developmental tasks in adolescence.

Adaptive development in adolescence refers to mastering developmental, age-related competencies and tasks. Developmental tasks refer to expectations about behavior that arise in a social context and may vary by gender, culture, and historical period.[31] According to Havighurst,[32] a developmental task arises when an individual need is met by a social demand. If tasks are not achieved, development is viewed as off-time and can lead to difficulties in negotiating future age-related tasks. Developmental tasks in young adulthood are mainly related to family, work, and social life such as getting married, having a career, or being part of a friendship group although more recent research suggests adults postponing parenting and marriage.[33] The developmental tasks in adolescence can be grouped in five domains: academic achievement, conduct (rule breaking or rule abiding), romantic relationships, work, and social competence with peers.[31]

Developmental competence is closely related to developmental tasks and refers to effective adaptation to meet associated age-related tasks. Competencies refer to the ability to accomplish a broad range of cognitive emotional social, moral, and behavioral tasks at various developmental stages. Developmental competencies in adolescence can generally be organized to include cognitive and affective competencies (critical thinking skills, emotional processing and perspective taking skills), moral competencies (developing a coherent set of values and beliefs, identity development), social competencies (forming relationships that are close and supportive), and behavioral competencies (achieving goals, adaptability, self-discipline). Strengths are often discussed as developmental competencies by researchers studying adaptive developmental processes. For purposes of this discussion, developmental competencies and strengths will be used interchangeably.

Professionals who work with teens can use their knowledge of adolescent development to guide a discussion of strengths. Although it is useful to have a working knowledge of general psychological changes that occur in adolescence, it is especially helpful to be familiar with brain-related changes. Strengths and competencies develop through a complex interaction of biopsychosocial influences. Research in neuroscience over the last two decades has contributed to a much better understanding of how the brain influences behavior in some important ways during the teen years.

## ADOLESCENT DEVELOPMENT AND THE BRAIN

Among the many behavior changes that describe the adolescent years, the three that are most robustly identified across cultures are (1) increased novelty seeking, (2) increased risk-taking, and (3) increased interactions with peers.[34a] These behaviors have helped humans evolve to become more independent and less concerned with reliance on the family for survival.[34] Over the past two decades, these changes have been validated in neuroscience specifically related to advances in technology. Magnetic resonance imaging (MRI) methods, including structural MRI and functional MRI (fMRI), are now considered essential modalities to understand brain development and changes that occur over time.[35] These imaging technologies provide detailed pictures of the functional abilities associated with brain maturation at different ages.

During adolescence, the neural connections between the amygdala and cortices in the frontal lobe become denser. Because these connections integrate emotional and cognitive processes, the ability to regulate and interpret emotions becomes more refined over time.[34] It has been well established that increases in white matter reflect, in part, increased myelination, which might be associated with age-related improvements in cognitive processing. Neuroimaging studies suggest that the prefrontal cortex matures more slowly than other regions of the brain and provides a greater top-down modulation of activity within limbic regions associated with the processing of emotion.[36] Adolescents become gradually better at integrating memory and experience into their decision making. The evidence suggests that this integration process continues through the early twenties.[37]

Because of changes in pubertal status, early adolescence is marked by a heightened sensitivity to rewards. During adolescence, there is an increase in the activity of the neural circuits using dopamine, a neurotransmitter implicated in creating the drive for reward. The reward circuitry in the brain may lead to increased risk-taking for some teens because more emphasis is placed on the potentially positive aspects of the experience. The risk feels worth the consequence.[30] Researchers have hypothesized that the lag time between acquisition of social emotional competencies that occur early in adolescence and the competencies associated with executive functioning and reasoning skills that peak later in adolescence may explain why an increase in risk-taking is associated with this era.[38,39] Behaviors guided by the reward circuitry of the brain are not yet fully under the control of the more logical and abstract cognitive functions.

Although executive functioning and competencies related to critical thinking and logical reasoning develop over time, these processes do not fully control actions linked to risk. Some teens although not all, are drawn to thrill-seeking experiences that test limits and may lead to impulsive actions such as binge drinking, driving too fast, or shoplifting on a dare. Because relating to peers is also an important developmental task, trying out behaviors involving risk is even more likely to be entertained if peers are involved.[40]

Behaviors that are viewed as reckless and impulsive from an adult perspective are simply not being perceived by the teen in the same way. Parents may find themselves moving between setting hard limits and consequences to actively trying to buffer their adolescents from taking any risks at all. Both strategies may end up being more frustrating than helpful for both the teen and his parents. However, identifying strategies for engaging strengths to help navigate this period can be helpful and lead to increased well-being for the adolescent and reduced conflict with parents.[30]

Siegel[30] points out that parents and other adult models can be actively involved but in ways they may not have considered. One area of involvement is helping teens manage high intensity emotions. Moodiness and irritability can be framed adaptively by helping the teens discover the upside of emotions. Finding passion and zest in day-to-day activities can help offset anxiety and rumination. Adults can help teens to find goals that are meaningful and encourage the pursuit of them. Another area that can be adaptively construed is social engagement. Although adolescents may be vulnerable to peer pressure, they can also use time with peers to refine social skills and work through conflict. Perceived failure or rejection can be a positive experience if it is framed in the context of leaning into adversity and learning from it. Adults can provide perspective by acknowledging hurt feelings when appropriate while encouraging teens to consider the types of relationships they want to develop. Rather than fearing peer rejection and isolating oneself, adolescents have an opportunity to deepen emotional connections through seeking out positive relationships.

Finally, with regard to risk, novelty seeking leads teens to explore and try out new behaviors and experiences. This brain-related function of seeking out novelty can also lead to the development of resilience and independence by encouraging natural differentiation from caregivers and affiliation with peers. Helping the adolescent channel risk-taking in positive ways can promote self-efficacy and confidence in trying out new things. At the same time, becoming aware of one's own impulses and desires through reflection and contemplation can simultaneously put a pause on actions that might otherwise be questionable or dangerous. Finding the appropriate amount of risk directed toward an appropriate but challenging experience can be a way to engage the adolescent in a discussion of risk and reward.

Professionals who work with teens can use information about how adolescents develop in the assessment process to create better channels of communication between the adolescent and family. Adults can foster the development of adolescents' sense of competence. Although parents often feel that they have little influence during the teen years, research has found that feelings of competence in both adolescent boys and girls are directly linked to feeling emotionally close and accepted by parents.[41]

As Siegel[30] notes, the skills that emerge in adolescence are a prelude to the complex competencies needed to navigate adulthood. Parents and other significant adults in the adolescent's life can help them channel these emerging capabilities by reinforcing positive behaviors, collaborating with them to solve problems and encouraging them to think through choices.

## THE SOCIAL ECOLOGICAL CONTEXT IN ADOLESCENCE

In addition to the biological and neurological changes in development, researchers who study developmental pathways in adolescence point out the importance of context in the development of competencies. Individual adaptation is a function of the combination and interaction of multiple contexts and experiences.[42,43] Pathways that support a successful transition to young adulthood are strongly linked with social class, outside resources, and the support and care of the family.[44,45] The traditional developmental milestones of independence from family, autonomy and self-direction, and achievement in work and school contexts are associated with strong parental relationships and close emotional bonds with significant caregivers.[46] In most cases, a supportive, encouraging adult and caring environment in general increases the likelihood that individual assets will be maximized.[47]

In contexts associated with low socioeconomic status, poverty and family disruption may cause young people to not have the extra boost needed to move out of the home and support themselves at an early age. Poverty is related to parental unemployment and single parent households and can be linked to parental drug addiction and other mental illness.[48] The effects of poverty can lead adolescents to interrupt their academic plans and limit opportunities for stable careers and family relationships[49] thus constraining their ability to achieve tasks related to typical developmental norms. From a developmental perspective, these early, nonnormative transitions have the potential to derail healthy coping, burden family supports and resources, and lead to choices that confound successful long-term outcomes.[50]

The adolescent's growing competencies and strengths are closely linked to environmental supports. When capable, caring and consistent caregivers are available, adolescents have more opportunities to activate their natural assets and unique capabilities. When families cannot provide opportunities for growth, external systems of support must help to create the conditions for strengths to flourish.

### Using a Developmental Framework to Assess Youths' Strengths

Based on the previous discussion, using a strength-based approach in adolescent assessment and treatment is most effective if consideration is given to assessing and identifying resources that can support the teen's developing competencies while also helping adolescents to identify and utilize current strengths that can be used to meet ongoing developmental tasks. Even though transitions are a normal part of development, adolescents are still likely to encounter extra stress in this transitional period of their lives.[51] Strengths can be conceptualized and integrated into the assessment process and treatment plan in three ways.

#### *Using strengths to accomplish normative developmental tasks*

First, strengths can be viewed as part of the developing capacities and capabilities that the youth exhibits in everyday contexts. If environments are supportive, development will flourish and a youth's strengths can be called upon to assist in navigating normative developmental tasks. For example, as adolescents mature, the behaviors indicating the development of an asset or strength will likely change. A sign of growing independence in a younger adolescent, for example, might be trying out a new practice that breaks with family traditions such as becoming a vegan or changing political views that might not be shared with other members of the family. As the teen gains experience in problem solving and managing decisions, the competency of independence may emerge in increasingly sophisticated ways. Leaving home for college is a task that requires additional sophistication in self-reliance because it calls on increasing responsibilities in self-direction and more opportunities to make one's own choices. Each new gradation in social demands faced by the adolescent requires added specialization in the strengths needed to be successful in task resolution.

### *Generalizing strengths to other contexts*

Second, adolescent strengths can be generalized to other more challenging contexts. The transition to adulthood involves interactions, interconnections, and mutual influences among such life domains as education, employment, and parenting.[50,52] Finding out how youth are using strengths in different domains of living and assessing the degree to which they are supported in each context provides a glimpse into the developmental pathways for promoting youths' natural assets. For example, the developmental tasks of gaining autonomy and increasing self-efficacy may come through successful work experiences. Asking adolescents about the skills and preparation required to do their work can lead to a discussion of how to use the same skills, competencies, and motivations in meeting academic goals. Rather than focusing on academic deficits and associated behaviors as the starting point, the focus can start with assessing where skills and developmental tasks are aligned in other contexts. How might these same skills and competencies be generalized to academic pursuits and what resources might be used to amplify the strength? Conversely, if in applying for college admittance an adolescent is able to draw on self-efficacy and discipline in meeting application deadlines, how might these same developmental competencies be applied to getting a summer job?

### *Using strengths to overcome adversity*

As outlined earlier, if environments are toxic or neglectful, strengths and competencies may be delayed. For example, children and teens affected by trauma and/or poverty may have hidden strengths and resiliencies that are not readily identified or discussed. There is no current diagnosis to capture the range of difficulties exhibited among youth with complex trauma, and both researchers and clinicians share the concern that youth may be mislabeled, receive one or more diagnoses not connected to their trauma, and as a result receive treatment or services that are not trauma informed.[53]

Responding to the effects of trauma on the developing brain may lead to underemphasizing strengths and only responding to behaviors that need immediate attention. Knowledge of how stress impacts development helps to reframe the source of negative or challenging behaviors leading to more productive channels of communication between teens, caregivers, and mental health professionals.

During a strength assessment, normalizing the teen's experience while pointing out the multiple ways self-protective strategies were used to meet challenges and adversity can shift the context from a focus on deficits to engagement of positive assets. For example, a strength may be viewed as a deficit limiting by medical professionals reviewing a teen's history because they fail to make the connection between the context in which the behavior develops and the teen's response to trauma. A trauma-informed practitioner may view the same behavior as an underdeveloped strength that served as an important protection against further pain. The clinician may then develop a treatment plan that includes refining the strength through appropriate modeling and coaching so that it can be called upon to serve a more adaptive role.

## STRENGTHS-BASED APPROACHES WITH AT-RISK YOUTH

Although most adolescents are able to manage both the social transitions and psychological changes occurring during this era, it is estimated that one in five teens have a serious mental disorder at some point in their lives[54] and about half of lifelong mental disorders begin by age 14.[55] The 12-month prevalence of Major Depressive Episode (MDEs) increased from 8.7% in 2005 to 11.3% in 2014 in adolescents.[56] In 2014, an estimated 2.8 million adolescents (11.4%) reported at least one major depressive episode in the year before being surveyed with higher percentages reported for White and Hispanic adolescents than Black adolescents.[57]

Because of misdiagnosis and the cascading effect of poverty, African-American youth are disproportionately diagnosed with conduct-related problems.[58,59] Minority racial groups are more likely to experience multidimensional poverty than their White counterparts.[60] In the United States, 39% of African-American children and adolescents and 33% of Latino children and adolescents are living in poverty, which is more than double the 14% poverty rate for non-Latino, White, and Asian children and adolescents.[61] American Indian/Alaska Native, Hispanic, Pacific Islander, and Native Hawaiian families are more likely than Caucasian and Asian families to live in poverty.[62] In 1 year, 39% of children between the ages of 12 and 17 years reported witnessing violence, 17% reported being a victim of physical assault, and 8% reported being the victim of sexual assault.[63]

Even though at-risk youth experience high levels of distress, research suggests that problem-oriented treatments and interventions designed to address diagnosed mental disorders have not been as effective in treating symptoms especially related to structural inequities. Without a focus on policies to address social conditions and support for individual and community resources, structural deficits are often overlooked in treatment planning.[64] Assessments designed only to focus on pathology and individual symptoms fail to address the larger systemic barriers affecting mental health. Diagnostic labels are so stigmatizing and difficult to remove that adolescents may begin to define themselves by these organizing frames leading to low self-esteem and self-efficacy that extends into adulthood.

Clearly, a change is needed in how to intervene with this target group. Although a specific diagnosis can lead to appropriate treatment in some cases, medicalizing a condition does not take the place of highlighting assets. The natural strengths and resiliencies that adolescents already possess should be considered in the assessment process and the development of treatment goals.[53] More work needs to be done in identifying programs that are rigorous and lead to effective outcomes.[7]

Additionally, finding out more about youths' systems of care is important as individual and family strengths are often tied to community networks and affiliations.[65] In general, capitalizing on the relationship between strengths and mental health can lead to well-designed prevention strategies and more positive interventions and treatment planning.[66,67] Mental health professionals conducting psychosocial assessments should consider how youth in high-risk environments might benefit from incorporating strengths in the assessment process.

### What Is Strength-Based Assessment?

A strength-based paradigm recognizes that all children have internalized strengths, but may not have had the opportunities to identify and develop these strengths.[21] What is known is that understanding and cultivating these strengths has been shown to play an integral role in enhancing treatment protocols for children and adolescents.[68] To use strengths effectively, research needs to explore ways to measure and operationalize strengths in every day practice.

As noted earlier, some researchers view strengths as individual traits, while researchers who study resilience more often view strengths as developmental and psychological competencies or as social processes that appear within a cultural and ecological context. One way to address these distinctions is to acknowledge that strengths may be viewed as both an individual attribute or trait and competency that develops in the context of loving and supportive families.

With that in mind, researchers have developed their own definitions of the assessment process. Strengths-based assessment, according to Epstein and Sharma,[19] *is a measurement of the emotional and behavioral skills, competencies, and characteristics that foster a sense of personal accomplishment, contribute to supportive and satisfying relationships with family members, peers, and adults, enhance one's ability to cope with challenges and stress, and promote one's personal, social, and academic development (p. 3)*. Their definition draws together the literature from positive psychology, positive youth development, and resilience theory. The authors point to the interrelated processes that define assets and strengths in these different contexts.

Saleebey[15] broadens this definition pointing to the importance of recognizing that strengths extend beyond the individual to the group, family, and community. Strengths are related to talents and individual abilities as well as caregiver and community resources and should be identified during the assessment process.[65] A strength-based assessment broadens the range of information received, providing a more comprehensive picture of clients and their environments.[69]

Although a clinical assessment can include a section on strengths, how much this information gets conveyed as important in treatment recommendations depends on the degree to which the clinician adopts a strength-based perspective. In a 2006 study, Cox found that a strength-based assessment is not necessarily effective if the assessor does not model an attitude that embraces the strength perspective. Believing in strengths as an intervention and conveying this to clients is an important part of modeling a strength-based approach.

## INFORMAL ASSESSMENT: SCREENING FOR STRENGTHS

Both informal and formal assessments can be used to incorporate strengths into the overall assessment process. If choosing to conduct a clinical interview that does not include the use of formal assessment tools, practitioners can learn to listen and identify strengths and positive emotions that may not be recognized by the adolescent.[69,70] Including strengths as an integral part of the assessment process offers a more proactive, balanced, and collaborative path to building rapport.[8,17,71] Although there may be many approaches to engaging teens in a discussion of strengths, five general guidelines for establishing an effective strength-based alliance are discussed below.

## RECOMMENDATION ONE: BE KNOWLEDGEABLE IN TRAUMA-INFORMED CARE

Practitioners who conduct strength-based assessments should have knowledge and skills in conducting strength screens that are trauma informed and culturally sensitive. Trauma-informed care embraces a perspective that highlights adaptation over symptoms and resilience over pathology.[72] A trauma-informed organization and staff are invested in creating a culture that views safety and trust as core principles that align with a strength-based perspective. Educating staff and clients about trauma and how trauma symptoms may manifest emotionally and behaviorally is an important first step in helping to create a safe environment. Education in trauma-specific interventions and how to refer to other services when needed can be useful when a referral is the appropriate choice.

Youth may not be accustomed to discussing sensitive and potentially revealing areas of their lives. They may not have yet identified the ways trauma impacts their behaviors and may not want to discuss information because of potential consequences to others in their system of care. Allowing teens to take the lead in what they share sends a message of mutual interest in wanting what is best for them. Cultural and familial norms may also play a role in what is discussed. In some cultures, discussing intimate personal information or emotions in general is not considered appropriate. Cultural humility and sensitivity to worldview should be modeled and care taken to create conditions for building a positive alliance with the teen and his or her family. Information gathered about strengths initially can be used to guide and enhance conversations with adolescents and caregivers about ways to support stabilization, build positive coping strategies, and support partnerships within the community.[53]

## RECOMMENDATION TWO: BUILD RAPPORT AND TRUST

In addition to creating a trauma-informed culture, each opportunity for interviewing youth should start with a focus on building the relationship. Mental health counselors and other professionals are equipped with a range of screening tools to choose from but may feel pressure to rule out symptoms of a mental disorder without adequately building a collaborative and trusting relationship first. Additionally, there may be a stigma attached to being seen for psychological concerns, and teens may have preconceived ideas about what the assessment process is designed to do. Questions that start with a focus on problems fail to address all facets of the youth's experience. Teens may not feel safe to self-disclose if asked too soon about areas that make them feel inadequate or vulnerable.

Basic listening skills that track youths' needs and concerns and show authentic interest in their lives are essential to creating a positive therapeutic alliance. Starting with strengths sets a positive tone and typically allows adolescents to feel more comfortable in discussing their hopes and fears. However, it is natural that there may be moments of discomfort or disengagement when discussing ways to address goals.

One approach that is useful in building rapport and developing a collaborative context for engagement comes from the field of Motivational Interviewing. Motivational Interviewing is an evidence-based, person-centered approach focused on helping the client resolve ambivalence about change.[73,74] The approach has been used in multiple treatment contexts and works well with clients who want to improve health-related behaviors.[75]

One of the initial strategies for developing a collaborative context is learning to use core skills known as OARS. OARS (open questions, affirmation, reflective listening, and summarizing) includes four active listening skills that can be integrated into the assessment process. It should be noted that the intent here is to provide a framework for a brief discussion of how active listening using OARS can be used to evoke strengths in an informal assessment. For a detailed discussion of how to use MI in practice, the reader is referred to the work of Miller and Rollnick.[73,74,76] Studies conducted with general healthcare providers demonstrated positive learning and application in the skills of Motivational Interviewing (MI).[77] For practitioners who want to gain expertise in this area, there are training opportunities and other resources available to support the integration of MI in behavioral health and other clinical settings.[78,79] For purposes of this review, using OARS can be helpful in highlighting skills that can be used in developing a collaborative relationship with teens.

Open-ended questions invite elaboration and thinking more deeply about an issue. Finding out about the teen's interests and goals conveys a willingness to learn more about the youth's experiences. Closed questions can be useful if specific information is warranted but open questions can create the momentum needed to explore the potential for change. Examples of open-ended questions are "Tell me more" or "What else do you see as important" or "How has this affected you?" In each case, the interviewer is asking for input that adds useful details about the teen's experience and invites their exploration of the area being discussed.

Affirmations are statements that recognize the teen's strengths. These listening skills are useful in setting a tone for collaboration that highlights strengths and competencies as a valued part of the overall assessment. To be effective, statements must be genuine and focused on behaviors that promote the teen's self-efficacy and confidence. Affirmations may also be used to reframe behaviors or concerns as evidence of positive client qualities. For example, reframing vulnerability as a strength when appropriate sets up an opportunity for discussing challenges in a nonthreatening way. Examples of affirmations are "I appreciate your openness to discuss this ..." or "You clearly have a strong desire to overcome this". Affirmations can also emphasize past experiences as a way to demonstrate strengths such as "You handled yourself well when faced with the disappointment of not getting in the play" or "You were able to draw on your creativity and communication to coordinate the food drive. How might you use those same strengths now?" A reframing response that is affirming could be "Although you mention feeling embarrassed about coming in today, your actions show your commitment and persistence to move through challenges. That says a lot about you."

Reflective listening is a basic set of skills used in any active listening approach. Reflections involve not only skill in listening to the content of a client's message but the feelings and emotion that accompany the client's story. Once the information is understood, the interviewer rephrases what was just heard and the dialogue continues. In Mi, reflective listening is used to guide the client toward making changes directed toward appropriate goals. The therapist guides the client toward resolving ambivalence by focusing on the negative aspects of the status quo and the positive aspects of making a change.

Summaries are used to open and close a session or transition between content areas. Summaries call attention to important themes and patterns discussed during the interview. This skill can serve to highlight specific topics for further exploration or action. In MI, summaries can highlight both sides of the client's ambivalence about change promoting discrepancy with an ultimate goal of promoting positive behavior change. Ultimately, building rapport creates a sense of alliance and cooperation leading to better outcomes and compliance with goals of treatment.[80]

## RECOMMENDATION THREE: INTEGRATE STRENGTH-BASED QUESTIONS

Once rapport has been established and trust is beginning to form, the clinician can explore interests and strengths in more depth. Knowledge of adolescent development and typical behaviors of developing teens will aid in making decisions about what areas to address. Strengths can be viewed developmentally as part of the maturing capacities and capabilities that the youth exhibits in everyday contexts. Questions might focus on how the adolescent's strengths are being used effectively with their social, academic, and home life. The clinician can listen for, inquire about, and point out strengths that occur naturally and are associated with everyday use. For example, an adolescent named Sasha may report volunteering with an after-school reading program for ESL students. Using OARS and listening for specific developmental competencies and strengths, the clinician might start with an open-ended question asking about what she most enjoys in the volunteer experience. Social engagement focused on broadening her sphere of friendships, and service to others may be pointed out as strengths. The conversation may then continue on how to use these same strengths in other domains of living promoting a sense of positive well-being and engagement in the interview process.

For some adolescents, strengths may not be as readily identified. Competencies may still be developing or viewed by others as liabilities because of association with risk-taking. As noted earlier, finding ways to ask about experiences the adolescent enjoys even in areas of high risk can be an opportunity for educating about how to use their strengths to maximize the upside and minimize the downside. Rather than using the interview as an opportunity to lecture about the hazards of associating with negative peer influences, the clinician can listen for what the experience provides the teen.

For example, on intake, Juan, a 15-year-old male who recently had to appear before the juvenile court, reports ambivalence in trying to decide whether to continue to associate with a group of peers who were charged with using drugs and shoplifting. Rather than noting how involvement with gangs is dangerous, the practitioner can acknowledge the importance of feeling part of a group in trying to build interpersonal competence. Using the OARS technique of affirmation, the clinician might point out Juan's strength of loyalty to his peers and not wanting to let his friends down as part of the motivation for a recent shoplifting charge. Rather than asking why he shoplifted, which might appear to be a logical question but not well timed for the adolescent's developmental goals, it might be more appropriate to ask what needs are getting met by being in the group. Juan may have felt peer pressure or excitement about trying something new that pushed the limits of anything he had done before. The clinician might ask whether the consequences such as getting caught and going to jail would be worth the risk of being part of the group. Highlighting the ambivalence Juan feels in staying with a group that has a clear downside could be beneficial. This could lead to a discussion of how joining other prosocial peer groups that offer new experiences and challenges could be equally rewarding. A prosocial group and mentoring could strengthen his interpersonal competencies and channel his drive for novelty. A new group might also have a high challenge but with less downside and risk of getting in trouble. Joining a karate team at school or being part of an outward-bound experience set up by a local youth agency where Juan lives could be explored.

Meeting Juan where he is and understanding his perspective rather than identifying the behaviors as deficient can lead to more productive outcomes and more open lines of communication. By integrating strengths as a natural part of the interview, the mental health professional is taking an exploratory rather than accusatory stance and recognizing the adolescent's competencies beyond his or her presenting concerns and diagnostic profile.[81]

## RECOMMENDATION FOUR: COLLABORATE ON GOALS

Once strengths have been recognized and linked to positive outcomes, collaborating with adolescents and when possible their support system on using their strengths to meet appropriate goals, increases the likelihood that areas targeted for change will be addressed.[82,83] To avoid the potential for miscommunication, goals should be stated in language and with objectives that are clear and manageable. Discussing how actions will be taken to achieve valued outcomes may increase motivation. Anticipating potential obstacles can pave the way to overcome the challenges that arise. Brainstorming strategies and activities the teen can do to increase a sense of flow and connection can decrease anxiety and rumination.[69] Teens may feel more empowered to take an active role in choices they make because of collaborating to meet goals.[8,66]

## RECOMMENDATION FIVE: INCLUDE OUTSIDE SUPPORTS AND RESOURCES WHEN AVAILABLE

Using a strength-based approach in assessment is most effective if consideration is given to assessing and identifying resources that can support the teen's developing competencies.

For example, work experience may be valuable if it promotes the development of positive values and skills but if association with peers or adults in the workplace leads to introducing negative behaviors such as drinking or delinquency, it can have the opposite effect on performance.[84] Broadening the scope of screening questions to include a focus on family and community resources can uncover positive environmental strengths and supports. Asking adolescents and their families about not only the teen's strengths but also the family's strengths can create a more positive alliance with caregivers who can in turn be effective in modeling a strength-based relationship in the home.[9,11] Asking about other natural support systems such as extended family, school resources such as teachers, peers, counselors, or coaches, and community-based youth groups and support networks can lead to new alliances. Mentoring programs and other community programs that support teens should be enlisted where possible.[14]

## FORMAL ASSESSMENTS AND STRUCTURED INVENTORIES

Empirical validation of strength instruments has historically not kept pace with deficit-oriented assessments[8,85] but in the last decade, the gap seems to be narrowing as several inventories that focus on strengths are now available. The following section describes screening and assessment tools that are strength-based and empirically validated. Four inventories are reviewed with recommendations for how results might be translated into strategies for supporting the adolescent's existing and developing strengths.

## POSITIVE PSYCHOLOGY AND THE VIA CLASSIFICATION OF STRENGTHS MODEL

Positive Psychology is associated with the scientific study of psychological health, well-being, and optimal functioning.[86] Rather than focusing on deficiencies or mental disorders, researchers are concerned with the way individuals maximize their strengths.[87] Although Positive Psychology is a relative newcomer to the field of nomothetic psychology, the breadth of studies providing an empirical basis for assessing universal strengths is notable.

The Values in Action (VIA) Classification of Strengths project provides a blueprint for systematically examining the study of character strengths and what constitutes good character.[4] One of the first efforts at classifying core human strengths was initiated by Chris Peterson and Martin Seligman[86] who published *Character Strengths and Virtues* describing the VIA Classification. Character strengths can be defined as the positive traits reflected in psychological processes of cognition, affect, behavior, and volition that contribute to well-being in self and other.[27] Character strengths have been empirically validated[87] and a number of inventories have been developed for use with different age groups.

The VIA Classification includes 24 character strengths, organized under six broad virtues. Several assessment instruments that focus on strengths, positive emotions, personal growth, and other related constructs are available for use with both youth and adults.

## VIA INVENTORY OF STRENGTHS FOR YOUTH SCALE

The VIA Inventory of Strengths for Youth (ages 10–17) is a self-report inventory for children and youth providing information about top character strengths and virtues. The VIA-Youth measures 24 character strengths and identifies the top five strengths known as signature strengths. Respondents are asked to rate the degree to which each statement is aligned with their preferences on a 5-point scale ranging from (1 = Strongly Disagree to 5 = Strongly Agree with a midpoint of 3 = Neutral/Undecided).

The original VIA-Youth consisted of 198 items but the VIA-Youth short form is now used widely in a variety of settings. The 96-question short form, which can typically be taken in 10–15 min, has been researched and empirically found to have comparable reliability and validity to the original instrument. Items in the latest version were also rewritten for ease of comprehension making the short form a more practical choice in most contexts.

## PSYCHOMETRIC PROPERTIES

Studies of the 96-item short form have found that internal consistency was fair to strong for all 24 character strength subscales (average Cronbach's alpha = 0.87, min = 0.69, max = 0.95). Based on the original 198-item form, test–retest reliability within a 6-month period was fair to strong for the subscales (mean test–retest correlation = 0.58, min = 0.46, max = 0.71).[4]

In reviewing validity, Park and Peterson[4] found support for four main types of character strengths. Additionally, the VIA-Youth Survey has established good psychometrics with positive convergence between parent and self-ratings.[4] In another review, five strength factors emerged and were independently associated with well-being and happiness.[88] In a study of South African learners, ages 13–17, criterion-related validity was supported by correlations in expected directions between VIA-Youth subscales and indices of psychological well-being and pathology.[89] The analysis found that the construct validity of the VIA-Youth is more homogeneous or unidimensional than multidimensional. Character strengths also have shown a positive relationship to school achievement.[90] Character strengths of the mind (e.g., self-regulation, perseverance, love of learning) were predictive of school success.[91]

## IMPLICATIONS FOR PRACTICE

Using strengths in practice has been associated with well-being and positive affect.[92] Researchers found positive education programming involving interventions using character strengths led to improved study skills and greater school engagement.[93] Character strengths may appear over time as part of the normal developmental trajectory of youth. For example, the least common strengths among young children and adolescents are those that require cognitive maturation: for example, appreciation of beauty and excellence, forgiveness, modesty, and open-mindedness.[4,4a] This research suggests that integrating the VIA Inventory of Strengths for Youth Scale (VIA-YS) as part of the ongoing assessment in schools and community settings has the possibility of increasing adherence to difficult tasks or assignments and lead in general to more positive affect and sense of overall well-being.

Some general guidelines can be summarized for using strengths in practice. First, using character strengths and in particular signature strengths should be encouraged. Using strengths in daily practice in one context can help to generalize learning to other domains.[20] Practitioners can engage adolescents collaboratively in pointing out assets, cultivating strengths, and determining strategies for reaching relevant goals. Programming that incorporates a strength vocabulary in classroom and extracurricular activities can help to create a culture that views strengths as a routine part of the academic experience.

## POSITIVE YOUTH DEVELOPMENT AND THE DEVELOPMENTAL ASSETS MODEL

Positive youth development is another area in research and practice that complements a strength-based focus. Positive youth development is based on the idea that it is not enough to notice areas of challenge for teens. It is also important to develop their talents and capabilities even in the face of adversity. Programs that incorporate this approach tend to promote adolescent development that is aligned with developmental stage, social and cultural expectations, and positive assets and resources. Positive youth development as a field is concerned with strengthening the family, school, and community bonds to achieve adaptive outcomes.[94] According to Scales,[95] early adolescence is a vulnerable period where many variables can impact a healthy developmental trajectory. Finding ways to build positive assets and channel energy away from negative influences can help to set in motion the possibility of future success even in the face of challenges that may arise.

An example of a framework that is based on the Positive Youth Development (PYD) philosophy is the 40 Developmental Assets framework. The framework[96] establishes a set of developmental experiences and positive assets that are linked to positive outcomes and correlated with developmental processes over time.[97–99] The framework was refined through input from a variety of stakeholders through the years before the final list of 40 assets was developed.

For over two decades, the Search Institute, a nonprofit organization dedicated to developing positive outcomes for youth, has continued to research the role of assets in promoting health and well-being for adolescents. Developmental assets represent the relationships, opportunities, skills, and values identified by the Search Institute as essential in promoting the positive development of all children and adolescents. These assets have the power to influence young people's developmental trajectories, protect them from a range of negative outcomes, and help them to become more productive, caring, and responsible citizens.[99] Among the 40 assets identified, 20 are external assets related to the positive developmental experiences in the youth's environment and 20 are internal assets identified as values and commitments that guide healthy choices and decisions (Search Institute, www.search-institute.org).

Research has shown that the more risk factors the child has and develops, the less chance to be successful[100] but the more assets a particular youth has, the more likely it is that she will make responsible lifestyle choices, do well in school, and avoid alcohol and other drugs.[97]

The assets model is based on a synthesis of multiple lines of inquiry aimed at identifying the building blocks of development that contribute to three types of healthy outcomes: the prevention of high-risk behavior, the enhancement of thriving behavior, and resilience identified as the capacity to function adequately in the face of adversity.[101]

## DEVELOPMENTAL ASSETS PROFILE: THE SEARCH INSTITUTE

The Developmental Assets Profile (DAP) survey (ages 11–18) is a self-report inventory designed to provide information about a youth's developmental assets within five social contexts: Personal, Social, Family, School, and Community. Additionally, the DAP assesses four External Asset Categories (Support, Empowerment, Boundaries and Expectations, Constructive Use of Time) and four Internal Asset Categories (Commitment to Learning, Positive Values, Social Competencies, and Positive Identity). The Developmental Assets Profile is one of four surveys created by researchers at the Search Institute that collects information on the strengths and assets of youth.

The DAP[102] (Search Institute, www.search-institute.org) consists of 58 strength items and can typically be completed in 10 min. Questions are rated on a 4-point scale from (Not at All or Rarely to Almost Always or Extremely). The DAP can be taken by hand or administered electronically.

## PSYCHOMETRIC PROPERTIES

In studies in the United States and internationally, the DAP has been found to be psychometrically sound showing strong reliability, validity, and stability in research conducted with a variety of youth populations (Search Institute, www.search-institute.org). The Search Institute reports the following summary of the DAP's psychometric properties. Internal consistency was 0.95 for internal assets, 0.93 for external assets, and 0.97 for total assets. Two-week test–retest reliability (sample 6th–12th grade, $n = 225$) averaged 0.86 for the total asset score, 0.86 for the internal assets score, and 0.84 for the external assets score. Concurrent validity was strong (0.82) for the correlation between the DAP total asset score and assets derived from the Attitudes and Behavior Survey. The asset framework appears to have comparable validity across demographic variables of gender, race, ethnicity, geographic background, and social economic status.[102a]

## IMPLICATIONS FOR PRACTICE

Research shows that of the 40 developmental assets studied, 76% of youth report having fewer than 30 assets while 41% possess only 11–20 assets (The Search Institute, www.search-institute.org). Search Institute research shows nine developmental assets consistently inform successful youth outcomes.[103] Internal assets include bonding to school, reading for pleasure, achievement motivation, and school engagement. External assets include a caring school climate, parent involvement, service to others, high expectations, and participation in high quality youth programs. These assets are being used to frame individual and community interventions.

Findings from the DAP survey can assist program coordinators, project leaders, teachers, and youth to discover what assets are needed in their particular environments and work toward building in assets to promote positive outcomes. Understanding what gaps exist and building assets into individual treatment plans, school curriculum, after school programming, or psychoeducation with families and community supports is an effective way to capitalize on youth strengths. Organizations that support positive youth development can use research informed by the DAP to write strategic plans. Additionally, the results from the DAP can empower youth to create their own opportunities by building on existing assets and seeking out positive assets in their homes, schools, and communities.

## THE STRENGTH-BASED ASSESSMENT MODEL

The Strength-Based Assessment Model can be used to guide practitioners in helping youth to cultivate undeveloped skills and competencies while also pointing to strengths that can be used to support existing capabilities. Epstein[10] noted that assessments in the area of emotional and behavioral disorders were created for the sole purpose of identifying and measuring children's deficits and yet there were no models emphasizing children's strengths. The Strength-Based Assessment Model assumes that a youth's background and life experiences may be directly related to the diagnosis of deficits that end up being the focus of treatment. Strengths may go unrecognized if environments are not supporting the assets needed to be successful.[19,104] By eliciting strengths in different domains, clinicians can form a more holistic picture of how teens are functioning across contexts.[10] The Behavioral and Emotional Rating Scale[19] was created to provide a balanced picture of youth functioning and a more comprehensive picture of youth strengths.

## BEHAVIORAL AND EMOTIONAL RATING SCALE SECOND EDITION

The Behavioral and Emotional Rating Scale, Second Edition (BERS-2)[19,105] measures the personal strengths and competencies of children and adolescents in five domains: Interpersonal Strength defined as the ability to control emotions and behaviors in a social situation; Involvement with Family describing participation and relationship with family; Intrapersonal Strength including an assessment of competence and accomplishment; Affective Strength identified as ability to express feelings toward others and to accept affection from others; and School Functioning defined as competence in school and classroom tasks.

Information about the adolescent can be gathered from self-report, parents, and teachers, or other professionals. The two observer forms, the BERS-2 Parent Rating Scale and Teacher Rating Scale, can be used to assess youth ages 5–18. The Youth Rating Scale can be used with children and adolescents ages 11–18. The advantage of the BERS assessment system is the ability to assess youth strengths across different domains of functioning. Any of the instruments can be used individually although there is added benefit in getting multiple perspectives.

The BERS-2 consists of 52 items, and the instrument takes less than 15 min to complete. Each item is rated on a 4-point scale of 0–3 from (Not at All Like to Very Much Like). In addition, there are eight open-ended questions on each version that ask about personal, academic, social, athletic, family, and community strengths. The questions should only be used by outside raters who have had enough interaction with the child or adolescent to be reliable informants.

## PSYCHOMETRIC PROPERTIES

Multiple studies have examined the BERS content, construct, and criterion-related validity. Internal reliability and test–retest reliability were found to be good.[19,106] Studies of the convergent validity of the BERS-2 have been done with students with special needs, elementary students as well as Hispanic and African-American youth. The instrument has been found to adequately operationalize the construct of behavioral and emotional strengths. The BERS-2 demonstrated moderate-to-high correlations with the Social Skills Rating Scale and negative correlations with deficit-oriented scales.[106,107]

The internal consistency reliability of the BERS-2 subtests was established with children without disabilities and with children who had emotional disabilities Coefficients were found to be strong for each subtest and for the overall score. Detailed reviews are included in the test manual including information on demographic variables.

## IMPLICATIONS FOR PRACTICE

Because the strength-based perspective assumes that all youth, even those with diagnosable emotional and behavioral difficulties, have strengths, the BERS-2 is useful in evaluating children who might need specialized services.[18,106] Similar to other instruments discussed in this review, the BERS-2 can identify children and adolescents who might benefit from further development of their strengths. Results can be used to create more effective treatment plans, highlight strengths in individualized educational plans, and develop a holistic curriculum that includes a strength-based focus. The BERS-2 has been used in a variety of settings including schools, juvenile justice, mental health clinics, and local, state, and federal agencies to evaluate the outcomes of services for children with and without disabilities.[21,105]

## STRENGTH ASSESSMENT AND TREATMENT MODEL

Rawana and Brownlee[28] developed a strength-based model that also considers context as an important factor in identifying strengths in youth. Although the inner traits and attributes that define strengths are considered unique and part of the personal agency, strengths are also discussed as developing through interaction with others. How strengths are expressed depends on the context in which they occur. According to the authors, strengths are conceptualized as competencies embedded in culture and valued both by the individual and by society.[28] Strengths may be overlooked if the only frame for viewing is an individual report. Youth may not consider all the ways they use their strengths. Because adolescents may express strengths differently depending on context, it is useful to examine what cues may be different whether at home, school, or work. Each opportunity to observe adolescents in their natural settings becomes a source of information for recognizing how strengths may be supported or ignored. Understanding and cultivating adolescent strengths has been shown to play an integral role in developing interventions and treatment plans for children and adolescents.[68]

## STRENGTH ASSESSMENT INVENTORY

The Strength Assessment Inventory for Youth (SAI-Y) is a 124-item measure that provides a comprehensive assessment of individual strengths in children and adolescents between the ages of 10 and 18 years.[108] Strengths are categorized into contextual domains (peer, family, school, employment, community) and developmental domains (personality, personal and physical care, spirituality and cultural, leisure and recreation).[109]

The measure is simple to complete by either the youth themselves or with someone who is close to them. There is an observer version (SAI-O) for use by professionals such as teachers, parents, counselors, or other identified resources. The SAI-O contains the same items as the SAI-Y.[110] Items are rated on a 3-point scale and respondents are asked to indicate the frequency with which each strength item is present for them from (0 = not at all 1 = sometimes to 2 = almost always). The respondents can also indicate if a question does not apply.[111]

## PSYCHOMETRIC PROPERTIES

Evaluation of the psychometric properties of the SAI-Y (using prorated scale scores) has revealed moderate-to-strong internal consistency for ratings on all scales (except the supplementary scales), with estimates ranging from 0.60 to 0.87. The total strength score and total empirical strength score also showed strong internal consistency estimates, 0.96 and 0.95, respectively.[111] The SAI-Y ratings have demonstrated good test–retest reliability when used with a sample of 572 children and adolescents ages 9–19 years, with estimates ranging from 0.47 to 0.82.[111] The SAI-Y total scores also demonstrated good convergent (0.52–0.60) and divergent (0.40–0.45) validity with standardized instruments of strengths and emotional and behavioral functioning including the BERS-2.[105]

## IMPLICATIONS FOR PRACTICE

The SAI includes an assessment of how strengths change over time. Some strengths may vary by context.[28] For example, an adolescent may be able to relate well to peers and have strong interpersonal strengths but these are not being expressed in the home environment. This may lead to the discussion of age-related changes and the natural tendency at this age to move away from identification with parents to identification with friends.

The multiple domains for expression of strengths can also be useful in helping to identify strategies for addressing problems that may be connected to specific areas of functioning. The assessment process can help to determine whether an individual asset is needed to manage an area of difficulty or whether a more effective strategy would be to bolster family or community resources. Because the SAI includes subscales for each strength domain, more specific information can be used to discuss goals and strategies for strengthening personal and academic development. Questions can lead to a more in-depth discussion and exploration of the teen's specific strengths with an aim of generalizing to other contexts.

## SUMMARY

Despite the increasing popularity of strength-based approaches in adolescent assessment, many assessment tools and processes still emphasize diagnosing mental disorders rather than highlighting developmental competencies and strengths. Mental health professionals would be well served to reconsider ways in which strengths are integrated into the overall mission of their agency, school, or clinic. A strength assessment offers a more comprehensive profile of youth functioning and empowers youth to be collaborators in designing appropriate treatment goals. Ongoing training in the field should include interprofessional collaboration and discussion among healthcare and mental health providers on how to promote best practices that integrate a strengths perspective in assessment and intervention.

## REFERENCES


1. Friedman HL, MacDonald DA. Humanistic testing and assessment. *J Humanist Psychol.* 2006;46:510–529.
2. Huebner ES, Gilman R. Toward a focus on positive psychology in school psychology. *Sch Psychol Q.* 2003; 18(2):99–102.
3. Seligman MEP, Csikszentmihalyi M. Positive psychology: an introduction. *Am Psychol.* 2000;55:5–14.
4. Park N, Peterson C. Moral competence and character strengths among adolescents: the development and validation of the values in action inventory of strengths for youth. *J Adolesc.* 2006;29:891–909.

4a. Park N, Peterson C, Seligman MEP. Character strengths in fifty-four nations and the fifty US states. *J Posit Psychol.* 2006;1(3):118–129.

5. Masten A, Hubbard JJ, Gest SD, Tellegen A, Garmezy N, Ramirez M. Competence in the context of adversity: pathways to resilience and maladaptation from childhood to late adolescence. *Dev Psychopathol.* 1999;11:143–169.
6. Ricks N. The strengths perspective: providing opportunities for teen parents and their families to succeed. *J Fam Strengths.* 2016;15(1). Article 11. Available at: https://digitalcommons.library.tmc.edu/jfs/vol15/iss1/11.
7. Brownlee K, Rawana J, Franks J, et al. A systematic review of strengths and resilience outcome literature relevant to children and adolescents. *Child Adolesc Social Work J.* 2013;30(5):435–459. https://doi.org/10.1007/s10560-013-0301-9.
8. Tedeschi RG, Kilmer RP. Assessing strengths, resilience, and growth to guide clinical interventions. *Prof Psychol Res Pr.* 2005;36(3):230–237.
9. Cowger CD. Assessing client strengths: clinical assessment for client empowerment. *Social Work.* 1994;39: 262–268.
10. Epstein MH. The development and validation of a scale to assess the emotional and behavioral strengths of children and adolescents. *Remedial Spec Educ.* 1999;20: 258–262.
11. Harniss MK, Epstein MH, Ryser G, Pearson N. The behavioral and emotional rating scale: convergent validity. *J Psychoedu Assess.* 1999;17:4–14.
12. Jimerson SR, Sharkey JD, Nyborg V, Furlong MJ. Strength-based assessment and school psychology: a summary and synthesis. *Calif Sch Psychol.* 2004;9:9–19.
13. Kaplan H. Toward an understanding of resilience: a critical review of definitions and models. In: Glantz M, Johnson J, eds. *Resilience and Development: Positive Life Adaptations.* New York: Plenum; 1999.
14. Masten AS, Coatsworth JD. The development of competence in favorable and unfavorable environments: lessons from research on successful children. *Am Psychol.* 1998;53:205–220.
15. Saleebey D, ed. *The Strengths Perspective in Social Work Practice.* 4th ed. Toronto: Pearson; 2006.
16. Wieck A, Rapp C, Sullivan WP, Kisthardt S. A strengths perspective for social work practice. *Social Work.* 1989; 34:350–354.

16a. Seligman MEP. Positive psychology, positive prevention, and positive therapy. *Handbook Posit Psychol.* 2002;2: 3–12.

17. Rhee S, Furlong MJ, Turner JA, Harari I. Integrating strength-based perspectives in psychoeducational evaluations. *Calif Sch Psychol.* 2001;6:5–17.

17a. Laursen EK. Frontiers in strength-based treatment. *Reclaiming Child Youth.* 2003;12(1):12–17.

18. Epstein MH. Assessing the emotional and behavioral strengths of children. *Reclaiming Child Youth.* 1998;6: 250–252.
19. Epstein M, Sharma J. *Behavioral and Emotional Rating Scale: A Strengths-Based Approach to Assessment.* Austin, TX: PRO-ED; 1998.
20. Park N, Peterson C. Positive psychology and character strengths: application to strengths-based school counseling. *Prof Sch Couns.* 2008;12:85–92.

20a. Cowger CD, Snively CA. Assessing client strengths: Individual, family, and community empowerment. In: Saleebey D, ed. *The strengths perspective in social work practice.* 3rd ed. Boston: Allyn and Bacon; 2002:106–123.

21. Buckley JA, Epstein MH. The behavioral and emotional rating scale-2 (BERS-2): providing a comprehensive approach to strength-based assessment. *Calif Sch Psychol.* 2004;9:21–27.

22. Practicing the strengths perspective: everyday tools and resourcesSaleebey D, ed. *Fam Soc.* 2001;82:221–222.
23. Garmezy N. Vulnerability and resilience. In: Funder D, Parke RD, Tomlinson-Keasey C, Widaman K, eds. *Studying Lives through Time: Personality and Development.* Washington DC: American Psychological Association; 1993.
24. Kirby LD, Fraser MW. Risk and resilience in childhood: an ecological perspective. In: Fraser MW, ed. *Risk and Resilience in Childhood: An Ecological Perspective.* Washington, DC: NASW Press; 1997:10–33.
25. Masten AS, Burt KB, Coatsworth JD. Competence and psychopathology in development. In: Cicchetti D, Cohen DJ, eds. *Developmental Psychopathology: Risk, Disorder, and Adaptation.* Hoboken, NJ: John Wiley & Sons Inc; 2006:696–738.
26. Graves S, Sobalvarro A, Nichols K, et al. Examining the effectiveness of a culturally adapted social emotional intervention for African American males in an urban setting. *Sch Psychol Q.* 2017;32:62–74.
27. Park N, Peterson C, Seligman MEP. Strengths of character and well-being. *J Soc Clin Psychol.* 2004;23:603–619.
28. Rawana E, Brownlee K. Making the possible probable: a strength-based assessment and intervention framework for clinical work with parents, children, and adolescents. *Famil Soc.* 2009;90:255–260.
29. Kaczmarek P, Riva M. Facilitating adolescent optimal development: training considerations for counseling psychologists. *Couns Psychol.* 1996;24(3):400–432.
30. Siegel DJ. *Brainstorm: The Power and Purpose of the Teenage Brain.* New York: Random House; 2013.
31. Masten AS, Burt KB, Roisman GI, Obradovic J, Long JD, Tellegen A. Resources and resilience in the transition to adulthood: continuity and change. *Dev Psychopathol.* 2004;16(4):1071–1094.
32. Havighurst RJ. *Developmental Tasks and Education.* Chicago, IL: University of Chicago Press; 1948.
33. Bonnie RJ, Stroud C, Breiner H, eds. *Committee on Improving the Health, Safety, and Well-Being of Young Adults; Board on Children, Youth, and Families; Institute of Medicine; National Research Council.* Washington (DC): National Academies Press (US); January 27, 2015.
34. Johnson SB, Blum RW, Giedd JN. Adolescent maturity and the brain: the promise and pitfalls of neuroscience research in adolescent health policy. *J Adolesc Health.* 2009;45(3):216–221.
34a. Spear LP. The adolescent brain and age-related behavioral manifestations. *Neuro Biobehav Rev.* 2000;24:417–463.
35. Yurgelun-Todd D. Emotional and cognitive changes during adolescence. *Curr Opin Neurobiol.* 2007;17(2): 132–139. https://doi.org/10.1016/j.conb.2007.03.009.
36. Casey BJ, Galvan A, Hare TA. Changes in cerebral functional organization during cognitive development. *Curr Opin Neurobiol.* 2005;15:239–244.
37. Benes FM. Brain development, VII: human brain growth spans decades. *Am J Psychiatry.* 1998;155(11):1489. https://doi.org/10.1176/aip.155.11.1489.
38. Dahl RE. Affect regulation, brain development, and behavioral/emotional health in adolescence. *CNS Spectr.* 2001;6:60–72.
39. Steinberg L. Risk-taking in adolescence: new perspectives from brain and behavioral science. *Curr Direct Psychol Science.* 2007;16:55–59.
40. Albert D, Steinberg L. Judgment and decision making in adolescence. *J Res Adolesc.* 2011;21:211–224.
41. Ohannessian CM, Lerner RM, Von Eye A. Perceived parental acceptance and early adolescent self-competence. *Am J Orthopsychiatry.* 1998;68(4):621–629.
42. Cicchetti D, Cohen DJ. Perspectives on developmental psychopathology. D.J. In: Cicchetti D, Cohen DJ, eds. *Theory and Methods In Developmental Psychopathology.* Vol. 1. New York: Wiley; 1995:3–20.
43. Sroufe AL. Psychopathology as an outcome of development. *Dev Psychopathol.* 1997;9(2):251–268.
44. Cohen P, Kasen S, Chen H, Hartmark C, Gordon K. Variations in patterns of developmental transitions in the emerging adulthood period. *Dev Psychol.* 2003;39(4): 657–669.
45. Osgood DW, Ruth G, Eccles JS, Jacobs JE, Barber BL. Six paths to adulthood: fast starters, parents without careers, educated partners, educated singles, working singles, and slow starters. In: Settersten Jr RA, Furstenberg Jr FF, Rumbaut RG, eds. *On the Frontier of Adulthood: Theory, Research, and Public Policy.* Chicago, IL: University of Chicago Press; 2005:320–355.
46. O'Connor TG, Allen JP, Bell KL, Hauser ST. Adolescent-Parent relationships and leaving home in young adulthood. In: Graber JA, Dubas JS, Semon J, eds. *Leaving Home: Understanding the Transition to Adulthood.* San Francisco: Jossey-Bass; 1996:39–52.
47. Csikszentmihalyi M, Schneider BL. *Becoming Adult: How Teenagers Prepare for the World of Work.* New York: Basic; 2000.
48. Copeland WE, Shanahan L, Costello EJ, Angold A. Childhood and adolescent psychiatric disorders as predictors of young adult disorders. *Arch Gen Psychiatry.* 2009;66: 764–772.
49. Goldscheider FK, Goldscheider C. The effects of childhood family structure on leaving and returning home. *J Marriage Fam.* 1998;60(3):745–756.
50. Maughan B, Champion L. Risk and protective factors in the transition to young adulthood. In: Baltes PB, Baltes MM, eds. *Successful Aging: Perspectives from the Behavioral Sciences.* New York: Cambridge University Press; 1990:296–331.
51. Niwa M, Lee RS, Tanaka T, Okada K, Kano S, Sawa A. A critical period of vulnerability to adolescent stress: epigenetic mediators in mesocortical dopaminergic neurons. *Hum Mol Genet.* 2016;25(7):1370–1381.
52. Gore S, Aseltine R, Colten ME, Lin B. Life after high school: development, stress, and well-being. In: Gotlib I, Wheaton B, eds. *Stress and Adversity Over the Life Course: Trajectories and Turning Points.* New York: Cambridge University Press; 1997:197–214.

53. Kisiel C, Summersett-Ringgold F, Weil LEG, McClelland G. Understanding strengths in relation to complex trauma and mental health symptoms within child welfare. *J Child Fam Stud*. 2017;26(2):437–451.
54. National Institute of Mental Health, 2017 Available from: https://www.nimh.nih.gov/health/statistics/major-depression.shtml.
55. Substance Abuse & Mental Health Services Administration. *Key Substance Use and Mental Health Indicators in the United States: Results from the 2016 National Survey on Drug Use and Health*; 2017. Retrieved from: https://www.samhsa.gov/data/sites/default/files/NSDUH-FFR1-2016/NSDUH-FFR1-2016.pdf-PDF.
56. Mojtabai R, Olfson M, Han B. National trends in the prevalence and treatment of depression in adolescents and young adults. *Pediatrics*. 2016;138(6). https://doi.org/10.1542/peds.2016-1878.
57. Substance Abuse and Mental Health Services Administration. *Behavioral Health Barometer: United States, 2015*. Rockville, MD: Substance Abuse and Mental Health Services Administration; 2015. HHS Publication No. SMA–16–Baro–2015.
58. Gonzalez MJ. Access to mental health services: the struggle of poverty affected urban children of color. *Child Adolesc Social Work J*. 2005;22(3–4):245–256.
59. Mizock L, Harkins D. Diagnostic bias and conduct disorder: improving culturally sensitive diagnosis. *Child Youth Serv*. 2011;32:243–253. https://doi.org/10.1080/0145935X.2011.605315.
60. Reeves R, Rodrigue E, Kneebone E. *Five Evils: Multidimensional Poverty and Race in America*; 2016. Available from: https://www.brookings.edu/wp-content/jploads/2016/06/ReevesKneeboneRodrigue_Multidimensional-Poverty_FullPaper.pdf.
61. Kids Count, Data Center, Children in Poverty; 2014. Available from: https://www.apa.org/pi/ses/resources/publications/factsheet-erm.pdf.
62. U.S. Census Bureau. (2014). U.S. Poverty Report. Available from: https://www.census.gov/population/projections/data/national/2014.html.
63. Finkelhor D, Turner HA, Ormond R, Hamby S, Kracke K. *Children's Exposure to Violence: A Comprehensive National Survey*. Washington, DC: U.S. Department of Justice; 2009.
64. McWhirter JJ, McWhirter BT, McWhirter AM, McWhirter EH. *At-Risk Youth: A Comprehensive Approach*. 2nd ed. Pacific Grove, CA: Brooks/Cole; 1998.
65. Early TJ, GlenMaye LF. Valuing families: social work practice with families from a strengths perspective. *Social Work*. 2000;45(2):118–130.
66. LeBuffe PA, Shapiro VB. Lending "strength" to the assessment of preschool social-emotional health. *Calif Sch Psychol*. 2004;9:51–61.
67. Suldo SM, Thalji-Raitano A, Kiefer S, Ferron J. Conceptualizing high school students' mental health through a dual-factor model. *Sch Psychol Rev*. 2016;45:434–457.
68. Oswald DP, Cohen R, Best AM, Jenson CE, Lyons JS. Child strengths and the level of care for children with emotional and behavioral disorders. *J Emot Behav Disord*. 2001;9(3):192–199.
69. Rashid T, Ostermann RF. Strength-based assessment in clinical practice. *J Clin Psychol*. 2009;65(5):488–498.
70. Duncan PM, Garcia AC, Frankowski BL, et al. Inspiring healthy adolescent choices: a rationale for and guide to strength promotion in primary care. *J Adolesc Health*. 2007;41:525–535.
71. Reid R, Epstein MH, Pastor DA, Ryser GR. Strengths-Based assessment differences across students with LD and EBD. *Remedial Spec Edu*. 2000;21(6):346–355. https://doi.org/10.1177/074193250002100604.
72. Elliott DE, Bjelajac P, Fallot RD, Markoff LS, Reed BG. Trauma-informed or trauma-denied: principles and implementation of trauma-informed services for women. *J Community Psychol*. 2005;33:461–477.
73. Miller WR, Rollnick. *Motivational Interviewing: Preparing People for Change*. 2nd ed. New York: Guilford Press; 2002.
74. Miller WR, Rollnick S. *Motivational Interviewing: Helping People Change*. 3rd ed. New York: Guilford Press; 2013.
75. Rollnick S, Miller WR, Butler C. *Motivational Interviewing in Health Care: Helping Patients Change Behavior*. New York: Guilford Press; 2008.
76. Miller WR, Rollnick S. Ten things that motivational interviewing is not. *Behav Cogn Psychother*. 2009;37(2):129.
77. Söderlund LL, Madson MB, Rubak S, Nilsen P. A systematic review of motivational interviewing training for general health care practitioners. *Patient Educ Couns*. 2011;84(1):16–26.
78. Miller WR, Mount KA. A small study of training in motivational interviewing: does one workshop change clinician and client behavior? *Behav Cogn Psychother*. 2001;29(4):457–471.
79. Miller WR, Moyers TB. Eight stages in learning motivational interviewing. *J Teach Addict*. 2006;5(1):3–17.
80. Clark MD. Strength-based practice: the ABC's of working with adolescents who don't want to work with you. *Fed Probat*. 1997;62(1):46–53.
81. Saleebey D. The strength perspective in social work practice: extensions and cautions. *Social Work*. 1996;41:296–305.
82. Cowger CD, Snively CA. Assessing client strengths: individual, family, and community empowerment. In: Saleebey D, ed. *The Strengths Perspective in Social Work Practice*. 3rd ed. Boston: Allyn & Bacon; 2002:106–123.
83. Rapp C. *The Strengths Model with People Suffering from Severe and Persistent Mental Illness*. New York, NY: Oxford Press; 1998.
84. Mortimer JT, Harley C, Aronson PJ. How do prior experiences in the workplace set the stage for transitions to adulthood? In: Booth A, Crouter AC, Shanahan MJ, eds. *Transitions to Adulthood in a Changing Economy: No Work, No Family, No Future?* Westport, CT: Praeger; 1999: 131–159.
85. Levitt JM, Saka N, Romanelli LH, Hoagwood K. Early identification of mental health problems in schools: the status of instrumentation. *J Sch Psychol*. 2007;45: 163–191.

86. Peterson C, Seligman MEP. *Character Strengths and Virtues: A Classification and Handbook*. New York: Oxford University Press; 2004. Washington, DC: American Psychological Association.
87. Seligman MEP, Steen TA, Park N, Peterson C. Positive psychology progress: empirical validation of interventions. *Am Psychol*. 2005;60(5):410–421. https://doi.org/10.1037/0003-066X.60.5.410.
88. Toner E, Haslam N, Robinson J, Williams P. Character strengths and wellbeing in adolescence: structure and correlates of the values in action inventory of strengths for children. *Pers Individ Differ*. 2012;52(5):637–642.
89. van Eeden C, Wissing MP, Dreyer J, Park N, Peterson C. Validation of the values in action inventory of strengths for youth (VIA-Youth) among South African learners. *J Psychol Afr*. 2008;18(1):143–154. https://doi.org/10.1080/14330237.2008.10820181.
90. Weber M, Wagner L, Ruch W. Positive feelings at school: on the relationships between students' character strengths, school-related affect, and school functioning. *J Happiness Stud*. 2016;17:341–355. https://doi.org/10.1007/s10902-014-9597-1.
91. Weber M, Ruch W. The role of a good character in 12-year-old school children: do character strengths matter in the classroom? *Child Indic Res*. 2012;5(2):317–334.
92. Wood AM, Linley PA, Maltby J, Kashdan TB, Hurling R. Using personal and psychological strengths leads to increases in well-being over time: a longitudinal study and the development of the strengths use questionnaire. *Pers Individ Differ*. 2011;50:15–19. https://doi.org/10.1016/j.paid.2010.08.004.
93. Seligman MEP, Ernst RM, Gillham J, Reivich K, Linkins M. Positive education: positive psychology and classroom interventions. *Oxford Rev Education*. 2009;35(3):293–311. https://doi.org/10.1080/03054980902934563.
94. Lerner RM, Dowling EM, Anderson PM. Positive youth development: thriving as a basis of personhood and civil society. *App Dev Sci*. 2003;7:172–180.
95. Scales PC. The role of family support programs in building developmental assets among young adolescents: a national survey of services and staff training needs. *Child Welfare*. 1997;76(5):611–635.
96. Benson PL. *The Troubled Journey: A Portrait of 6th–12th Grade Youth*. Minneapolis, MN: Search Institute; 1990.
97. Scales PC, Leffert N. *Developmental Assets: A Synthesis of the Specific Research on Adolescent Development*. Minneapolis, MN: Search Institute; 1999.
98. Scales PC, Leffert N. *Developmental Assets: A Synthesis of the Scientific Research on Adolescent Development*. 2nd ed. Minneapolis: Search Institute; 2004.
99. Scales PC, Benson PL, Leffert N, Blyth DA. Contribution of developmental assets to the prediction of thriving among adolescents. *App Dev Sci*. 2000;4:27–46.
100. Chew W, Osseck J, Raygor D, Eldridge-Houser J, Cox C. Developmental assets: profile of youth in a juvenile justice facility. *J Sch Health*. 2010;80(2):66–72.
101. Mannes M. *Research on and Evidence for the Developmental Assets Model*. Search Institute; 2006. Available from: http://www.searchinstitute.org/sites/default/files/aGTO_AppendixB_ Compressed.pdf.
102. Scales PC. Youth developmental assets in global perspective: results from international adaptations of the developmental assets profile. *Child Indic Res*. 2011;4:619–645. https://doi.org/10.1007/12187R011R9112R8. Advance online publication.
102a. Benson PL, Scales PC, Roehlkepartain EC, Leffert N. *A Fragile Foundation: The State of Developmental Assets Among American Youth*. Minneapolis, MN: Search Institute; 2011.
103. Scales PC, Benson PL. *Texas Instructional Leader*. 2007;20(3):1–3, 8–10, 12.
104. Epstein MH, Dakan E, Oswald DP, Yoe JT. Using strengths-based data to evaluate children's mental health programs. In: Hernandez M, Hodges S, eds. *Systems of Care for Children's Mental Health. Developing Outcome Strategies in Children's Mental Health*. Baltimore, MD: Paul H Brookes Publishing; 2001:153–166.
105. Epstein MH. *Behavioral and Emotional Rating Scale: A Strength-Based Approach to Assessment*. 2nd ed. Austin, TX: PRO-ED; 2004.
106. Epstein MH, Mooney P, Ryser G, Pierce CD. Validity and reliability of the behavioral and emotional rating scale (2nd edition): youth rating scale. *Res Soc Work Pract*. 2004;14:358–367.
107. Epstein MH, Nordness PD, Nelson JR, Hertzog M. Convergent validity of the behavioral and emotional rating scale with primary grade-level students. *Top Early Child Spec Ed*. 2002;22(2):114–121.
108. Rawana E, Brownlee K, Hewitt J. *Strength Assessment Inventory for Children and Adolescents*. Thunder Bay, ON: Department of Psychology, Lakehead University; 2006.
109. Brownlee K, Rawana E, MacArthur J, Probizanski M. The culture of strengths makes them valued and competent: aboriginal children, child welfare, and a school strengths intervention. *Child Fam Rev*. 2009;4(2):106–113.
110. Rawana E, Brownlee K. *The Strengths Assessment Inventory Manual*. Thunder Bay, ON: Centre of Excellence for Children and Adolescents with Special Needs; 2010.
111. Brazeau JN, Teatero ML, Rawana EP, Brownlee K, Blanchette LR. The strengths assessment inventory: reliability of a new measure of psychosocial strengths for youth. *J Child Fam Stud*. 2012;21(3):384–390.

## FURTHER READING

1. Cox KF. Investigating the impact of strength-based assessment on youth with emotional or behavioral disorders. *J Child Fam Stud*. 2006;15:287–301.
2. Roberts C, Scales PC. Developmental assets and academic achievement. In: *Miniplenary Session Presented at Annual Healthy Communities, Healthy Youth Conference, Dallas, TX November 2005*; 2005. Available at: www.search-institute.org.

CHAPTER 18

# Screening for Screen Time

## Screen Time and Your Child's Health

LESLIE GREENBERG, MD, FAAFP • DAVID KURTMEN, MD

## INTRODUCTION

The world has changed dramatically in the last generation. Technology advances impact health, challenging both clinicians and parents. Nothing has changed this landscape more than the spread of screens—from the theater to the home and now in everyone's pocket. Information accessibility is vast and everchanging, at a pace that is hard to keep pace with. Today, nearly 75% of US teenagers own a smartphone, with nearly one-third admitting to feeling a need to be constantly connected to the internet. Social media has exploded over the past 15 years to the point that many adolescents and teens spend most of their time on various social media sites.[1] This raises a myriad questions regarding the health and safety of media content. How much time is healthy? What types of media are harmful? How does a child's age affect health and screen time? Can web-surfing habits predict behavioral or emotional problems? Adolescence in the context of this new environment poses unique challenges as teens are striving for independence in a digital world. There is research highlighting certain health trends in media usage while other areas need further study. Undoubtedly, screening for unhealthy media use in adolescents is of growing importance.

Media content and quantity has a huge impact on the developing young mind of children through adolescence. Research suggests a U-shaped distribution comparing mental health and internet usage, in which very high and very low users tend to have the highest rates of depression.[2] This suggests that too much or too little internet use may have an association with depression, in this particular study the researchers found that adolescents deemed as high internet users, those that used the internet for >2 h per day, and those that used <1 h a week or not at all were more likely to report higher depression scores. This does not mean causation, but it may help clinicians identify patients at greater risk of depression. Not only do the amount and the type of media exposure matter, but also the way in which it is viewed. Adolescents who passively viewed social media posts reported reduced life satisfaction while those who interacted with the posts that they viewed, such as liking, commenting, or sharing, did not report that same trend.[3]

Previous generations were confined to watching media on home television sets. Multimedia exists everywhere today. Content has expanded and evolved in a way that makes it difficult to study and screen for the effects of media use. The invention of the smartphone combined with almost universal use of social media has dramatically changed viewed content and the way that people use media. A recent study found that American teens (13–17) recorded ~9 h of media use a day.[4]

Research on social media use has shown differences in health perceptions based on the amount of and the way in which media is viewed. We should consider the perception of one's health in regards to the effects of screen time. Research has shown that adolescents who were active and did not exceed recommended screen time limits (2 h for adolescents), perceived their health better than their peers.[5]

## WHAT SCREEN TIME, SEARCH PATTERNS, AND SOCIAL MEDIA CAN PREDICT ABOUT HEALTH

It seems obvious that media use in adolescents has a major impact on the development of the adolescent mind, but what specifically is the impact? What time or content limits should be set? The challenge for parents and physicians is to determine the effects of media content and quantity on adolescent patients. The goal of creating improved screening tools is to provide better advice for patients and parents alike regarding healthy media practices. Interactive media yields community

Adolescent Health Screening: An Update in the Age of Big Data. https://doi.org/10.1016/B978-0-323-66130-0.00018-1

involvement and engagement opportunities and may help with school and workplace collaboration. Technology allows geographically separated individuals to stay in contact.[6] Tele-medicine may allow greater access to care and younger patients report media as a beneficial adjunct to medical visits with health professionals.[7]

Social media with its varied content of new ideas and information may lead to greater tolerance of diversity. Social media gives historically marginalized groups a platform to find local and online support. Transgender communities are known to use social media to discuss needs and health issues.[8] Social media can allow people suffering from mental illness to connect to other people with similar problems.[9]

Social media use transcends most socioeconomic barriers, different from former technologies.[10] Social media has the potential to target specific health outcomes such as smoking cessation, substance abuse, and weight loss.

## POTENTIAL NEGATIVES OF MEDIA USE BY ADOLESCENTS

As previously described, media use may alter viewer behavior. Research from both the United States and the United Kingdom indicates that most alcohol brands maintain a strong presence on Facebook, Twitter, and YouTube.[11,12] Adolescents are more likely to imitate behaviors they see on multimedia platforms.[13] In fact, studies have shown that adolescents exposed to media depictions engage in similar pursuits at a younger age than without media exposure: earlier alcohol ingestion,[11,14] tobacco use,[15] and sexual behavior.[16,17] Adolescents who reported very high media usage had modest increases in ADHD symptoms at 2 years later.[18] It is unclear, however, whether adolescents who have ADHD are more likely to use more media or vice versa; either way, the association is worth considering.

Adolescents may see social media content posted by their peers as normative, more so than when viewing general media or nonpeer content. This has the potential for both positive and negative consequences, depending on the content of the media in question.[19,20] Adolescents not only view social media but are major producers of it, often portraying high-risk behaviors including substance abuse, sexual behavior, self-injury, or eating disorders.[21–24]

With regard to parent and child/adolescent interactions, there is an *opportunity* for benefit in the form of platforms such as video chat to connect parents with their geographically separated children. In contrast, studies have shown that in younger children when a parent is on a media device, the amount of interaction between a parent and the child can reduce. It seems reasonable to extrapolate this to adolescents and their parents as well, meaning that adolescent/parent interaction may be diminished when media is used as a means of contact.[25–27] It may, therefore, be prudent to include screening questions addressing media use by other members of the household.

Although social media companies offer safeguards to protect the user's privacy, there are inherent and unavoidable risks of publishing information online.[28,29] Adolescents vary in their understanding of privacy practices and while many do not believe these practices will actually work, others are not aware of the "long-term" nature of their social media posts.[30,31]

## MEDIA USE WHILE DRIVING

Media use while driving, specifically texting, is a growing problem. Research has shown that texting while dramatically increases the risk of collisions, according to the national safety council, there is an increased risk of at least fourfold[32] making texting riskier than driving under the influence of alcohol. Many states have enacted laws to target texting and distracted drivers. Between 25% and 75% of high school teens report texting while driving depending on the state surveyed.[33] Although the rates of teen fatalities because of drunk driving are on the decline, the overall number of teen deaths resulting from car collisions is not. Data are currently lacking regarding whether interventions by primary care providers will reduce this trend, but given the prevalence and risk, it would be reasonable to screen for media use while driving.

## MEDIA USE AND OBESITY

It has long been hypothesized that media use is a major cause and predictor of a sedentary lifestyle and obesity. A study from 1996 found that adolescents who watched more than 5 h of TV daily were five times more likely to be obese compared with those who watched 0–2 h.[34] Given that media use requires the low expenditure of calories, children and adolescents are not performing other activities that are higher energy expenders while using media. Having a TV in the bedroom increased association with obesity.[35] Exposure to television food advertisements targeting children (6–11) has been found to have a positive correlation with childhood obesity, and increased media use has been found to have a positive correlation with caloric intake.[36] It is reasonable to conclude that the link between childhood obesity and screen time is multifactorial and includes both increased caloric consumption as well as reduced activity.[37]

## MEDIA USE AND SLEEP

A reasonable segue into asking about screen time is to question patients about their sleep hygiene and sleep patterns. This creates an opportunity for both sleep disorder screening and intervention by primary care providers. Screen time has a strong impact on sleep, and there are specific behaviors tied to poor sleep hygiene. Adolescents sleep less and report worse sleep habits when media devices are either in physical or temporal proximity to the bedroom and bedtime. Media use after 9:00 p.m. is associated with worse sleep. There is a negative association between quality of sleep and increasing number of media devices in a bedroom.[38] Lack of sleep is more likely when parents or children had electronic devices in the bedroom. The American Academy of Pediatrics suggests children and adolescents should not have TVs, smartphones, or tablets in the bedroom after bedtime. This strong association between social media use and sleep disturbance continues in young adults.[39] There are a number of theories for these associations. One small laboratory study found that people exposed to the type of light that digital screens emit report less feelings of drowsiness and have reduced levels of urine melatonin compared to when not exposed to digital screen light before bedtime.[40] This implies that screen time around bedtime is a physiologic contributor to insomnia in addition to the behavioral cause classically thought of with sleep hygiene.

## PROBLEMATIC INTERNET USE AND INTERNET GAMING DISORDER (DSM-V)

There are two screen-based DSM-V psychiatric diagnoses: problematic internet disorder and internet gaming disorder. Addictive behaviors due to either specific content or excessive use lead to negative consequences.[41,42] As with most addictive disorders, the consequences do not stop the behavior. Up to 8.5% of US youth between 8 and 18 years old meet criteria for "internet gaming disorder."[43] Both of these disorders are associated with high likelihood of depression, substance abuse, and aggressive behaviors and is present in approximately 4% of US high school aged children. Although these addictions are clearly a problem, and worthy of addressing, more research is needed to identify risk factors, further classify of these disorders, and delineate a treatment plan.

Adolescents will often think that they can effectively multitask like doing computer homework while chat messages populate the screen.[44] Conversely, multitasking with multimedia has been found consistently to reduce overall productivity (e.g., comprehension, grades, and GPA).[44] Electronic media use in particular when used during academic settings (e.g., study, class, homework) is a negative predictor of performance.[45]

## A NEW SPACE FOR OLD PROBLEMS

The central theme of social media is the creation of a digital world for people to connect and interact. These connections span almost any barrier imaginable. This allows people to connect for good reasons as well as provides a new platform for abuse. Cyberbullying, "sexting," and online solicitation are of special concern among adolescents.

## CYBERBULLYING

Cyberbullying is a form of bullying with social media. Overlap exists between cyberbullying and real-world bullying.[46] Cyberbullying has been shown to lead to both short- and long-term effects for both the perpetrator and the victim.[47] Specific concerns regarding cyberbullying are that it provides anonymity to the abuser as well as provides a fast medium for information to spread.[48] Bullies may post more hurtful content and be more vicious with an infinite audience because they feel protected by the perceived anonymity of social media. There is also the distinction that, different from typical bullying, cyberbullying has the potential to follow victims home.[49] Research has well established the short- and long-term harms that bullying can have on young people. More longitudinal research is currently needed to better assess the specific long-term effects of cyberbullying. There are early signs from research that cyberbullying may be more harmful regarding certain outcomes, for example, one study found it to be more closely linked to substance abuse and depression.[50] Healthychildren.org suggests that primary care providers inquire with the following questions: "How are things going at school?" "What do you think of the other kids?" "Does anyone get picked on or bullied?" Screening should also address cyberbullying because of its proven harm and prevalence and because newer interventions targeted against cyberbullying seem to be helpful.[51]

## SEXUAL ABUSE AND MEDIA USE

Social media users are at risk for online solicitation further studies are needed. Social media give sexual predators a vehicle to contact potential victims.[52] An estimated 12% of 10–19-year-olds have sent a nude photo to someone else. Children who engage in sexting or admit to sending or receiving nude photos report an earlier age of engaging in sexual activity themselves.[53]

## HOW TO SCREEN FOR EXCESSIVE OR UNSAFE SCREEN TIME

Screen time has the potential to disrupt the lives of children during a time already fraught with developmental challenges. The goal of screening for screen time is to reliably identify areas that are both potentially harmful and changeable. There have been several tools developed to create uniformity when screening. The Problematic and Risky Internet Use Screening Scale (PRIUSS) is a tool used to identify problematic internet use. There are two specific tools: the PRIUSS-18 screening tool comprises 18 questions that span three domains related to problematic internet use, social impairment, emotional impairment, and risky/impulsive internet use. The PRIUSS-3 is a shorter version designed as an initial screening test that when positive would require further screening with PRIUSS-18, akin to the current depression screening tools of PHQ-2 and PHQ-9. The PRIUSS-3 addresses the following three questions: "(1) anxiety when away from the internet, (2) loss of motivation when on the internet, and (3) feelings of withdrawal when away from the internet" and was found to have a sensitivity of 100% and a specificity of 69% for problematic internet use.[54] Limited early evidence is promising regarding the PRIUSS or two-step PRIUSS for screening for problematic internet use but further studies are needed to evaluate for efficacy and generalizability of these tools.[55]

Other tools were developed and tested before screen time, the way we know it today existed. Likely the most widely used adolescent screening tool is the Home environment, Education and employment, Eating, peer-related Activities, Drugs, and Sexuality, Suicide/depression, and Safety from injury and violence (HEADSSS) questionnaire. This addresses the major causes of morbidity and mortality among adolescents. HEADSSS was revised in 2014 to include media use under their home section and bullying and solicitation under safety.[56] Other researchers have advocated that the HEADSSS questionnaire is adapted even further to specifically address media use.

Whatever the screening tool is used, we suggest that all adolescents be screened for unsafe screen time. Discuss with patients the types of media used and media content. Ask about whether adolescents feel safe online. While addressing media, screen children and adolescents for adequate physical activity (1 h per day) and for adequate sleep (≥8 h/day). Encourage parents to role model healthy media use and engage in coviewing. Encourage family members to interact with adolescents online and on social media, thereby fostering a community of safe adults online. Just like when screening adolescents for abuse, drug use, or sexual activity, ask all adolescents specifically about cyberbullying, sexting, and online solicitation remembering to screen for both victims as well as potential perpetrators.

### Blue Boxes

1. AAP (American Academy of Pediatrics) recommendations for families
   a. Recommend that families come up with a plan that places consistent limits on time spent on media devices. Families should discuss types of media content that are appropriate for given age groups and ways to monitor this.
   b. Consider creating areas and times that are designated "media free" for both parents and children.
   c. Suggestions should include no devices in bedrooms an hour before bed or as part of the bedtime routine, or at the dinner table at mealtimes.
   d. Parents and providers should "have ongoing communication about online citizenship and safety, including treating others with respect online and offline."
2. Parental screen time
   a. Parental media use reduces parent–child interaction and may even increase the potential for parent–child conflict. In addition, there is a positive correlation between parental media use and child media use, therefore reducing parental screen time and role modeling is important.
3. Texting while driving
4. Media use plan
   a. We agree with AAP recommendations that all families devise a media use plan that consistently sets limits on time and type of media used by each child. We encourage providers to help review media use plans with patients and parents.
   b. https://www.healthychildren.org/English/media/Pages/default.aspx

## REFERENCES


1. Lenhart A. *Teens, Social Media & Technology Overview 2015.* Washington, DC: Pew Internet and American Life Project; 2015.
2. Bélanger RE, Akre C, Berchtold A, Michaud PA. A U-shaped association between intensity of Internet use and adolescent health. *Pediatrics*. 2011;127(2):e330–e335. pmid: 21242218.
3. Kross E, Verduyn P, Demiralp E, et al. Facebook use predicts declines in subjective well-being in young adults. *PLoS One*. 2013;8(8):e69841. pmid:23967061.
4. Jiang J. *Pew Research Center, Internet and Technology, How Teens and Parents Navigate Screen Time and Device Distractions*. August 2018.
5. Herman KM, Hopman WM, et al. Physical activity, screen time and self-rated health and mental health in Canadian adolescents. *Preventative Medicine*. 2015;73:112–116.
6. *Media Use in School Aged Children and Adolecents, Pediatrics*. From the American Academy of Pediatrics, Policy Statement; October 2016.
7. Briones R. Harnessing the web: how e-health and e-health literacy impact young adults' perceptions of online health information. *Med 2 0*. 2015;4(2):e5.
8. Krueger EA, Young SD. Twitter: a novel tool for studying the health and social needs of transgender communities. *JMIR Ment Health*. 2015;2(2).
9. Naslund JA, Aschbrenner KA, Marsch LA, Bartels SJ. The future of mental health care: peer-to-peer support and social media. *Epidemiol Psychiatr Sci*. 2016;25(2):113–122. pmid:26744309.
10. Chou WY, Hunt YM, Beckjord EB, Moser RP, Hesse BW. Social media use in the United States: implications for health communication. *J Med Internet Res*. 2009;11(4): e48. pmid:19945947.
11. Winpenny EM, Marteau TM, Nolte E. Exposure of children and adolescents to alcohol marketing on social media websites. *Alcohol Alcohol*. 2014;49(2):154–159. pmid: 24293506.
12. Jernigan DH, Rushman AE. Measuring youth exposure to alcohol marketing on social networking sites: challenges and prospects. *J Public Health Policy*. 2014;35(1):91–104. pmid:24284473.
13. Klein JD, Brown JD, Childers KW, Oliveri J, Porter C, Dykers C. Adolescents' risky behavior and mass media use. *Pediatrics*. 1993;92(1):24–31. pmid:8516081.
14. Robinson TN, Chen HL, Killen JD. Television and music video exposure and risk of adolescent alcohol use. *Pediatrics*. 1998;102(5):E54. pmid:9794984.
15. Dalton MA, Beach ML, Adachi-Mejia AM, et al. Early exposure to movie smoking predicts established smoking by older teens and young adults. *Pediatrics*. 2009;123(4): e551–e558. pmid:19336346.
16. Ashby SL, Arcari CM, Edmonson MB. Television viewing and risk of sexual initiation by young adolescents. *Arch Pediatr Adolesc Med*. 2006;160(4):375–380. pmid: 16585482.
17. Titus-Ernstoff L, Dalton MA, Adachi-Mejia AM, Longacre MR, Beach ML. Longitudinal study of viewing smoking in movies and initiation of smoking by children. *Pediatrics*. 2008;121(1):15–21. pmid:18166552.
18. Ra CK, Cho J, et al. Association of digital media use with subsequent symptoms of attention-deficit/hyperactivity disorder among adolescents. *JAMA*. 2018;320(3):255–263.
19. Litt DM, Stock ML. Adolescent alcohol-related risk cognitions: the roles of social norms and social networking sites. *Psychol Addict Behav*. 2011;25(4):708–713. pmid: 21644803.
20. Moreno MA, Briner LR, Williams A, Walker L, Christakis DA. Real use or "real cool": adolescents speak out about displayed alcohol references on social networking websites. *J Adolesc Health*. 2009;45(4): 420–422. pmid:19766949.
21. Hinduja S, Patchin JW. Personal information of adolescents on the Internet: a quantitative content analysis of MySpace. *J Adolesc*. 2008;31(1):125–146. pmid:17604833.
22. Moreno MA, Parks MR, Zimmerman FJ, Brito TE, Christakis DA. Display of health risk behaviors on MySpace by adolescents: prevalence and associations. *Arch Pediatr Adolesc Med*. 2009;163(1):35–41. pmid:19124701.
23. McGee JB, Begg M. What medical educators need to know about "Web 2.0". *Med Teach*. 2008;30(2):164–169. pmid: 18464141.
24. Moreno MA, Ton A, Selkie E, Evans Y. Secret Society 123: understanding the language of self-harm on Instagram. *J Adolesc Health*. 2016;58(1):78–84. pmid:26707231.
25. Fiese BH. Family mealtime conversations in context. *J Nutr Educ Behav*. 2012;44(1):e1. pmid:22243981.
26. Jago R, Thompson JL, Sebire SJ, et al. Cross-sectional associations between the screen-time of parents and young children: differences by parent and child gender and day of the week. *Int J Behav Nutr Phys Act*. 2014;11:54–62. pmid:24758143.
27. Radesky J, Miller AL, Rosenblum KL, Appugliese D, Kaciroti N, Lumeng JC. Maternal mobile device use during a structured parent-child interaction task. *Acad Pediatr*. 2015;15(2):238–244. pmid:25454369.
28. Tsukayama H. *Facebook Draws Fire From Privacy Advocates Over ad Changes*. The Washington Post; June 12, 2014. Available at: https://www.washingtonpost.com/news/the-switch/wp/2014/06/12/privacy-experts-say-facebook-changes-open-up-unprecedented-data-collection/.
29. Hoadley CM, Xu H, Lee JJ, Rosson MB. Privacy as information access and illusory control: the case of the Facebook news feed privacy outcry. *Electron Commer Res Appl*. 2010; 9(1):50–60.
30. Marwick A, Boyd D. Networked privacy: how teenagers negotiate context in social media. *New Media Soc*. 2014; 16(7):1051–1067.
31. Madden M, Lenhart A, Cortesi S, et al. Teens, Social Media, and Privacy. Available at: http://www.pewinternet.org/2013/05/21/teens-social-media-and-privacy/. Accessed September 2, 2016.

32. Annual Estimate of Cell Phone Crashes 2013. National Safety Institute.
33. Li L, Shults RA, Andridge RR, Yellman MA, Xiang H, Zhu M. Texting/emailing while driving among high school students in 35 states, United States, 2015. pii: S1054-139X(18)30250-30257 *J Adolesc Health.* August 17, 2018. https://doi.org/10.1016/j.jadohealth.2018.06.010 [Epub ahead of print] PubMed PMID: 30139720.
34. Gortmaker SL, Must A, Sobol AM, Peterson K, Colditz GA, Dietz WH. Television viewing as a cause of increasing obesity among children in the United States, 1986–1990. *Arch Pediatr Adolesc Med.* 1996;150(4): 356–362. pmid:8634729.
35. Borghese MM, Tremblay MS, Katzmarzyk PT, et al. Mediating role of television time, diet patterns, physical activity and sleep duration in the association between television in the bedroom and adiposity in 10 year-old children. *Int J Behav Nutr Phys Act.* 2015;12:60–70. pmid:25967920.
36. Goris JM, Petersen S, Stamatakis E, Veerman JL. Television food advertising and the prevalence of childhood overweight and obesity: a multicountry comparison. *Public Health Nutr.* 2010;13(7):1003–1012. pmid:20018123.
37. Blass EM, Anderson DR, Kirkorian HL, Pempek TA, Price I, Koleini MF. On the road to obesity: television viewing increases intake of high-density foods. *Physiol Behav.* 2006; 88(4–5):597–604. pmid:16822530.
38. Bruni O, Sette S, Fontanesi L, Baiocco R, Laghi F, Baumgartner E. Technology use and sleep quality in preadolescence and adolescence. *J Clin Sleep Med.* 2015;11(12): 1433–1441. pmid:26235161.
39. Levenson JC, Shensa A, Sidani JE, Colditz JB, Primack BA. The association between social media use and sleep disturbance among young adults. *Prev Med.* 2016;85(Jan): 36–41. pmid:26791323.
40. Wahnschaffe A, Haedel S, Rodenbeck A, et al. Out of the lab and into the bathroom: evening short-term exposure to conventional light suppresses melatonin and increases alertness perception. *Int J Mol Sci.* 2013;14(2): 2573–2589. pmid:23358248.
41. Moreno MA, Jelenchick L, Cox E, Young H, Christakis DA. Problematic Internet use among US youth: a systematic review. *Arch Pediatr Adolesc Med.* 2011;165(9):797–805. pmid:21536950.
42. Liu TC, Desai RA, Krishnan-Sarin S, Cavallo DA, Potenza MN. Problematic Internet use and health in adolescents: data from a high school survey in Connecticut. *J Clin Psychiatry.* 2011;72(6):836–845. pmid:21536002.
43. Gentile D. Pathological video-game use among youth ages 8 to 18: a national study. *Psychol Sci.* 2009;20(5):594–602. pmid:19476590.
44. Carrier LM, Rosen LD, Cheever NA, Lim AF. Causes, effects, and practicalities of everyday multitasking. Special issue: living in the "net" generation: multitasking, learning, and development. *Dev Rev.* 2015;35:64–78.
45. Jacobsen WC, Forste R. The wired generation: academic and social outcomes of electronic media use among university students. *Cyberpsychol Behav Soc Netw.* 2011;14(5): 275–280. pmid:20961220.
46. Waasdorp TE, Bradshaw CP. The overlap between cyberbullying and traditional bullying. *J Adolesc Health.* 2015; 56(5):483–488. pmid:25631040.
47. Vaillancourt T, Brittain HL, McDougall P, Duku E. Longitudinal links between childhood peer victimization, internalizing and externalizing problems, and academic functioning: developmental cascades. *J Abnorm Child Psychol.* 2013;41(8):1203–1215. pmid:23907699.
48. Raskauskas J, Stoltz AD. Involvement in traditional and electronic bullying among adolescents. *Dev Psychol.* 2007; 43(3):564–575. pmid:1748.
49. Slonje R, Smith PK. Cyberbullying: another main type of bullying? *Scand J Psychol.* 2008;49(2):147–154. pmid: 18352984.
50. Mitchell KJ, Wolak J, Finkelhor D. Trends in youth reports of sexual solicitations, harassment and unwanted exposure to pornography on the Internet. *J Adolesc Health.* 2007; 40(2):116–126. pmid:17259051.
51. Del Rey R, Casas JA, Ortega R. The impacts of the CONRED program on different cyberbullying roles [published online ahead of print 2015]. Aggress Behav. doi: 10.002/ab.21608.
52. Mitchell KJ, Finkelhor D, Wolak J. Youth Internet users at risk for the most serious online sexual solicitations. *Am J Prev Med.* 2007;32(6):532–537. pmid:17533070.
53. Temple JR, Choi H. Longitudinal association between teen sexting and sexual behavior. *Pediatrics.* 2014;134(5): e1287–e1292. pmid:25287459.
54. Moreno MA, Arseniev-Koehler A, Selkie E. Development and testing of a 3-item screening tool for problematic internet use. *J Pediatrics.* 2016;176. https://doi.org/10.1016/j.jpeds.2016.05.067.
55. Jelenchick LA, Eickhoff J, Zhang C, Kraninger K, Christakis DA, Moreno MA. Screening for adolescent problematic internet use: validation of the problematic and risky internet use screening scale (PRIUSS). *Acad Pediatr.* 2015;15(6):658–665. pmid:26547545.
56. Klein D, Goldenring J, Adelman W. HEADSSS 3.0: the psychosocial interview for adolescents updated for a new century field by media. *Contemp Pediatrics.* January 1, 2014: 16–28.

CHAPTER 19

# Putting It All Together: A Role for Big Data in Health and Adolescent Health Screening

VINCENT MORELLI, MD • NICHOLAS CONLEY, MD

## INTRODUCTION

There is no question that we are now fully grounded in the age of "big data." A recent International Data Corporation study[1] predicted that the world's digital data repository will reach 44 zetabytes (1 zetabyte = 1 billion terabytes = 1 trillion gigabytes) by 2020. The study anticipated that 37% of this data would be useful in various applications and innovative businesses including healthcare.

In the preceding chapters, we have presented much information relevant to adolescent health screening, behaviors, and health outcomes. Questions now arise. How to put this deluge of "academic" information to practical use? How to translate scholarship into clinically useful screening and prevention and thus contribute to a healthier society. Obviously, ours is not a knowledge problem. There is enough knowledge siloed throughout the literature. What we have instead is a technology problem—a big data problem—and we need to know how best to tame and integrate the continual onslaught of information that surrounds us.

In this, the final chapter, we will first (1) give a brief history of big data; (2) discuss data as they are currently being used; and (3) postulate how big data might be used in the future, particularly with respect to adolescent health screening.

However, first, we provide a definition. The term "big data" refers to extremely large data sets that may be analyzed computationally to reveal patterns, trends, and associations, especially relating to human behavior and interactions.[2] Obviously, such information is useless without a proper way to analyze, interpret, and utilize it. Thankfully, technology is now at a point—in terms of both computational power and data storage—where these data can begin to be utilized. Advancement will be dependent on the ability of creative innovators to envision new ways of utilizing this fantastic resource.

## HISTORY OF BIG DATA

The history of big data can be traced all the way back to John Graunt, in 1663.[3] Although Mr. Graunt did not utilize Google as a predictive model of human interests, he did study the bubonic plague using statistics, and he is credited as the first person to use statistical data analysis, the foundation of our current big data. Later, in 1880, the United States census data had become unmanageable, and workers predicted that it would take 8 years to finish recording the results. They envisioned the 1890 census would take at least 11 years. Just then, an American inventor, Herman Hollerith, realized that data could be recorded electromechanically by placing and utilizing holes on paper cards. Thus, necessity, once again the mother of invention, prompted Mr. Hollerith to invent the forerunner of the modern punch card.[4] The 1890 census would go on to be finished 2 years faster than the 1880 census.[5] Hollerith found multiple companies including the Computing–Tabulating–Recording Company, which would later be renamed IBM.

The 20th century would see many instrumental developments creating the basis for the big data we see today. In 1927, Austrian-German engineer Fritz Pfleumer developed a method of storing information on tape magnetically.[6] The British would build on this to create the first data processor, Colossus, during

Adolescent Health Screening: An Update in the Age of Big Data. https://doi.org/10.1016/B978-0-323-66130-0.00019-3

World War II to aid in deciphering Nazi Codes.[7] Colossus could scan 5000 characters a second, reducing the person-hours needed to decipher codes from weeks to hours.

Following the end of the war, in 1952, the US government created the National Security Agency, which was tasked with decrypting ensuing cold war messages. Throughout the Cold War, the US government would build on these early pillars of big data to establish the true foundation of the concept.

In 1969, ARPANET, a precursor to the internet, was founded as part of the Advanced Research Projects Agency. This innovation allowed for the networking of machines and laid the foundations of cloud-based processing power.[8] In addition, in the 1960s, the US government created its first data center, storing millions of fingerprint sets and tax returns.[3] Already, people were seeing the value of biometric data and records.

The development of big data would take a tremendous leap forward in the 1970 and 1980s with the introduction and popularization of personal computers. Later, in 1990, Tim Berners-Lee developed the concept of a "World Wide Web" that fostered the networking of these personal computers, thus augmenting computational power and allowing for the efficient sharing of information utilizing a hypertext system and IT commands.[9] At the same time, advances in data storage have complemented the rise in data acquisition and computational power. Early magnetic storage devices (e.g., discs, hard drives) have given way to the more efficient and less costly cloud storage.[3] Big data as its being used now is discussed:

1. Big data as a cost saver

The National Health Expenditure Accounts, the official estimate of total health care spending in the United States, grew by 4.3% in 2016, reaching $10,348 per person, or a total of 3.3 trillion dollars. This accounts for 17.9% of the Gross Domestic Product of the United States.[10,11] (Roughly twice that of other OEDC countries.) Traditional fee for service, while reimbursing providers for work performed, has also incentivized repeat testing, led to the excessive performance of procedures, and has left many providers more invested in treatment rather than prevention.[12] Big data, with its ability to monitor many health factors in an ongoing fashion—blood sugar, blood pressure monitoring, daily activity, sleep/wake cycles—may offer one way to promote prevention rather than treatment with great cost-saving benefits. Preventing diabetes, for example, would not only benefit patients but would be significantly financially rewarding for a nation's health system. Clearly, a model of healthcare prevention is advantageous to the current model.

Thus, to optimize patient health and healthcare delivery, research must continue to explore ways to accurately predict factors placing patients at risk for disease, while also providing insights into the ways PCPs may influence or change unhealthy behaviors. Big data will play a significant role in both of these areas both enhancing individual health and reducing systemic costs.

The health-promoting and cost-saving benefits gained from linking, coordinating, and incorporating big data into prevention and treatment have already saved the Kaiser Permanente/Health Connect system over a billion dollars. Savings have resulted from a reduction in office visits, a reduction of unnecessary or duplicate testing and presumably improved compliance and outcomes.[13]

As we move away from a strict fee for service model toward a system that is more results-oriented (e.g., MACRA, MIPS), big data will play an increasingly important role. It will aid in preventing disease and enhancing treatment efficiency, while at the same time augmenting physician reimbursement with policies that reward better patient outcomes and more efficient utilization of healthcare resources.

2. Big data as a more efficient research tool.

The term "evidence-based medicine" has been a hot topic in healthcare for quite some time. However, the concept was notable even in ancient times, perhaps hitting a renaissance in the 17th century with the widespread use of personal journals and textbooks.[14,15] With the advent of computers, data storage, and information sharing, a second renaissance has been underway. Utilizing big data makes possible a third renaissance in evidence-based medicine. For example, big data's ability to vastly increase sample size could help to decrease selection bias and improve study sensitivity and specificity. An example of this can be seen in the Genome-Wide Association studies where large data sets/meta-analyses of individual basic measurements, such as BMI and hip-waist ratio, provided more useful health information than small, hypothesis-driven data collection.[16]

Such utilization of big data will force a paradigm shift in experimental design, not only in terms of sample size but also of the incorporation of more fluid (constantly changing) variables.[16,17]

Another advantage big data offers is the incorporation of information into studies of human behavior. Big data promises a much more accurate and nuanced analysis of our complex behaviors—specifically those with untoward health effects. This is made possible by our newfound ability to incorporate heretofore-immeasurable parameters (e.g., amount of sleep, heart rate, wearable tech data, location data) and correlating them with disease risk and disease prevention.

Up until this point, statistics have allowed researchers to maximize the impact of small data sets; however, with the colossal data sets now provided by big data, the traditional means of analyzing data may not be as useful. Going forward, new analytical methods will be required to cull and maximize the impact of useful information found in our vast and ever-expanding pool of data.

Although traditionally research has involved determining a hypothesis, designing an experiment, testing the hypothesis, and revisiting that hypothesis, big data offers a way to change and improve this paradigm. By tradition, data are used to evaluate the hypothesis and, if possible, prove it true or false.[18] With sufficiently large data stores, such as seen in big data, this process could fundamentally change. Enough input would not only allow for the answering of specific hypotheses, but also offer a way to address, and improve, the very way the question is asked. The way big data could accomplish this paradigm shift is through machine learning—a method of data analysis, which presupposes that systems can identify patterns in data and make decisions with little to no human interaction. In the context of big data machine learning shifts from an abstract concept to a reimagining of study design itself—quite novel and quite an aid in the creative process. Machine learning systems have existed for over 40 years, but only recently able to take advantage of the massive volumes of data and adequate computing power.[19] The process, of course, would still need human oversight, as the machine would have no way to intrinsically know the usefulness of the data parameters it was refining, thus not replacing the researcher but instead serving as a powerful investigative tool. In addition, such systems would not prove or disprove a hypothesis but instead would create hypotheses themselves from the learning process. This would transform research into a truly inductive process—taking specific data and making broad generalizations from it. (As it is now, research is a deductive process whereby researchers make a general hypothesis and tries to make conclusions applicable to specific cases.) Furthermore, machine learning could be used to determine even more appropriate hypotheses to further test and refine. In many ways, the purpose itself shifts from merely answering questions to also generating more hypotheses.[20]

Thus, utilization of big data and machine learning could find and examine innovative data streams (e.g., from wearable tech), glean new health impacting insights, formulate a creative new hypothesis and allow scientists to better understand the world at large.[20]

3. Examples of how some companies are currently using big data

Blue Shield of California has partnered with Nanthealth to develop an integrated technology system, allowing insurers, hospitals, and doctors to deliver more coordinated, personalized evidence-based care.[21] They believe this will improve both illness outcomes and disease prevention. Although currently the partnership is focused mainly on linking Electronic Medical Record (EMRs), sharing medical information between physicians, and facilitating coordination between insurance and billing companies, the idea is that such a system would incorporate future health-related parameters and several big data streams including those focused on the emerging field of precision medicine.

AstraZeneca, the pharmaceutical company, has partnered with HealthCore, to conduct real-world studies examining treatment outcomes and cost-effectiveness of various disease treatments.[22] HealthCore is focused on helping several medical players (e.g., pharmaceutical, biotech, insurance) pursue their research goals. Such services will naturally include the incorporation of big data into their researched solutions.

Google researchers attempted to track the spread of flu in the United States using Centers for Disease Control data and they developed a model using Internet search behaviors as proxies to track flu symptom.[17] The study tested 50 million frequent search terms and 450 million combined terms, then used machine learning to allow for the refinement of algorithms with time. Despite an early dip in result accuracy, machine learning eventually facilitated more accurate results and more precise flu tracking. Thus, the possibility of incorporating this type of big data into disease tracking was clearly illustrated.

A final example may be seen in MindStrong Health, where the frequency and manner in which smartphone owners use their phones are captured in "digital big data" and then used to correlate to mental health symptoms.[23]

The earlier are just a few examples of uses of big data in healthcare. Other businesses from Netflix to NASA to Nike are also actively engaged in the use of bid data to improve their services their bottom lines.

4. How might big data be used in the future?

We have already alluded to several ways in which big data can be used in medicine. This final section will expound on this idea proposing additional ways in which big data may be used in the future to benefit patient health and health care system efficiency. In a final paragraph, we will propose how big data might be used specifically to improve adolescent health risk screening, giving primary care providers the ability to offer early prevention and to more effectively promote health in our youthful population.

As touched upon earlier, big data's utility, enhanced by machine learning, will give us an augmented ability to predict disease, create predictive models of human behavior, and inform early prevention—all of which can impact compliance and health outcomes. For example, incorporating information from wearable tech (e.g., real-time physical activity, blood pressure, pulse, EKGs) into the medical record will be immensely helpful. Although healthy but at-risk adolescents might spend little time with a provider (possibly showing up just once per year for an annual school physical), wearable tech and other healthcare applications might greatly expand a provider's knowledge of risk, thus enabling earlier access to healthcare, more frequent visits, and earlier prevention if needed. One of the likely advantages of capturing this type of data is that self-monitoring capabilities will likely enhance patient engagement and self-motivated healthful actions. Through providing such parameters to patients, patients will begin to "own" their health and feel more connected to it. Another benefit is that such an approach will allow providers to spend less time "fishing" for relevant health issues and more time focused on addressing them. Such data-dependent approaches have been found effective by physicians and associated with higher levels of parent and adolescent satisfaction, helping to prepare patients and parents for health visits and helping to facilitate doctor–patient communication.[24–28]

As we move forward into the future, monitoring the longitudinal habits of individuals and pooling data for entire populations will take on added importance, significantly augmenting both preventive and predictive healthcare.

Another area of prevention planning might be examining health issues on a larger scale, which could help providers and city planner's direct resources toward more problematic areas (i.e., divert more exercise efforts toward more obese geographic areas). These types of analyses could also redirect patients to specific providers based on need, thereby increasing the amount of time a patient is in front of the healthcare provider best suited to their individual needs. An example of this type of data usage might be seen in companies such as OPTUM labs, where 200 million deidentified lives containing linked data from administrative claims, medical records, and self-reported health information have been harnessed using artificial intelligence, to focus on disease prevention, best treatments, and improved quality.

In addition to big data's ability to affect individual patients, it will also affect future research, redefining how study outcomes are measured and analyzed, and indeed even changing how hypotheses are generated and how research itself is conducted (as discussed in the previous section).

Another fascinating addition to the current "siloed" use of big data is that of knowledge integration across disciplines. Such integration promises to create further imaginative insights and cascading systems improvements. For example, after big data have performed its function of early identification of patients at medical risk, behavioral economic theories such as the Nudge Theory of Behavioral Economics,[29] might be employed to enhance patient compliance with prescribed preventive measures (e.g., dietary restraint, increased exercise, sleep, social interaction). The idea here is that *early* identification of patients (biomedical big data) would allow *early*-applied behavioral economic measures to be implemented (economic/behavioral big data-inspired intervention) and improve outcomes. In this "cross discipline" example, big data is necessary not only to identify *patients* at risk but also to identify *environments* fostering risk and to help establish healthful environmental alterations to improve patient behavior, nudging patients toward aligning their actions with their intentions. (A simple example of a "positive nudge" was discussed in a recent Journal of Public Health article,[30] showing a healthy eating choice change by placing fruit and other healthy options near the cash register and placing junk food in more remote areas of the store). Such behavioral nudging or "choice architecture"[29] could also be put to use in other areas of big-data-identified need, such as climate change, disease spread (e.g., HIV, malaria), and resource utilization.

## PUTTING IT ALL TOGETHER

There are countless possibilities for using big data in adolescent health. As such, we have a great opportunity to augment and update our current biopsychosocial model, where *physicians* gather most of the data relevant to assessing adolescent health risk, to a more collective "biopsychosocial-collaborative" model, where input from parents, teachers, adolescents themselves, and big data may be incorporated into more comprehensive adolescent health screening.

There is good evidence that such a comprehensive, holistic approach benefits both adolescent patients and PCPs as they interact in this critical life stage. Although the optimal frequency of caregiver visits is unknown—and obviously will vary depending on patient needs—a preannual-visit-holistic checklist has been proven to help PCPs spend less time asking historical questions and more time focused on addressing health needs.[28,31,32] Such previsit screenings have been viewed positively by parents, PCPs, and adolescents,[24–26] with adolescents, in particular, more comfortable participating in their own care and in reporting personal information via computer.[33,34] Studies have documented that adolescents feel computerized prescreens to be more confidential, enabled them to be listened to more carefully, and generally facilitated more satisfying visits.[27] Authors postulated that such patient-driven computerized prescreening helped adolescents approach subjects that were more difficult to raise in person and facilitated greater patient involvement in their own care, thus setting the stage for increased compliance, improving doctor–patient relationships, and moving adolescents toward more fulfilled and healthy adulthoods.[28] In our opinion, the goal of helping adolescents move toward actualized healthy adulthoods could be facilitated by discussions during at least three annual visits:

1. Initial visit (perhaps at their preschool physical exam). A holistic questionnaire given before the first visit can help identify the goals and expectation of guardians and adolescents and can help focus PCP attention on areas of need. The PCPs could start preliminary discussions of risk areas illuminated by the questionnaire.
2. Follow-up visit. A second visit should be used to follow-up on any deficits uncovered in the first visit, discuss aspects of adolescent health and thriving, and alert parents and patients to the available clinic and community resources if needed.
3. Final visit. A final visit should facilitate discussion of the past year's journey and allow for further questioning on relevant biopsychosocial topics. All three visits further a trusting patient/practitioner relationship so that health risks will continue to be sought and discussed in a collaborative fashion and that adolescents feel comfortable in approaching caregivers for health and wellness guidance.

In conclusion, we have constantly evolving health needs to address, new tools and technologies with which to address them, and an exciting chance to contribute and innovate. In the words of Steve Jobs, "If you give people tools, they'll do wonderful things with them." Adolescents are just 13% of our population,[35] but they are 100% of our future. It is incumbent on us to secure that future.

## REFERENCES


1. The Digital Universe of Opportunities: Rich Data and the Increasing Value of the Internet of Things. EMC Digital Universe with Research and Analysis by IDC. April 2014. https://www.emc.com/leadership/digital-universe/2014iview/high-value-data.htm.
2. https://www.dictionary.com/browse/big-data.
3. Foote, KD. Brief History of Big Data. www.dataversity.net/brief-history-big-data/.
4. Randell B, ed. *The Origins of Digital Computers, Selected Papers*. 3rd ed. Springer-Verlag; 1982. ISBN 0-387-11319-3.
5. Carrol D. *Report of the Commissioner of Labor in Charge of the Eleventh Census to the Secretary of the Interior for the Fiscal Year Ending June 30, 1895 Washington, D.D.* Wright Commissioner of Labor in Charge; July 29, 1895:9. You may confidently look for the rapid reduction of the forces of this office after the 1st of October, and the entire cessation of clerical work during the present calendar year. The condition of the work of the Census Division and the condition of the final report show clearly that the work of the Eleventh Census will be completed at least two years early than was the work of the Tenth Census.
6. Daniel ED, Mee CD, Clark MH, eds. *Magnetic Recording: The First 100 Years*. Piscataway, NJ: IEEE Press; 1999.
7. *A Brief History of Computing. Jack Copeland*. Alanturing.net; June 2000.
8. ARPANET: United states Defense Program. Kevin Featherly, Encyclopedia Britannica. https://www.britannica.com/topic/ARPANET.
9. Berners-Lee T, Fischetti M. *Weaving the Web: The Original Design and Ultimate Destiny of the World Wide Web by its Inventor*. Brittain: Orion Business; 1999.
10. https://www.cms.gov/Research-Statistics-Data-and-Systems/Statistics-Trends-and-Reports/NationalHealthExpendData/.
11. NationalHealthAccountsHistorical.html.
12. Doran T, Maurer KA, Ryan AM. Impact of provider incentives on quality and value of health care. *Annu Rev Public Health*. 2017;38:449–465.
13. Kayyali B, Knott D, Van Kuiken S. *The Big Data Revolution in Healthcare: Accelerating Value and Innovation*. McKinsey Report; April 2013. https://www.mckinsey.com/industries/healthcare-systems-and-services/our-insights/the-big-data-revolution-in-us-health-care.
14. Claridge JA, Fabian TC. History and development of evidence-based medicine. *World J Surg*. 2005;29(5):547–553.
15. Sackett DL, Rosenbert WMC, Gray JAM, Haynes RB, Richardson WS. Evidence based medicine: what it is and what it isn't. *BMJ*. 1996;312.
16. Locke AE, Kahali B, Berndt SI, et al. Genetic studies of body mass index yield new insights for obesity biology. *Nature*. 2015;518:197–206.

17. Lazer D, Kennedy R, King G, Vespignani A. Big data. The parable of google flu: traps in big data analysis. *Science*. 2014;343:1203–1205.
18. Popper K. *Conjectures and Refutations. The Growth of Scientific Knowledge*. London, UK: Routledge; 1963.
19. Mayer-Schönberger V, Cukier K. *Learning With Big Data*. Boston, MA: Houghton Mifflin Harcourt; 2014.
20. Mayer-Schonberger V, Ingelson E. Big data and medicine: a big deal? *J Intern Med*. 2017;283(5).
21. Blue of California. NantHealth and Blue Shield of California Form Proactive Healthcare Collaborative. https://www.blueshieldca.com/bsca/about-blue-shield/media-center/nant-100212.sp.
22. AstraZeneca and HealthCore Announce Real-World Evidence Data Collaboration in the U.S. https://www.businesswire.com/news/home/20110202006102/en/Astra Zeneca-HealthCore-Announce-Real-World-Evidence-Data-Collaboration.
23. Metz R. The smartphone app that can tell you're depressed before you know it yourself. *MIT Technol Rev*. 2018:56–61.
24. Zuckerbrot RA, Maxon L, Pagar D, et al. Adolescent depression screening in primary care: feasibility and acceptance. *Pediatrics*. 2007;119:101. e8.
25. Fein JA, Pailler ME, Barg FK, et al. Feasibility and effects of a web-based adolescent psychiatric assessment administered by clinical staff in the pediatric emergency department. *Arch Pediatr Adolesc Med*. 2010;164:1112. e7.
26. Slovin SR, Rowe TL, Mmari K, et al. Can you fill this out? Caregiver, clinician, and staff perspectives on pre-visit questionnaires prior to well-child care. *PAS*. 2014. ABS# 1509.119.
27. Olson AL, Gaffney CA, Hedberg VA, Gladstone GR. Use of inexpensive technology to enhance adolescent health screening and counseling. *Arch Pediatr Adolesc Med*. 2009; 163:172. e7.
28. Gadomski AM, Fothergill KE. Integrating mental health into adolescent annual visits: impact of previsit comprehensive screening on within-visit processes. *J Adolesc Health*. 2015;56:267–e273.
29. Thaler RH, Sunstein CR. *Nudge: Improving Decisions About Health, Wealth, and Happiness*. Yale University Press; April 8, 2018.
30. Kroese F, Marchiori D, de Ridder D. Nudging healthy food choices: a field experiment at the train station. *J Public Health*. 2016;38(2):e133–e137.
31. Majeed-Ariss R, Baildam E, Campbell M, et al. Apps and adolescents: a systematic review of adolescents' use of mobile phone and tablet apps that support personal management of their chronic or long-term physical conditions. *J Med Internet Res*. 2015;17(12):e287. Published online 2015 Dec 23.
32. Nagykaldi ZJ, Voncken-Brewster V, Aspy CB, Mold JW. Novel computerized health risk appraisal may improve longitudinal health and wellness in primary care. *Appl Clin Inform*. 2013;4:75e87.
33. Julian TW, Kelleher K, Julian DA, Chisolm D. Using technology to enhance prevention services for children in primary care. *J Prim Prev*. 2007;29:155–165.
34. Diamond G, Levy S, Bevans K, et al. Development, validation, and utility of internet-based, behavioral health screen for adolescents. *Pediatrics*. 2010;126:e163–e170.
35. US Department of Health and Human Services. The Changing Face of America's Adolescents. https://www.hhs.gov/ash/oah/facts-and-stats/changing-face-of-americas-adolescents/index.html.

# Index


**A**

Acceptance, motivational interviewing, 38
ACEs. *See* Adverse childhood experiences (ACEs)
Achievement gap
  nonheteronormative students, 83
  racial, 83
Acne, CAM therapy, 12
Actigraphy, 51
Acupressure, dysmenorrhea, 9
Acupuncture, atopic dermatitis, 13
Adaptive development, 228
AD/HD. *See* Attention deficit/hyperactivity disorder (AD/HD)
Adolescence Surveillance System for Obesity Prevention (ASSO), 37
Adolescents
  communities, 116
  developmental growth, 115
  developmental stages, 115
  development and brain
    adolescent channel risk-taking, 229–230
    behavior changes, 229
    critical thinking and logical reasoning, 229
    magnetic resonance imaging (MRI) methods, 229
    moodiness and irritability, 229
    neural connections, 229
    neuroimaging studies, 229
    pubertal status, 229
  development phases, 1
  exercise screening. *See also* Physical activity
    cardiorespiratory fitness, 65, 66f
    concurrent validity of physical activity, 63
    Exercise is Medicine (EIM), 64–65
    Kasch Pulse Recovery Test (KPR Test), 65
    test–retest reliability, 63, 64t
    VPA and 60-min MPA measures, 63–64, 64f
  health screening, 1
    benefits, 1
    biomedical model, 2
    detection screening, 1
    prevention screening, 1
    shortcomings, 1–2
    WHO screening, 1
Adolescents (*Continued*)
  obesity
    BMI status screening, 36–37
    food frequency questionnaire, 36–37
    healthcare providers, 37
    life stressors, 35–36
    motivational interviewing, 37–38
    parental eating behaviors, 36
    USPSTF screening, 36
  personal identity and autonomy, 116
  psychosocial development, 115–116
  young adolescents, 116
Adolescent Sleep Hygiene Scale (ASHS), 49
Adolescent Sleep–Wake Scale (ASWS), 48
Adolescent spirituality
  identity formation and making meaning, 210
  as a multidimensional construct
    Daily Spiritual Experience Scale (DSES), 212, 215t
    forgiveness, 215–218
    meaning/purpose, 212, 213t–214t
    MMRS scale, 211–212, 218
    Organized Religiousness, 212–214
    Private Religious Practices, 212–214, 216t–217t
    RCOPE scale, 214–215
    Religious Support, 212–214
    Spiritual Well-Being Scale, 218
  screening tools, 210
  as a single construct
    caveats, 211
    mental and behavioral health, 210–211
    physical health, 211
    positive youth development, 211
  spiritual care, 220
  United States, 210
Adult spirituality
  analytic, 208–209
  JCAHO, 208
  multidimensional spirituality, 209–210
  "single construct", 208–209
  spiritual history instruments, 208
Advanced sleep phase syndrome, 46
Adverse childhood experiences (ACEs), 3, 191–192
  adverse outcomes, 75, 76t
Adverse childhood experiences (ACEs) (*Continued*)
  Behavioral Risk Factor Surveillance System (BRFSS), 76–77
  Building Community Resilience (BCR) model, 80
  categories of, 77f
  cohort of participants, 77–78
  common community resources, 80t
  community trauma, 80–81
  early childhood adversities and mental health, 75
  intervention resources, 80t
  nonnormative traumatic events, 75
  screening tools, 76, 79t
  sexual abuse, 75, 77f
  trauma-informed approach, 78–80
  trauma-informed care (TIC), 78
  Urban Networks to Increase Thriving Youths (UNITY), 80–81
Affective strength, 238
Affirmations, motivational interviewing, 38
Aggression, 126t
Alcohol use disorder (AUD), 165, 173
American Academy of Child and Adolescent Psychiatry (AACAP), 142
Anorexia nervosa (AN), 153–154
ARPANET, 252
Ask Suicide-Screening Questions (ASQ), 141–142
Atopic dermatitis, CAM therapy, 12–13
Attention deficit/hyperactivity disorder (AD/HD)
  CAM therapy, 11
  CHADIS platform, 111
  diagnosis, 107
  DSM-5 criteria, 108
  electronic health records (EHR), 111
  NICHQ Vanderbilt Assessment Scales, 110
  Pediatric Symptoms Checklist 17 (PSC-17), 110–111, 110t
  screening measures, 107
  symptoms, 108t, 109
Autism spectrum disorder (ASD), 26


*Note:* Page numbers followed by "f" indicate figures, "t" indicate tables.

## B

Balneotherapy, atopic dermatitis, 13
BAQ. *See* Body Attitudes Questionnaire (BAQ)
BAT. *See* Body Attitudes Test (BAT)
BCR model. *See* Building Community Resilience (BCR) model
BEARS questionnaire, 49
Beck Scale for Suicidal Ideation (BSSI), 140
Behavioral and Emotional Rating Scale, Second Edition (BERS-2)
  advantage, 238
  domains, 238
  implications for practice, 239
  observer forms, 238
  psychometric properties, 238–239
Behavioral Risk Factor Surveillance System (BRFSS), 76–77
BERS-2. *See* Behavioral and Emotional Rating Scale, Second Edition (BERS-2)
Big data
  advantage, 252–253
  ARPANET, 252
  AstraZeneca, 253
  "biopsychosocial-collaborative" model, 254
  Blue Shield of California, 253
  Centers for Disease Control data, 253
  as a cost saver, 252
  data-dependent approaches, 254
  definition, 251
  early identification of patients, 254
  evidence-based medicine, 252
  fee for service model, 252
  health-promoting and cost-saving benefits, 252
  history, 251–254
  holistic approach, 255
  machine learning systems, 253
  magnetic storage devices, 252
  MindStrong Health, 253
  paradigm shift, 253
  patient-driven computerized prescreening, 255
  prevention planning, 254
  statistics, 253
  wearable tech, 254
  "World Wide Web", 252
Binge eating disorder (BED), 153–154
Biomedical model, 2
"Biopsychosocial-collaborative" model, 254
Biopsychosocial (BPS) model
  in adolescent medicine
    comorbid conditions, 2
    HEEADSSS assessment, 3
    pain management, 3
  evidence-based practices, 2
  general systems theory, 2
  Ghaemi's criticism, 2
  limitations, 4
BMMRS. *See* Brief Multidimensional Measure of Religiousness/Spirituality (BMMRS)
Body Attitudes Questionnaire (BAQ), 156
Body Attitudes Test (BAT), 156
Body image concerns
  Body Attitudes Questionnaire (BAQ), 156
  Body Attitudes Test (BAT), 156
  Body Satisfaction Scale, 156
  Body Shape Questionnaire (BSQ), 156
  Contour Drawing Rating Scale, 157
  cultural considerations, 158
  cultural diversity, 152
  and eating disorders, 153
  gender differences, 152–153
  "ideal" body type, 153
  physical reality, 151
  puberty, 152
  Rosenberg Self-Esteem Scale (RSES), 157
  sociocultural pressures, 152
  Thought–Shape Fusion Body Questionnaire, 157
  "traumatic sexualization", 151
  Western cultures, 152
Body perceptions pathway, 153
Body Satisfaction Scale, 156
Body Shape Questionnaire (BSQ), 156
Bovine lactoferrin, acne, 12
BRFSS. *See* Behavioral Risk Factor Surveillance System (BRFSS)
Brief Multidimensional Measure of Religiousness/Spirituality (BMMRS), 210
Brief Negotiated Interview (BNI), 171
Brief RCOPE scale, 214–215, 217t
Building Community Resilience (BCR) model, 80
Bulimia nervosa (BN), 153–154
Bullying, 117–118

## C

Caffeine, 15
  insufficient sleep, 45
CAM therapy. *See* Complementary and alternative medicine (CAM) therapy
Cannabis, substance use, 165
CASQ. *See* Cleveland adolescent sleepiness questionnaire (CASQ)
Catathrenia, 47
CD-RISC. *See* Connor-Davidson Resilience Scale (CD-RISC)
Celiac disease, 24–25
Center for Epidemiologic Studies Depression Scale (CES-D), 137
Child and Adolescent Needs and Strengths (CANS), 185
Child Health and Development Interactive System (CHADIS) platform, 111
Childhood obesity, 33, 60–61
Childhood Trauma Questionnaire-Short Form (CTQ-SF), 157–158
Child-on-child violence, 118
Child Protective Services, 155
Children's Eating Attitudes Test (ChEAT), 157
Chinese herbal medicine (CHM), 9
Chronic sleep loss, 45
Circadian rhythm, 43–44
Circadian rhythm sleep disorders, 46
Cleveland adolescent sleepiness questionnaire (CASQ), 48
Coconut oil, atopic dermatitis, 13
Cognitive and affective competencies, 228
Columbia Depression Scale (CDS), 136–137
Columbia Suicide Screen (CSS), 141
Columbia-Suicide Severity Rating Scale (C-SSRS), 141
Community Reinforcement and Family Training (CRAFT), 172
Community trauma, 80–81
Community violence, 126t
Compassion, motivational interviewing, 37–38
Complementary and alternative medicine (CAM) therapy
  acne, 12
  "ARMED", 8
  atopic dermatitis, 12–13
  attention-deficit/hyperactivity disorder, 11
  depression, 10
  dysmenorrhea, 8–9
  ethnic variations, 8
  generalized anxiety disorder, 11
  headache, 12
  National Center for Complementary and Integrative Health, 8
  NHIS data, 7
  obesity and eating disorders, 13
  parental use, 7–8
  performance-enhancing substances, 14–16
  preparticipation physical examination, 8
  psychiatric disorders, 9
  sleep disorders, 11
  supplements, 7
Conduct disorder
  age of onset, 111
  assessment system, 111–112
  DSM-5 criteria, 108–109
  etiology, 111
  gender difference, 111
  pediatric symptom checklist, 112
  self-report screening measures, 111
Connor-Davidson Resilience Scale (CD-RISC), 197

Consensus Sleep Diary, 48
Contour Drawing Rating Scale, 157
Couple violence, 126t
CRAFT. *See* Community Reinforcement and Family Training (CRAFT)
Creatine, 14
Criminal violence, 117
"Crisis of medicine", 2
Cyberbullying, 118, 247
Cyber-victimization, 92

**D**
Daily Spiritual Experience Scale (DSES), 212, 215t
Dairy consumption, 25
DAP survey. *See* Developmental Assets Profile (DAP) survey
Dating violence, 118
Dehydroepiandrosterone (DHEA), 14–15
Delayed sleep phase insomnia, 45
Delayed sleep phase syndrome (DSPD), 46
Delinquency, 126t
Depression. *See also* Suicide screening
  CAM therapy, 10
  insufficient sleep, 45
  major depressive disorder. *See* Major depressive disorder (MDD)
  nutrition, 21–22
  screening tools, 138t–139t
Detection screening, 1
Developmental assets model, 237
Developmental Assets Profile (DAP) survey, 237
  implications for practice, 238
  psychometric properties, 237
  social contexts, 237
Developmental-ecological model, 124
DHA Oxford Learning and Behavior (DOLAB) study, 24
Dietary screening
  celiac disease, 24–25
  dairy consumption, 25, 28
  epigenetics, 27–28
  fast foods, 24, 28
  microbiome
    colonization, 25
    diet components, 25–26
    gut–brain axis, 26
    immune cells, 25–26
    lower bacterial diversity, 25–26
    and personalized nutrition, 26–27
  "one-size-fits-all" diets, 22
  processed foods, 23–24, 28
  substance abuse, 22–23, 27–28
  sugar consumption, 23, 28
Dieting and fad diets, 22
Dilute bleach baths, atopic dermatitis, 13
Disorganized communities, 122
Drugs of abuse (DOA), 23
"Drunkorexia", 23
Dysmenorrhea, CAM therapy, 8–9

**E**
Eating Among Teens (EAT) study, 22
Eating Attitudes Test (EAT), 156–157
Eating disorder inventory (EDI), 157
Eating disorder inventory for Children (EDI-C), 157
Eating disorders
  in adolescence, 154
  anorexia nervosa, 153–154
  binge eating disorder (BED), 153–154
  biological and genetic factors, 151–152
  body dissatisfaction, 151–152
  and body image concerns, 153
  Children's Eating Attitudes Test (ChEAT), 157
  cultural considerations, 158
  Eating attitudes test (EAT), 157
  eating disorders not otherwise specified (EDNOS), 154
  prevalence and severity, 154
  subclinical, 151–152
Eating disorders not otherwise specified (EDNOS), 154
Electronic health records (EHR), 111, 142
Emollients, atopic dermatitis, 13
Emotional regulation, 36
Ephedra, 15
Epigenetics, 27, 33
Epworth sleepiness scale (ESS), 48–49
Evocation, motivational interviewing, 38
Executive function (EF), 193
Exercise. *See also* Physical activity
  benefits, 58t
  definition, 57
Exercise deficit disorder (EDD), 61, 66, 67f

**F**
Family Health History Questionnaire (FHH), 76
Fast foods, 24
Fetal alcohol spectrum disorders (FASD), 174
5-hydroxytryptamine [5-HT], 26
Follicle-stimulating hormone (FSH), 57–58
Food frequency questionnaire (FFQ), 36–37
Forgiveness, 215–218
Fragile Families and Child Wellbeing Study, 22
FRAMES model, 171
Fructose, 23

**G**
Gang violence, 119
Garcinia, obesity and eating disorders, 13–14
Generalized anxiety disorder, CAM therapy, 11
General systems theory (GST), 2
Genomic imprinting, obesity screening, 33
Get Self Help Sleep Diary, 48
Gluten intolerance, 25
Glyphosate
  celiac disease, 25
  depression and functional dyspepsia, 25
  obesity and and autism, 25
Gonadotropin-releasing hormone (GnRH), 57–58
Green tea, obesity and eating disorders, 13–14
Growth mind-set theory, 92
Guarana, obesity and eating disorders, 13–14
Guidelines for Adolescent Depression for Primary Care, (GLAD-PC) Toolkit, 137–140
Gut–brain axis, 26

**H**
Headache, CAM therapy, 12
Health Appraisal Questionnaire (HA), 76
Home, Education/Employment, Eating, Activities, Drugs and Alcohol, Sexuality, Suicide and Depression, Safety (HEEADSSS)
  assessment, 3, 248
  substance use screening, 169
  youth violence, 127
Homicide, 117, 120
*Hoodia gordonii*, 13–14
β-Hydroxy-β-methylbutyrate (HMB), 15
Hypnosis, insomnia, 11

**I**
Individual resilience, 192–193
Insomnia, 45
  CAM therapy, 11
Insufficient sleep
  caffeine effect, 45
  chronic sleep loss, 45
  circadian rhythm disturbance, 44–45
  depression, 45
  National Sleep Foundation survey, 44
Internet gaming disorder, 247
Interpersonal strength, 238
Intrapersonal strength, 238

**J**
Joint Commission on Accreditation of Healthcare Organizations (JCAHO), 208
Juvenile criminality/recidivism
  community risk factors, 181
  "crossover" risk factors, 179
  cumulative and grouping of risk factors, 181
  family/peer risk factors, 181
  individual risk factors, 180–181

Juvenile criminality/recidivism (*Continued*)
intervention programs, 185–187
juvenile justice system (JJS), 179
needs assessment
"age appropriate interpretation", 183–184
dynamic factors, 183
dynamic needs, 184
lack of clarity, 184
property recidivism, 184
shortcomings, 184
superficial needs assessment, 183–184
tools, 185
prevention programs, 187
protective factors, 181–182
risk assessment, 179–183
risk assessment tools
Juvenile Sanctions Center (JSC), 183
limitations, 183
Youth Assessment and Screening Instrument (YASI), 182–183
school/workplace risk factors, 181
Juvenile justice system (JJS), 179
Juvenile Sanctions Center (JSC), 183

**K**

Kasch Pulse Recovery Test (KPR Test), 65
Kola nut, obesity and eating disorders, 13–14

**L**

Lactose intolerance, 25
Learning disabilities (LD)
behavioral indicators, 84
neurodevelopmental disorders
biological stressors, 85–86
developmental deficits, 84
DSM-5 classifications, 84–85
etiology, 85
gender difference, 85
traumatic brain injury, 85
psychosocial risk factors
behavioral challenges, 87
caregiver educational attainment and involvement, 90
childhood trauma, 89
community factors, 91–92
earlier school challenges, 89
foster or adoptive status, 90
gender identity and sexuality concerns, 88
juvenile justice system, 88
lack of school engagement, 86–87
low motivation and negative school attitude, 86
low participation in extracurricular activities, 88–89
low socioemotional competence, 88

Learning disabilities (LD) (*Continued*)
parental divorce and separation, 89–90
parental education and low family income, 90
peer factors, 91
permissive/authoritarian parenting style, 89
poor academic self-concept, 86
school factors, 91
sociocultural factors, 91
substance use, 88
technology factors, 92
work factors, 91
Lesbian, gay, bisexual, transgender, and questioning (LGBTQ) adolescents, 173
Loughborough Sleep Research Center, 48
Low-glycemic-load diet, acne, 12
Low motivation and negative school attitude, 86
Luteinizing hormone (LH), 57–58

**M**

Machine learning systems, 253
Maintenance of wakefulness test (MWT), 51
Major depressive disorder (MDD)
depression-specific questionnaires, 135
diagnostic criteria, 135
parent checklists, 135
primary care providers (PCPs), 135
screening instruments, 135
screening tool
Center for Epidemiologic Studies Depression Scale (CES-D), 137
challenges, 137–140
Columbia Depression Scale (CDS), 136–137
GLAD-PC toolkit, 137–140
Hamilton Depression Rating Scale, 136
Massachusetts Youth Screening Instrument (MAYSI), 137
Mood and Feelings Questionnaire (MFQ), 137
Patient Health Questionnaire (PHQ), 136
Pediatric Symptom Checklist (PSC), 137
self-report questionnaires, 136
Strengths and Difficulties Questionnaire (SDQ), 137
Well-Being Index (WBI-5), 137
USPSTF screening, 135
Massachusetts Youth Screening Instrument (MAYSI), 137
MedicineWise Sleep Diary, 48
Melanocortin 4 receptor (MC4R) gene, 33–34
Melatonin, 11, 198

Metabolic equivalent of task (MET), 57
Model Youth and Family Assessment of Needs and Strengths, 185
Moderate-intensity physical activity (MPA), 57, 58t
Moderate-to-vigorous physical activity (MVPA), 59
Modified Scale for Suicide Ideation (MSSI), 140
Mood and Feelings Questionnaire (MFQ), 137
Moral competencies, 228
Motivational interviewing (MI)
acceptance, 38
affirmations, 38
compassion, 37–38
evocation, 38
open-ended questions, 38
partnership, 38
reflections, 38
substance use, 171
summary statements, 38
Multidimensional Measure of Religiousness/Spirituality (MMRS), 210
Multidimensional spirituality, 209–210
Multiple Sleep Latency Test (MSLT), 51
Music therapy, insomnia, 11

**N**

National Center for Complementary and Integrative Health (NCCIH), 8
National Eating Disorders Association (NEDA), 154
National Initiative for Children's Health-care Quality (NICHQ) Vanderbilt Assessment Scales, 110, 110t
National Sleep Foundation, 48
Neighborhood poverty, 91
Neighborhood violence, 92
Neurodevelopmental disorders
learning disabilities
biological stressors, 85–86
developmental deficits, 84
DSM-5 classifications, 84–85
etiology, 85
gender difference, 85
traumatic brain injury, 85
Neurogenesis, 59
Nicotine, substance use, 165
Nightmares, 47
Nitric oxide boosters, 15
Nocturnal enuresis, 47
Nonalcoholic fatty liver disease (NAFLD), 23
Nonrapid eye movement (NREM) sleep, 43
North Carolina Assessment of Risk (NCAR), 182

Nudge Theory of Behavioral Economics, 254
Nutrition
- and depression, 21–22
- dieting and fad diets, 22
- neurocognitive effects, 21
- and obesity, 22
- and violent and aggressive behaviors, 22

## O

Obesity screening
- childhood and adolescent obesity
  - BMI status screening, 36–37
  - cardiovascular effects, 35
  - food frequency questionnaire, 36–37
  - genetic causes, 33–34
  - healthcare providers, 37
  - life stressors, 35–36
  - metabolic complications, 35
  - motivational interviewing, 37–38
  - parental eating behaviors, 36
  - psychosocial concerns, 35
  - race and ethnicity, 34–35
  - socioeconomic status, 34
  - USPSTF screening, 36
- NHANES analysis, 33
- prevalence, 33
- and social media, 246–247

Obstructive sleep apnea (OSA), 45–46
Ohio Youth Assessment System (OYAS), 182
Olive oil, atopic dermatitis, 13
Open questions, affirmation, reflective listening, and summarizing (OARS) skills
- affirmation, 234
- open-ended questions, 233–234
- reflective listening, 234
- summaries, 234

Opioids, substance use, 165
Opportunity gap, 83
Oppositional defiant disorder
- age of onset, 111
- assessment system, 111–112
- DSM-5 criteria, 108–109
- etiology, 111
- gender difference, 111
- pediatric symptom checklist, 112
- self-report screening measures, 111

Organized Religiousness (OR), 212–214

## P

Parasomnias, 46–47
Parental divorce and separation, 89–90
Parental eating behaviors, 36
Parental substance use, 173
Parent empowerment framework, 92
Partnership, motivational interviewing, 38
Patient Health Questionnaire (PHQ), 136
Patient Safety Screener-3 (ED-SAFE screener), 142
Pediatric daytime sleepiness scale (PDSS), 49
Pediatric sleep questionnaire (PSQ), 49–50
Pediatric Symptom Checklist (PSC), 137
Pediatric Symptoms Checklist 17 (PSC-17), 110–111, 110t
Peer victimization, 91
Performance-enhancing substances
- β-hydroxy-β-methylbutyrate, 15
- creatine, 14
- nitric oxide boosters, 15
- prohormones, 14–15
- stimulants, 15

Permissive/authoritarian parenting style, 89
Philadelphia ACE Survey (PHLACES), 77–78
Physical activity
- adolescent development
  - academic and cognitive performance, 59
  - adolescence to adulthood transition, 58–59
  - child-to-adolescent transition, 57–58
  - exercise training adaptations, 57
  - motivation, 57
  - multiple systems and health outcomes, 57, 58t
  - neurogenesis, 59
  - normal neuroendocrine changes, 59
- childhood obesity, 60–61
- definition, 57
- exercise deficit disorder (EDD), 61, 66
- expectation, 59
- overweight children, 60–61
- racial bias, obesity, 60–61
- reality
  - Healthy People 2020 Objectives, 60t
  - moderate-to-vigorous physical activity, 59–60
  - NHANES data, 60

Physical Activity Vital Sign (PAVS), 65
Physical fitness, 57
Physical inactivity, 61
Pittsburgh Sleep Diary, 48
Pittsburgh sleep quality Index (PSQI), 50
Polysomnography (PSG), 50–51
Polyunsaturated fatty acids (PUFAs), 11
Poor academic self-concept, 86
Poor teacher–student relationship, 91
Positive Achievement Change Tool (PACT), 185
Positive psychology movement, 235–236
Positive youth development (PYD), 211, 237
Preadolescent nutritional insults, 26
Pregnancy, substance use, 173–174
Prevention screening, 1
Primary lactase deficiency, 25
Primary youth violence prevention activities, 124–125
Private Religious Practices (PRP), 212–214, 216t–217t
Problematic and Risky Internet Use Screening Scale (PRIUSS), 248
Processed foods, 23–24
Prohormones, 14–15
Property recidivism, 184
Protein powders, 15
Psychiatric disorders, CAM therapy, 9
Psychologic difficulties pathway, 153
Psychophysiological insomnia, 45

## R

Rapid eye movement (REM) sleep, 43
- behavior disorder, 46

Reasons for Living Questionnaire (RLQ), 141
Religiosity, 207
Religious Coping (RCOPE) scale, 210, 214–215
Religious Support (RS), 212–214
Resilience
- definition, 193
- enhancement programs, 192–193, 197–200
  - at-risk youths, 198
  - broad-based policy interventions, 198
  - family and parenting factors, 198
  - intervention programs, 199
  - mentoring programs, 198
  - promotion and intervention, 197–198
  - resilience promotion, 199–200
  - screening tools, 198
  - self-efficacy, 198
- environmental factors, 192–193
- future research, 200
- individual, 192–193
- individualist viewpoint, 193
  - combat veterans, 194
  - executive function (EF), 193
  - factors affecting, 194
  - mental health outcomes, 194
  - neurologic and cognitive basis, 194
  - protective factors, 195
  - Resiliency Scale for Children and Adolescents, 194–195
- interactionist viewpoint, 193
  - community influences, 196
  - family's role, 195–196
- research perspectives, 193
- resilient survivors, 191
- screening, 196–197

Resilience (*Continued*)
trauma
adverse childhood experiences, 191–192
events, 191
physical and mental health, 192
prevalence, 191–192
Resiliency Scale for Children and Adolescents (RSCA), 194–195, 197
Response-to-Intervention (RtI) method, 84
Resveratrol gel, acne, 12
Risk of Suicide Questionnaire (RSQ), 141–142
Rosenberg Self-Esteem Scale (RSES), 157

**S**

S-adenosyl-L-methionine (SAMe), 10
SAI-Y. *See* Strength Assessment Inventory for Youth (SAI-Y)
School engagement
behavioral engagement, 86–87
cognitive engagement, 86–87
correlational and longitudinal studies, 87
disengaged students, 87
educational outcomes, 87
emotional engagement, 86–87
Scoring Atopic Dermatitis (SCORAD) scale, 12–13
Secondary youth violence prevention programs, 125
Serotonin, 21–22, 26
Sexual abuse
and body image concerns/ED, 155–156
Childhood Trauma Questionnaire-Short Form (CTQ-SF), 157–158
Child Protective Services, 155
child sexual abuse, 154–155
cultural considerations, 158
factors contributing, 155
and social media, 248
Trauma History Profile (THP), 158
Sexual violence, 119
Sibling violence, 118–119
"Single-construct spirituality", 208–209
Sleep
and age, 44
architecture, 43
circadian and homeostatic systems, 43–44
objective assessment
actigraphy, 51
maintenance of wakefulness test (MWT), 51
Multiple Sleep Latency Test (MSLT), 51
polysomnography (PSG), 50–51
and social media, 247
subjective assessment
sleep diary, 48
Sleep (*Continued*)
sleep history, 47–48
sleep questionnaires, 48–50
Sleep diary, 48
Sleep-disordered breathing (SDB), 45–46
Sleep disorders
CAM therapy, 11
circadian rhythm disorders, 46
insomnia, 45
insufficient sleep
caffeine effect, 45
chronic sleep loss, 45
circadian rhythm disturbance, 44–45
depression, 45
National Sleep Foundation survey, 44
parasomnias, 46–47
screening for, 47
sleep-disordered breathing, 45–46
Sleep Disturbance Scale for Children (SDSC), 50
Sleep habits survey (SHS), 50
Sleep paralysis, 46–47
Sleep related hallucinations, 47
Sleep–wake cycle, 43–44
Slow-wave sleep (SWS), 43
"Social bond", 122
Social capital, 122–123
Social competencies, 228
Social disorganization theory, 122
Social ecological context
individual adaptation, 230
poverty, 230
youths strengths assessment
adversity, 231
challenging contexts, 231
normative developmental tasks, 230–231
Social media, 92
cyberbullying, 247
health outcomes, 246
interactive media, 245–246
internet gaming disorder, 247
mental health and internet usage, 245
negatives of, 246
and obesity, 246–247
problematic internet use, 247
reduced life satisfaction, 245
and sexual abuse, 248
and sleep, 247
smartphone, 245
tele-medicine, 245–246
transgender communities, 246
unsafe screen time, 248
while driving, 246
Soft-drink consumption, 23
Spirituality
adolescent. *See* Adolescent spirituality
behavior mechanisms, 208
noncommunicable diseases, 208
physical mechanisms, 208
Spirituality (*Continued*)
psychologic and emotional mechanisms, 208
screening
nature and nurture, 207
shortcomings, 207
social mechanisms, 208
Spiritual Well-Being Scale (SWBS), 210, 218, 219t
Stimulants, 15
St. John's wort
adverse drug interactions, 10
Cochrane review, 10
pharmacologic antidepressant, 10
S-adenosyl-L-methionine (SAMe), 10
ω-3 fatty acids, 10
Strength Assessment Inventory for Youth (SAI-Y)
contextual domains, 239
developmental domains, 239
implications for practice, 239–240
observer version, 239
psychometric properties, 239
Strength-based assessment
at-risk youth, 231–232
Behavioral and Emotional Rating Scale, Second Edition (BERS-2)
advantage, 238
domains, 238
implications for practice, 239
observer forms, 238
psychometric properties, 238–239
benefits, 227
collaborative goals, 235
definition, 227
developmental assets model, 237
Developmental Assets Profile (DAP) survey
implications for practice, 238
psychometric properties, 237
social contexts, 237
developmental competencies and tasks
adaptive development, 228
cognitive and affective competencies, 228
domains, 228
moral competencies, 228
problematic behaviors, 228
social competencies, 228
emotional and behavioral disorders, 227–228
formal assessments and structured inventories, 235
implications for practice, 236
informal assessment, 232–233
outside supports and resources, 235
positive psychology movement, 227, 235–236
positive youth development, 237
psychometric properties, 236–237
psychopathology, 228
rapport and trust building
basic listening skills, 233

Strength-based assessment (*Continued*)
motivational interviewing, 233
OARS, 233
social ecological context
adversity, 231
challenging contexts, 231
normative developmental tasks, 230–231
Strength Assessment Inventory for Youth (SAI-Y)
contextual domains, 239
developmental domains, 239
implications for practice, 239–240
observer version, 239
psychometric properties, 239
Strength-Based Assessment Model, 238
trauma-informed care, 233
treatment planning, 228
VIA Inventory of Strengths for Youth
implications for practice, 236
psychometric properties, 236
Strengths and Difficulties Questionnaire (SDQ), 137
Stress, 191
Stress Inoculation Training (SIT), 199–200
Substance use
brief interventions
Brief Negotiated Interview (BNI), 171
FRAMES model, 171
motivational interviewing, 171
co-occurring disorders, 174
epidemiology
alcohol, 165
cannabis, 165
family and economic stress, 166
nicotine, 165
opioids, 165
peer experiences, 166
poly-drug use, 166
fetal alcohol spectrum disorders, 174
and LGBTQ adolescents, 173
parental substance use, 173
and pregnancy, 173–174
primary care follow-up and management
alcohol and opioid use disorders, 173
preventive health care, 172
tobacco use disorders, 172–173
referral to treatment, 171–172
school engagement, 88
screening
anticipatory guidance, 170
binge drinking, 166
confidentiality, 169
CRAFFT Interview, 166, 167t
evidence-based screens, 169–170
HEEADSSS, 169
illicit drugs, 166–167
parental requests for drug testing, 169
Substance use (*Continued*)
routine primary care visits, 166
tools, 168t
Suicidal Behaviors Questionnaire (SBQ), 140–141
Suicidal Ideation Questionnaire (SIQ), 141
Suicide Risk Screen (SRS), 141
Suicide screening, 143t
AACAP recommendations, 142
artificial intelligence surveillance of social media, 142
Ask Suicide-Screening Questions (ASQ), 141–142
Beck Scale for Suicidal Ideation (BSSI), 140
clinical interview, 140
Columbia Suicide Screen (CSS), 141
Columbia-Suicide Severity Rating Scale (C-SSRS), 141
emergency departments, 140
history of depression, 142
Modified Scale for Suicide Ideation (MSSI), 140
Patient Safety Screener-3 (ED-SAFE screener), 142
Reasons for Living Questionnaire, 141
Risk of Suicide Questionnaire (RSQ), 141–142
Suicidal Behaviors Questionnaire (SBQ), 140–141
Suicidal Ideation Questionnaire (SIQ), 141
Suicide Risk Screen (SRS), 141
universal screening, 142
Sun-flower seed oil, atopic dermatitis, 13

**T**

Taurine, obesity and eating disorders, 13–14
Tea tree oil, acne, 12
Tele-medicine, 245–246
Test–retest reliability, 63
Thought–Shape Fusion Body Questionnaire, 157
Trauma History Profile (THP), 158
Trauma-informed care (TIC), 78, 233
Traumatic brain injury (TBI), 85
"Traumatic sexualization", 151
Type 2 diabetes mellitus (T2DM), 35

**U**

Ultraprocessed foods, 23
Unrefined Chinese rapeseed oil, 24
Urban Networks to Increase Thriving Youths (UNITY), 80–81

**V**

Valerian root, 11
VIA Inventory of Strengths for Youth Scale (VIA-YS), 236
Videogaming and mobile device, 92
Vigorous-intensity physical activity (VPA), 57
Violent Crime Index, 117

**W**

ω-3 fatty acids
attention-deficit/hyperactivity disorder, 11
depression, 10
Washington State Juvenile Court Assessment (WSJCA), 185
Well-Being Index (WBI-5), 137

**Y**

Yoga, obesity and eating disorders, 13
Youth Assessment and Screening Instrument (YASI), 182–183
Youth Risk Behavior Survey, 120
Youth violence
bullying, 117–118
community factors, 121–123
community-level protective factors, 123–124
criminal violence, 117
cyberbullying, 118
dating violence, 118
family factors, 121
family-level protective factors, 123
fighting, 118–119
gang violence, 119
healthcare providers
developmental-ecological model, 124
primary care providers, 127
primary prevention activities, 124–125
secondary prevention programs, 125
tertiary prevention interventions, 125
violence screening, 125–127
hyperactivity, 120
individual characteristics, 120
individual-level protective factors, 123
interpersonal violence, 116
peer factors, 121
peer-level protective factors, 123
poor academic achievement and school failure, 120
before puberty, 116
public health perspective
health objectives, 119
homicide, 120
primary prevention, 120
secondary prevention, 120
tertiary prevention, 120
Youth Risk Behavior Survey, 120
risk and protective factors, 116–117
school-aged children and adolescents, 116
school connectedness, 123
sexual violence, 119